KEYGUIDE TO INFORMATION SOURCES IN

Veterinary Medicine

KEYGUIDE TO INFORMATION SOURCES IN

Veterinary Medicine

Mike Gibb

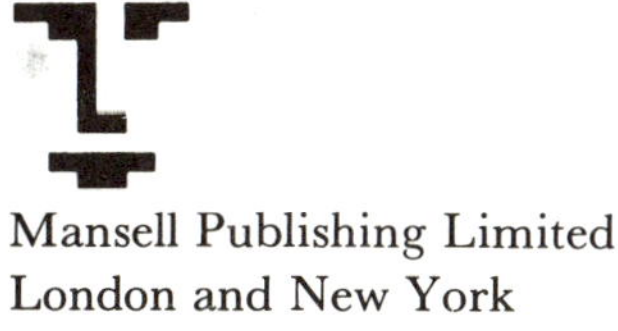

Mansell Publishing Limited
London and New York

First published 1990 by
Mansell Publishing Limited, *A Cassell Imprint*
Artillery House, Artillery Row, London SW1P 1RT, England
125 East 23rd Street, Suite 300, New York 10010, U.S.A.

British Library Cataloguing in Publication Data
Gibb, Mike, *1952–*
    Keyguide to information sources in veterinary medicine.
    1. Veterinary medicine. Information sources
    I. Title
    636.089′07

    ISBN 0–7201–2018–7

Library of Congress Cataloging-in-Publication Data applied for

Printed and bound in Great Britain by
Biddles Ltd, Guildford and King's Lynn

For Mum and Dad, Susan and Katherine

Contents

Introduction   xi
Acknowledgements   xii
Abbreviations   xiii

PART I   Survey of veterinary medicine and its literature   1

1   The history and scope of veterinary medicine   3
1.1   Historical introduction   3
1.2   The scope of veterinary medicine today   7
1.3   Organization of the subject field   9
1.4   Statutory and professional bodies   13
1.5   Education   18

2   Veterinary information: its origins and utilization   23
2.1   Journals   23
2.2   Books   24
2.3   Utilization of the literature   25
2.4   Literary style   29
2.5   Veterinary libraries   30
2.6   Classification schemes and subject headings used in libraries   33

3   Who, what, where?   37
3.1   General directories   37
3.2   Directories of individuals   38
3.3   Organizations and institutions   40

3.4   Research   41
3.5   The animal health industry   46

4   Keeping up to date with current information   52
4.1   Introduction   52
4.2   *Index veterinarius* and *Veterinary bulletin*   53
4.3   *Veterinary update*   56
4.4   *Quarterly index* and *Small animal abstracts*   60
4.5   Other CAB International journals   60
4.6   VETDOC   62
4.7   Contents lists and current awareness services   62
4.8   Information on new books   66
4.9   Trade literature   67
4.10   Conferences and continuing education events   68

5   Finding out about the literature   71
5.1   Guides to the literature and bibliographies   71
5.2   Reviews   72
5.3   Abstracting and indexing services   73
5.4   Computerized information retrieval systems   75

6   The literature of veterinary medicine   82
6.1   Original contributions   82
6.2   Reference books   85
6.3   Textbooks and monographs   87

7   Sources of special information   89
7.1   Government publications   89
7.2   Intergovernmental publications   91
7.3   Legislation   93
7.4   Standards   94
7.5   Patents and trade marks   95
7.6   Statistical data   98
7.7   Audiovisual materials   99

8   Language problems   101

PART II   Bibliography   105

9   General works   107
General sources   107
Reference works   156
Multivolume works and series   157
General veterinary books   165

Materials for ancillary personnel   166

10 Large animals   169
General   169
Cattle   171
Buffaloes   180
Deer   181
Sheep   184
Goats   190
Pigs   194
Camelids   199
Horses   201

11 Small animals   211
General   211
Cats   223
Dogs   225
Rabbits   231
Laboratory animals   234
Poultry and cage birds   241
Amphibians and reptiles   247
Exotic pets, zoo and wild animals   249
Fish   255
Invertebrates   241

12 Specialities   263
Anaesthesia   263
Anatomy and histology   265
Animal husbandry and production   267
Bacteriology   270
Behaviour   271
Dentistry   273
Epidemiology and preventive medicine   274
Haematology, cytology and clinical chemistry   275
History   278
Immunology   280
Laboratory manuals   282
Legislation and regulatory matters   283
Microbiology   286
Mycology and mycotoxicoses   288
Neurology   290
Nutrition and digestion   290
Oncology   296
Ophthalmology   297

Parasitology   298
Pathology   307
Physiology and metabolism   309
Practice management   311
Protozoology   312
Public health (including zoonoses) and hygiene   314
Radiology   317
Reproduction and genetics   318
Surgery   322
Therapeutics, pharmacology and pharmaceutics   324
Toxicology   328
Tropical veterinary medicine   331
Virology   334
Welfare   337
Miscellaneous subjects   339

PART III   Directory of organizations   341
Selected list of veterinary libraries   343
National veterinary associations   348
Veterinary associations and societies   363
Online systems   410
Online databases   414
Publishers and booksellers   418

Index   429

Introduction

Information about the care of animals, the diseases they are prone to, and the treatment of those conditions is required by many people: veterinary practitioners and researchers, teachers and students of veterinary medicine, agricultural scientists, farmers and pet owners. As veterinary medicine is such a vast subject, it seemed useful to summarize details of the major information sources in a single volume.

Part I presents a narrative survey of the kinds of information resources available with some discussion of their use in practice. Each chapter has a list of appropriate documentation studies. This section will be of most value to those unfamiliar with the subject field itself or with the methods of information transfer within the discipline.

Part II is an annotated bibliography of reference sources, and has entries for the key works on veterinary medicine in general, and for those devoted to particular species and specialities. The lists are not intended to be comprehensive but the major and most recent texts are included. Standard works on animal husbandry and also included. For monographs and textbooks the emphasis is on English-language works. For journals the core titles and the major specialist periodicals in a variety of languages are noted.

Part III is an address directory with details of national veterinary associations, other associations and societies, and selected libraries, online systems, online databases and publishers. Addresses and other contact dctails for organizations alter frequently but the directory was correct at the time of going to press.

Acknowledgements

I am grateful to many people who have helped during the preparation of this book, in particular my colleagues within the Information Department at Coopers Animal Health. Thanks are due to the staff of the libraries of the Royal College of Veterinary Surgeons and of the Royal Veterinary College for allowing me to use their resources. I am grateful to the BVA's External Affairs Department (Ms Chrissie Nichols and Ms Helena Cotton) for assistance in compiling details on British associations. J. P. Jetté of the University of Montreal provided details of some of the libraries listed in Part III. Finally, thanks are due to Louise Collyer who word-processed, again and again, my scrawls. I hope my efforts have been worthy of hers.

Abbreviations

AAHA	American Animal Hospital Association
AFRC	Agricultural and Food Research Council
AHI	Animal Health Institute
AVMA	American Veterinary Medical Association
BSAVA	British Small Animal Veterinary Association
BVA	British Veterinary Association
BVNA	British Veterinary Nursing Association
CAB	Commonwealth Agricultural Bureaux now C·A·B International
CwVA	Commonwealth Veterinary Association
FAO	Food and Agriculture Organization of the United Nations
IEMVT	Institut d'Élevage et de Médecine Vétérinaire des Pays Tropicaux
ILCA	International Livestock Centre for Africa
ILRAD	International Laboratory for Research on Animal Diseases
MAFF	Ministry of Agriculture, Fisheries and Food (of the UK)
NOAH	National Office of Animal Health
OIE	Office International des Épizooties
RCVS	Royal College of Veterinary Surgeons
UFAW	Universities Federation for Animal Welfare
WHO	World Health Organization of the United Nations
WVA	World Veterinary Association

PART I

Survey of Veterinary Medicine and Its Literature

1 The History and Scope of Veterinary Medicine

1.1 HISTORICAL INTRODUCTION

Man has held animals in high regard since prehistoric times; the representations of wild animals dating from the palaeolithic period testify to this. However it would not have been until the domestication of animals that man became concerned with their health and well-being. The dog was the first animal to be domesticated: a recent archaeological discovery is of a tomb in northern Israel in which the remains of a human and dog were buried together. This apparently dates from around 10000 BC. The domestication of the dog was followed by that of the common food animals, first goats and sheep, then cattle. Horses were domesticated comparatively recently (Mason, 1984 [1653]*; Clutton-Brock, 1988).

The early practitioners of veterinary medicine were as much priests as animal healers and their art would have relied on sympathetic magic and prayer, techniques which are still components of the modern art! Then, as now, good husbandry and the sensitive care of animals were of prime importance in promoting health. The first animal healer known by name is a Sumerian priest–healer, or *azu*, *Urlugaledinna* (*Figure 1.1*). Similar priest–healers existed in early Egyptian and Greek civilizations. There are very early records of the veterinary art; the Babylonian Code of Eshnunna (*c.* 1900 BC) describes the dehorning of oxen, and the Code of Hammurabi (*c.* 1750 BC) has a code of laws prescribing a scale of fees for doctors of oxen and asses. The Egyptian papyrus of

*Numbers in square brackets refer to entries in the bibliography (Part II)

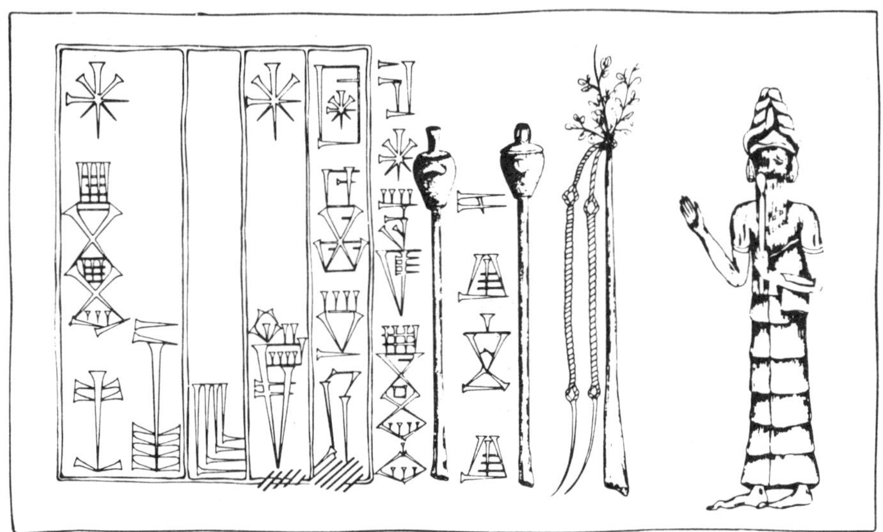

Figure 1.1   Cylinder seal from the Mesopotamian city of Lagash (*c.* 2200 BC). Depicts *Urlugaledinna* and items of his trade: bovine obstetrical cords hanging from a medicinal plant and two urns for drugs or fragrances.
(Reproduced with permission from C. W. Schwabe, *Veterinary medicine and human health*, 3rd edition, © 1984, Williams & Wilkins, Baltimore).

Kahun (1800 BC) has the oldest written account of detailed veterinary procedures. Many early writings in Sanskrit survive from the Vedic period of India (1800 to 1200 BC). These indicate that there was already specialization in veterinary practice (Smithcors, 1978). Later on King Asoka (*c.* 265–238 BC) established veterinary hospitals all over India.

Both Greece and Rome were agricultural communities and the veterinary medicine of farm animals was important. However in both civilizations veterinarians concentrated on equine medicine and surgery. Practitioners were known as *hippiatroi* in Greece and *equarius medicus* in Rome. Later on in Rome doctors of animals were called *veterinarius* (from the Latin *veterinae* – pertaining to cattle). Progress was made in equine veterinary practice during the Roman Empire and during this period Publius Vegitius Renatus (*c.* AD 450–500) wrote a treatise, *Books of the veterinary arts, or digests of the art of curing the diseases of mules*. Another text on equine medicine, the *Hippiatrika*, dates from Byzantine times, the major contributor being Apsyrtus of Nicomedia (*c.* AD 340), chief *hippiatros* in the army of Constantine the Great. The *Hippiatrika* was prepared at the instigation of Constantine the Seventh in the tenth century AD and is a compilation of the works of the most important Greek and Latin authors. It provided the basis for most of the scientific study of veterinary medicine during the Middle Ages. Interest in the study of the early texts was reawakened by the publication of editions in Latin of Publius Vegetius Renatus' work (1528) and the *Hippiatrika* (1530) but the first modern scientific work, Carlo Ruini's *Anatomia del cavallo, infirmita et suoi rimedii*

(*Anatomy of the horse, diseases and treatment*) did not appear until 1598 (Dyce and Merlen, 1953).

Although the Greek and Roman writings were studied at medical schools and universities during the Middle Ages veterinary medicine made little progress. Some indications of a professional organization were apparent but much of the practice of veterinary medicine remained in the hands of the farriers. (The term farrier derives from the Latin, *ferrarius*, used by the Romans to refer to individuals who fitted and forged horseshoes.) By the fourteenth century practitioners in Britain were called 'Marshals' and the Master Marshals of London had formed a trade guild. The title Marshal is a contraction or corruption of French and Italian words for horsemaster. The Marshals originally functioned as heads of the military veterinary services. After this period the art declined and there was little control over the level of knowledge or skill required by someone to practise veterinary medicine.

By the eighteenth century the profession had fallen into disrepute. This was one reason for the founding of the early veterinary colleges. Another was the growth of interest in veterinary science as a separate discipline from human medicine. The most important factor, however, was the intensification of animal husbandry during the eighteenth century which resulted in many serious outbreaks of disease. In Europe between 1710 and 1760 over 200 million cattle died from rinderpest. Contagious pleuropneumonia in cattle and distemper in dogs were also major problems. The concern was such that the French government appointed Claude Bourgelat (1712–79) to establish a veterinary school. This was founded at Lyons in 1762 and a second college followed at Alfort in 1765. Schools were also set up in Turin (1769), Vienna (1767), Copenhagen (1773), Skara (1778), Hanover (1778) and Berlin (1787). By 1825 there were thirty veterinary schools in twelve countries. England was one of the last European countries to found a veterinary college. The Royal Veterinary College was created in 1791 by a Frenchman, Charles Vial de Saint-Bel (De Wailly, 1985). A second school, the Dick Veterinary College, was founded in Edinburgh in 1823.

Education in countries outside Europe took some time to develop. The first Canadian school was founded in Guelph in 1862 and the first American school to produce graduates, the Boston Veterinary Institute was founded in 1854. There was little widespread disease among animals in the United States until the mid-nineteenth century, by which time bovine pleuropneumonia, hog cholera and Texas cattle fever were important diseases. In response to the threat of these diseases the US Congress established the Bureau of Animal Industry within the USDA in 1884. The BAI and USDA were extremely successful and bovine pleuropneumonia was eradicated within eight years and since then a further twelve diseases have been eradicated from the United States. The State Veterinary Service in Britain was founded in response to a similar need, the Veterinary Department of the Privy Council being created following an outbreak of cattle plague in Britain in 1865. During its existence the State Veterinary Service has eradicated fourteen serious diseases from farm stock.

Once the veterinary schools were established the graduates realized that some form of official body should be responsible for administering the profession. The national associations were thus created to advance the standing of the profession and to control standards. The first was the Gesellschaft Schweizerischer Tierärzte in 1813; the Danish Veterinary Association was formed in 1849; the Royal Netherlands Veterinary Association in 1862; and the Société Vétérinaire Pratique de France in 1878. In Britain the graduates petitioned for a Royal Charter. This was granted in 1844 and incorporated the Royal College of Veterinary Surgeons. A number of supplementary charters have been issued over the years. The first Royal Charter established veterinary medicine as a profession and gave members of the College the sole and exclusive right to practise the art and to be be distinguished by the name of veterinary surgeon. (The first veterinarians were called farriers and the English term 'veterinary surgeon' was coined by the British Army to distinguish them from human surgeons.) Originally the RCVS held all the professional examinations. Since the Veterinary Surgeons Act of 1948 these have been conducted by the universities. Associations have now been founded in most countries (e.g. Australia, 1921; India, 1922; New Zealand, 1928; and Canada, 1948).

Although there are now many women in the profession their entry is a recent phenomenon; the first female to qualify was probably Fraulein Stephanie Kruszewska, who (*The veterinary journal* noted) graduated with distinction from the Zurich Veterinary Institute in 1889 (Pattison, 1984 [1326]). The first female veterinary surgeon to qualify in Britain, Aleen Cust, completed her veterinary education in 1900 yet was only allowed to take the RCVS examinations in 1922 (Ford, 1985). The first female graduate in North America was Dr Elinor McGrath who obtained her degree from Chicago Veterinary College in 1910. In America and the United Kingdom men and women now enter the profession in approximately equal numbers. Of 1,472 graduates in the United States in 1988 who responded to a survey 49 percent were women (Wise, 1988b) and in 1986–7 a break-down of the total enrolment in veterinary medical degree programmes was 46.2 percent male and 53.8 percent female. In other countries, however, the profession is predominantly male. For example, in New Zealand only 18 percent of registered veterinarians are female (Boland and Morris, 1988).

For most of recorded history veterinary medicine has been primarily concerned with the horse. Initially this was because of the importance of the horse as a military animal. In more recent centuries the horse has been the principal form of transport and the most important work animal in Europe. In the nineteenth century, a veterinary surgeon's workload would have mainly been with horses and cattle. Cats and dogs have been domesticated for many thousands of years but it is only in the twentieth century that companion animals have become important recipients of veterinary care. Small animal practice, which is now such a feature of the profession, is thus a very recent development.

The veterinary art has developed in tandem with advances in human medicine. Products and techniques have been introduced into veterinary medical practice shortly after their use in man. Thus after the use of ether and chloroform in the nineteenth century for anaesthesia in man these products were used with animals. Similarly the first UK radiographs were taken in 1896 only one year after the discovery of X-rays.

The pharmacological revolution which transformed medical practice in the early twentieth century also transformed veterinary practice and has replaced all the empirical remedies. Prontosil was discovered in 1935 and, as the first sulphonamide, was the first of the modern drugs developed by the pharmaceutical industry. A host of new chemical entities has followed. Other sulphonamides became available in the late 1930s, and then the natural and synthetic antibiotics in the 1940s. Nowadays, apart from antibacterials there is an enormous range of pesticides, anthelmintics, antifungals, cardiovascular drugs and agents with other pharmacological properties available to the veterinarian. An important development has been the availability of effective tranquillizers and anaesthetics: they have greatly assisted in the handling of animals during routine procedures and have allowed the full benefits of sophisticated surgical technique to be realized.

Preventive veterinary medicine is now very important; both chemo- and immunoprophylaxis are extensively used nowadays. Development of clinical chemistry is proceeding apace and there is increasing sophistication in the range of tests available to the veterinarian to diagnose disease. The greatest potential lies in animal health products derived from biotechnology.

Karasszon's work (1988) provides a modern survey of the history of veterinary medicine from earliest times to the beginning of the twentieth century.

1.2 THE SCOPE OF VETERINARY MEDICINE TODAY

Veterinary medicine is concerned with the scientific study of health and well-being in animals. Veterinarians strive to prevent disease and other health problems. Advising owners on their animals' care is an important aspect of this, as is the use of a planned animal health programme to prevent disease. Regular veterinary examination can detect health problems and when they are apparent a diagnosis will be made. Diagnosis can involve a range of investigative procedures including radiography and a battery of laboratory tests. When the disease is recognized then treatment is applied. This may involve relatively minor practices such as nail clipping or dental care, or it may involve major surgery. Drugs are used extensively to treat animal disease and the veterinarian must be familiar with the use of a large number of drugs in many species of animals. Once treatment is complete the veterinarian has a responsibility to ensure the rehabilitation of his patients.

Veterinary medicine makes an important contribution to the improvement of animal production throughout the world. The OIE estimates that losses caused by animal diseases worldwide average 20 percent of animal production. Estimates of

Table 1.1   Estimates of the cost of the principle diseases of animals in US$ millions

Diseases common to several species		Pigs	
Foot and mouth disease	50,000	Trichinellosis	2,500
Rift Valley fever	7,500	Gastroenteritis	1,800
		Aujeszky's disease	650
Cattle		Pasteurellosis	500
Mastitis	35,000		
Leptospirosis	4,500	**Horses**	
Brucellosis	3,500	Potomac fever	2,000
Shipping fever	3,000	Equine influenza	1,250
Bluetongue	3,000	Equine infectious	
Calf diarrhoea	1,750	anaemia	1,000
Enzootic bovine leucosis	900		
		Poultry	
		Avian retrovirus	
		infections	1,000
		Fowl cholera	200

Source: Technology Management Group Inc., 1986.

the major costs of the major epizootic diseases are shown in *Table 1.1*. The table omits the diseases principally affecting Asian and African countries, e.g. rinderpest, contagious bovine pleuropneumonia, haemorrhagic septicaemia etc.

The profession deals with both animals and their owners and thus needs a keen awareness of the social, behavioural and cultural interactions of animals and human beings. The animal rights movement and the long-standing involvement of the veterinarian in animal welfare put veterinarians in an important position in determining the way in which animals may be used in society. Serpell (1986) has discussed the relationships of man and animals in general terms and a wide-ranging examination of the situation of pet animals in society is given in *Companion animals in society* (1988). Pets play many roles in society and there is a vast literature on the benefits of pet-ownership and on the ethical, social and psychological issues involved (e.g. Allen, 1985; Bergler, 1986; Katcher and Beck, 1983).

The financial and research contributions that animal health and disease research has made to US agriculture are described by King (1981). He also outlines the major veterinary health problems requiring further research.

1.2.1 Relationships with Other Disciplines

The scope of the subject fields of veterinary medicine is indicated in *Figure 1.2*. Veterinary hygiene and preventive veterinary medicine hold central positions. The diagram also shows the overlapping neighbouring sciences. Medicine, biology and agriculture are vast subjects in their own right and all have information relevant to veterinary science. The veterinary sciences are closely related to human medicine and many of the techniques used in human medicine are directly applicable to the veterinary sciences. The veterinary scientist differs from the human clinician because of the variety of species he encounters and the lack of meaningful veterinarian–client communication. The veterinarian plays an important role in protecting public health via their work in veterinary inspection and in controlling zoonotic diseases. The basic non-clinical biomedical sciences are directly relevant to veterinary research and laboratory workers. The techniques, methods and modes of working of veterinary microbiologists, virologists, clinical pathologists etc. are essentially similar in both medical and veterinary areas. Veterinarians make significant contributions to livestock health and production and require a good knowledge of livestock husbandry and the agricultural sciences.

1.3 ORGANIZATION OF THE SUBJECT FIELD

1.3.1 Varieties of Veterinary Practice

Clinical veterinary medicine is primarily the preserve of individuals in private practice. The records of the American Veterinary Medical Association show that about 75 percent of US veterinarians are in private practice and another study has shown that a similar percentage of new graduates enter private practice (Wise, 1988a). The British Veterinary Association's figures show that in Britain 80 percent of veterinary surgeons are in private practice although there are only about 1700 veterinary practices in the UK.

Practices usually specialize in dealing with particular groups of animals. A division is usually recognized between large and small animal practice, often corresponding to those located in rural and urban areas respectively. In the USA about 49 percent of practitioners are in small animal practice, that is, treating pet animals, mostly cats and dogs. About 11 percent are in large animal practice, that is, caring for farm animals and horses. Veterinarians in large animal practice are increasingly concerned with planned health maintenance and with the management of the reproductive status of the animals in order to optimize productivity. Another 40 percent are in mixed or general practice dealing with all types of animals. Equine veterinary medicine is a speciality in itself and involves some of the most sophisticated veterinary medical care. Within each practice some veterinary surgeons may have particular expertise in certain disciplines, for

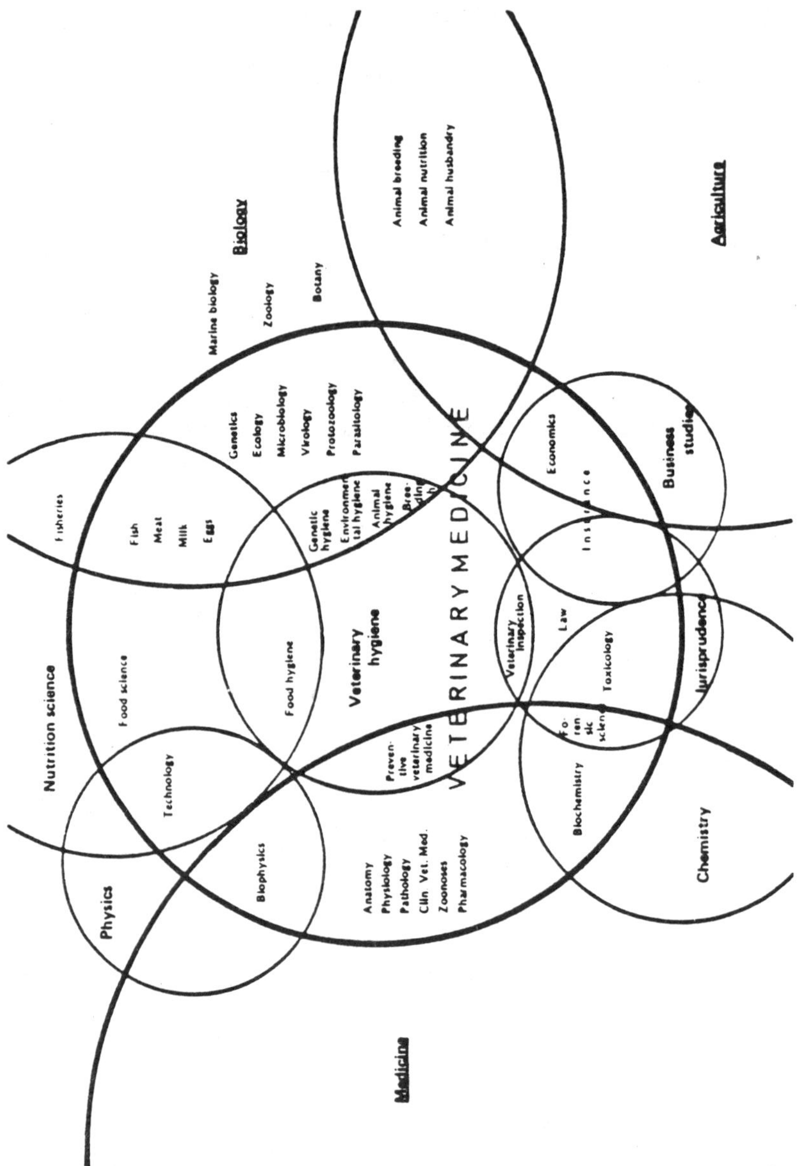

Figure 1.2   Relationship of veterinary medicine to other sciences.
(Brodauf *et al.*, 1977, *see* ref. Chapter 5).

example anaesthesia or ophthalmology, and may have specialist postgraduate training in these or other fields.

A survey of practices in the UK, the results of which were published in *Veterinary record* (**118** (1986): 600–3), indicated that 43 percent of practices were exclusively concerned with small animals, 17 percent exclusively with large animals and 43 percent with mixed practice. On average the small animal practices employed 2.54 veterinarians whereas the other types employed 4.08 and 4.1 veterinarians respectively. Most practices have a principal or principal partner and there may be several junior partners. These will together administer the practice. There may also be assistant veterinary surgeons employed by the practice. The larger practices may employ a practice manager, head nurse, other qualified nurses and trainees, and there may be unqualified lay staff assisting in animal care, other administrative staff and cleaners.

Although most veterinarians are engaged in private practice others are employed by central or local government (8 percent of total qualified personnel in the UK), veterinary schools and research institutes (6 percent), commerce and livestock breeding (4 percent) and welfare organizations (2 percent).

Government agencies are major employers. Government is a major financer of research and most countries have one or more veterinary research institutes. Veterinarians are involved in food hygiene in order to protect the consumer. They examine animals prior to slaughter to eliminate unfit animals and inspect carcasses at slaughter to ensure they are fit for human consumption. They are responsible for controlling the national and international movement of animals. In this case they are attempting to minimize the danger of the spread of disease and to ensure transport techniques are humane. Government veterinarians are also involved in the diagnosis and control of disease generally. Because of the danger to the public of animal diseases most countries have established regional and local veterinary offices which deal with cases locally. They investigate disease outbreaks, assist practising veterinarians in diagnosis and may be involved in research. Governments also actively promote health of farm animals. For example in the UK the State Veterinary Service has four voluntary Animal Health Schemes covering pigs, poultry, cattle and sheep and goats. They serve to promote health and welfare standards and improve productivity via the monitoring and control of disease. Most farm practitioners in Britain act in a part-time capacity as local Veterinary Inspectors of the Ministry of Agriculture. They carry out work testing for tuberculosis or brucellosis and may act as veterinary inspectors at markets looking after the animals' welfare and looking out for any notifiable diseases. Practitioners may also be involved in meat hygiene work in abbatoirs or poultry slaughterhouses. Veterinarians may also work full- or part-time for local government. Here they would be inspecting riding establishments, zoos, dog kennels, pet-shops etc., and may be involved in food hygiene work.

In the United States nearly 3,000 veterinarians are employed by Federal government. Nearly 2,000 of these are employed by the various arms of the USDA, the majority by the Food Safety and Inspection Service (FSIS) and by the

Animal and Plant Health Inspection Service (APHIS). FSIS ensures that all meat and poultry products are safe, wholesome and accurately labelled. APHIS is responsible for the control and eradication of disease, for preventing foreign animal diseases entering the country, for assuring safe and potent veterinary biologics and for ensuring the humane care and use of animals. The US Department of Defense is a major employer.

Academic veterinary medicine is concerned with the education and training of veterinary students. Full-time teaching staff are employees of the university and the majority of their time is spent on research and teaching. Over 3,000 of the veterinarians in the United States are involved in veterinary education.

Veterinarians are employed by industry and are involved in two industrial sectors. First there are the animal health companies which develop and market products for use as animal medicines or medicated feedstuffs. In this case the veterinarian could be involved in research, development, sales support or marketing. Second, there are pharmaceutical, chemical, pet-food, food and nutrition companies using animals in research and development. Veterinarians are required to supervise the health and care of these laboratory animals. Veterinarians may also be employed in commercial livestock breeding enterprises. A booklet outlining the responsibilities and rewards of working in industry has been issued by the Association of Veterinarians in Industry (1985).

Many veterinarians work for charitable institutions which are usually concerned with the welfare and well-being of companion animals. Thus in the UK the Royal Society for the Prevention of Cruelty to Animals, Blue Cross etc., employ many veterinarians. These practitioners are salaried and the organizations are funded by gifts, legacies and donations invited from pet owners. The People's Dispensary for Sick Animals is the largest veterinary practice in the UK. More than a million treatments are given every year at its fifty-seven Animal Treatment Centres and a further 150,000 pets are treated free by private veterinary surgeons participating in its Pet-Aid scheme.

Veterinarians can be involved in many other areas such as zoo animal medicine, fish farming and aquaculture, horse racing etc.

1.3.2 Ancillary Personnel

The veterinary surgeon is assisted in the care and treatment of their patients by a variety of ancillary staff who may also be involved with reception work, liaising with clients, admitting and discharging animals etc. Senior ancillary staff may play an important role in practice management.

In Britain there are now some 2,800 veterinary nurses and more than 5,000 trainees. The British Veterinary Nursing Association (BVNA) is the national body representing veterinary nurses. It was formed in 1965 and now has almost 800 members. The RCVS runs a training scheme for veterinary nurses and has published a guide, which includes the syllabus for the examinations, for those wishing to enter this field (RCVS, 1988). The BVNA can also supply useful information on the requirements and procedure for becoming a trainee veterinary nurse. The training and examinations are orientated to staff working in small animal practices. Both full- and part-time courses are available; practical experience is a prerequisite before applying for such courses. The BVNA can advise on other professional matters, including salaries and conditions. The Manpower Services Commission has produced brief guides which outline all the careers available working with animals (1986, 1984). A more detailed description of these careers is provided by Young and Donald (1983).

In other countries veterinary assistants and nurses may be called animal health technicians or veterinary technicians. As in the UK the national veterinary association is often involved in approving academic courses. The AVMA for example, in conjunction with the American Association of Veterinary Technician Educators, publishes a list of American schools offering accredited programmes in animal technology. This gives details of programmes in thirty-five states. The AVMA can supply a list of state and regional professional technician associations and provides a range of career advisory services including a job listing/placement service. Guides are available describing the training programmes and courses available in animal health technology and nursing (Giamattei and Anderson, 1985). Other guides describe careers as DVMs as well as in animal health technology and nursing (Lee and Lee, 1984; Simmons 1984).

In many of the developing countries much of the animal health care is provided by auxiliary animal health workers and not by professional graduate veterinarians.

1.4 STATUTORY AND PROFESSIONAL BODIES

There are three types of organizations involved in the running and development of the veterinary profession. The universities and their veterinary schools train veterinarians, and are discussed in the next section. The other two types are the statutory bodies, empowered by governments, and the professional organizations which may be international, national, local or speciality.

1.4.1 Statutory Bodies and Legislation

In most countries the practice of veterinary medicine is governed by national or regional government laws. A newly-qualified veterinarian must therefore register with the appropriate authority before beginning to provide treatment. Qualified persons are thereby entitled to perform surgical work on animals, to dispense drugs, and to work within a complex set of legislation relating to animal health and welfare. The statutory body is able to supervise the standards of veterinarians in these tasks and is able to monitor standards of professional conduct.

In Britain, for example, the veterinary profession is governed by the Royal College of Veterinary Surgeons (RCVS). The RCVS receives its powers from

Royal Charters, the most recent being the Supplemental Royal Charter of 1967, and from the Veterinary Surgeons Act, the most recent being passed in 1966. All practising veterinary surgeons are members of the RCVS. The RCVS deals with disciplinary matters and ethics, and is under a statutory obligation to maintain its *Registers* [206]. All veterinarians entitled to practise in the UK pay an annual fee to the RCVS and are thereby listed in the *Registers*. The RCVS's *Guide to professional conduct* (1987) outlines the responsibilities veterinary surgeons have and indicates standards for good practice in the execution of their duties. An important function of the RCVS is the maintenance of eduational standards. This involves close liaison with the universities in order to exercise its supervisory powers in relation to veterinary undergraduate education. The RCVS also awards its own postgraduate Diplomas and Certificates in some of the specialities.

British graduates may practise in other EEC countries and European nationals with approved qualifications may practise in Britain. Details of approved qualifications are given in the RCVS's *Registers*. Graduates from veterinary schools in Australia, New Zealand, Pretoria in South Africa, and Guelph and Saskatoon in Canada are also eligible to become RCVSs but they are not entitled thereby to practise in Europe. Graduates from other schools must pass a membership examination.

In the USA each state has its own licensing board, which issues its own regulations, and each state holds examinations to assess a veterinarian's competence. Most use the National Board Examination and Clinical Competency Test. Although there is some reciprocity between the states in recognizing the validity of the licences they issue, a veterinarian licensed to practise in one state would normally have to obtain a new licence to practise in another.

In Canada a graduate must be certified or licensed to practise in the various provinces by the appropriate provincial veterinary association. In Australia also, veterinarians register with the state or territory in which they wish to practise.

1.4.2 International Organizations

Veterinary medicine is practised worldwide, and practitioners, academics and policy-makers co-operate extensively in developing the profession. The diversity of veterinary practice has led to the creation of many special interest groups. These link people working in the same field, and may operate at national or international level. Most groups publish newsletters or journals as a service to their members; these are listed in Part II. The more important American, British and international specialist groupings are listed in the directory of organizations which forms Part III.

In most cases the international association for a speciality has been created from the merger of various national societies. The World Small Animal Veterinary Association (WSAVA) is a typical example. It now has some 30,000 members, most of whom are also members of one of the fourteen national associations and two international specialist study groups involved in small animal practice. The

World Association for Buiatrics is a similar international grouping and Rehkemper (1985) has written an account of its history and of that of the various national cattle veterinary associations which are members. The main functions of such international groups are to publish journals and newsletters, and to arrange international congresses. However they become involved in any activity which fosters international co-operation and collaboration; the WSAVA, for example, is currently engaged in a project on the international control of inherited disease in dogs.

Apart from the groups devoted to a speciality the two international bodies which have had the greatest impact on improving international collaboration and liaison are the Office International des Épizooties and the World Veterinary Association.

Office International des Épizooties

The Office International des Épizooties was founded in 1924 to improve world-wide co-operation in controlling contagious animal diseases. The history, objectives and working of the OIE have been described by Wrathall (1986). There are now 111 member countries. The activities of the OIE are guided by an International Committee which meets at a General Session annually. The delegates are generally the Chief Veterinary Officers from each country.

The OIE's most important role is to disseminate information on epizootics which endanger livestock or pose a hazard to human health. Information is central to the OIE's activities and it publishes several journals, monographs (in its Technical Series) and conference proceedings. Its publications on animal disease incidence are reviewed later on. The OIE has four Regional Commissions covering the Americas, Asia–Far-East–Oceania, Europe and Africa. Each Commission promotes regional co-operation in animal disease control, mainly by holding conferences, on average once every two years. The proceedings of these conferences, at which several topics of general interest are discussed are published. Apart from the Regional conferences the OIE also organizes symposia on specialist matters of topical interest and publishes the proceedings. The most recent are: 1986: *Foot and mouth disease – 17th Conference*; 1985: *Round Table on sanitary problems related to embryo transfer*; 1984: *Symposium on fish vaccination*; 1983: *Anabolics in animal production*. There are also four specialist Commissions: the Foot and Mouth Disease Commission; the Norms Commission (concerned with standards for diagnostic methods and vaccine production); International Zoo-Sanitary Code Commission (provides recommendations on the import/export of animals and animal products); Fish Diseases Commission. The work of the Norms and International Zoo-Sanitary Code Commissions is published in the *International zoo-sanitary code* [1366]. This provides guidelines which can be used by national veterinary services to compile statutory regulations for the international trade of animals and animal products. The code also includes standards for biological products, vaccines, for diagnostic tests, disinfection procedures and the transport of animals.

World Veterinary Association

The World Veterinary Association provides a central link for the exchange of information between the national associations. It is also able to co-ordinate international efforts in developing the profession's standing and in improving veterinary education and practice. It represents the interests of the profession in consultations with other international associations and organizations such as the various United Nations agencies. Most of the larger international and specialist veterinary associations are associate members of the WVA and there are national members, that is, national organizations or groups of national organizations, in seventy-two countries. There are also affiliated and honorary members.

The main activities of the WVA are the production of its *Bulletin* [326] and the organization of the quadrennial World Veterinary Congress. Indeed, the WVA, which was founded in 1959, is a continuation of the Permanent Committee for the International Veterinary Congresses which was created at the Ninth Congress (Budapest, 1905).

Other International Organizations

There are several other international federations of national veterinary associations apart from the WVA. The Commonwealth Veterinary Association (CwVA) [2148] is the largest. It was founded in 1967 and now has forty-two member countries and a membership of more than 50,000 veterinary surgeons. The Indian Veterinary Association is the largest national association in the CwVA having 22,000 members out of a total of 30,000 veterinarians in India. The CwVA is divided into six geographical regions. Regional conferences are organized at frequent intervals. A books project has been set up to provide textbooks to countries who have currency difficulties and a twinning project has been established linking BVA Divisions with Commonwealth associations. One of the most active regions in the CwVA is the Canada/Caribbean region. All the associations in the Caribbean are members of the Caribbean Veterinary Association which is a federation of fourteen local associations.

The Federation of Veterinarians of the EEC [2182] is a collection of twelve national veterinary associations with a further four associations having observer status. It has an important role in representing the views of the member associations at all levels within the EEC.

The main other regional associations are the Federation of Asian Veterinary Associations [2180], which now has twelve member organizations, the Nordic Committee for Veterinary Science Cooperation and the Panamerican Association of Veterinary Sciences (founded at the Pan American Congress of Veterinary Science 1988). These collaborative ventures allow the smaller associations to work together in tackling common problems and in developing their members' skills and professional interests. For example, associations in North Africa (Morocco, Algeria and Tunisia) formed the Maghreb Veterinary Associations Group and this sponsors a regional veterinary meeting (Journées Vétérinaires Maghrebines) and together they publish a quarterly journal (*Maghreb vétérinaire*).

1.4.3 National Associations

Most countries have their own professional veterinary society. These societies are the public face of the profession and promote the profession's views to the public, government, academic and other institutions. Registration with the appropriate statutory body is usually mandatory whereas membership of the national professional societies is optional; none the less most veterinarians become members, be they practitioners, students or academics. The national associations will protect their members' interests and offer personal assistance to individual members. They also become involved in developing ethical standards of veterinary medical practice. They usually produce a journal and/or a newsletter. These contain items of both local and international relevance. The associations often run courses to allow practitioners to develop their business skills and assist in continuing professional development. Many produce materials suitable for veterinarians to distribute to clients to aid client education or to assist the veterinarian in public relations activities.

National veterinary associations are useful sources of information on the profession in that country. Some representative bodies are described below; a complete list is given in Part III.

American Veterinary Medical Association

The AVMA was founded in 1863 and it is now the largest veterinary organization in the world with over 47,000 members. Over 99 percent of new graduates join the AVMA. It is a federation of over seventy state, territorial and allied veterinary medical groups. The association now has a full time paid staff of nearly sixty. Sixty percent of the operating budget comes from members' dues and most of the rest is generated from advertising in the Association's journals and from the sale of journals and convention exhibit space. The AVMA's *Directory* [211] contains detailed information about the Association's structure and its activities. News about the Association's work is reported in the *Journal of the American Veterinary Medical Association.*

British Veterinary Association

The BVA was founded in 1881 at a National Veterinary Congress as the British National Veterinary Association. It was formed from fifteen local associations and it still retains its regional roots and structure. There are now thirty-one territorial divisions and nineteen specialist divisions. The British Small Animal Veterinary Association (BSAVA) is the largest of the latter. The BVA is the focal point for all matters affecting veterinary surgeons in the United Kingdom and the association now has 8,400 members and 36 employees. The BVA promotes the advancement of veterinary science on a broad front. The wide range of the association's activities is summarized in its *Annual report*. It is the publisher of three important journals: *Veterinary record, Research in veterinary science* and *In practice*, a monthly news magazine for members, *BVA news*, and several journals for the divisions. The

Veterinary record is one of the most widely read journals having a circulation of about 11,000 copies. The BVA also publish a magazine for clients, *You and your vet*. A recent survey showed that 72 percent of small animal practices distribute this to clients.

1.4.4 Other Associations

Countries with large numbers of veterinarians often have networks of regional organizations and in most countries the national association is the best source of information about these. These groups provide a convenient local forum for practitioners to meet and exchange ideas. In the United States each state has its own association and there are regional and local veterinary medical associations in the major market areas. The *Media guide to veterinary sources and information* is a free publication produced annually by the AVMA's Public Affairs Division which gives contacts for each of these groups. In Britain the BVA has divisions in each region. Most advertise their meetings in *Veterinary record*. Canada too has regional societies.

1.5 EDUCATION

An international meeting on veterinary education was held in 1962 at which it was recommended that the minimum duration of undergraduate education should be five years. In some countries, for example Japan, students follow a six-year course. Usually the degree which is granted qualifies the individual to practise veterinary medicine although some countries still require practitioners to pass a national licensing examination. In most colleges of veterinary medicine the course-work is split so that students study the basic biomedical sciences first and then study clinical aspects of the subject. The latter section involves much practical work and experience. The schools run veterinary hospitals and have their own farms. They are thus able to provide students with all types of clinical training. The schools play an important role by acting as centres to which practising veterinarians can refer troublesome or interesting cases for further study.

Mexico and Brazil have the largest number of students and schools in relation to their populations. Mexico has thirty-six schools, Brazil has twenty-eight from which 2,000 veterinarians graduate each year; by 1991 Brazil will have more than 30,000 qualified personnel. There are thirty-nine veterinary schools in Europe and overall there are now between 360 and 370 veterinary schools in the world. The WVA has recently expressed concern at the proliferation of centres of veterinary education of inadequate standard.

About 2,200 veterinarians qualify each year in the USA and about 290 in Canada. In the United States and Canada students are awarded a Doctor of Veterinary Medicine degree. The AVMA *Directory* gives details of the veterinary colleges in North America including information on their accreditation status. To obtain a degree requires three years of preveterinary college education and four years of study at a veterinary school or college. A compilation of the admissions requirements of the US schools plus three in Canada is available (Sawyer, 1987) and a general guide has been published for students intending to study for a DVM (Crawford, 1987). There are several guides to careers in veterinary medicine in the United States (Swope, 1987; Duncan, 1988).

Many internship and residency programmes have been established and many new graduates take advantage of these. Wise (1988b) surveyed new graduates and found that 10.7 percent of men and 20.5 percent of women were engaged in advanced study. Information from the Association of Veterinary Medical Colleges shows that in 1986–7 820 students were following MS degrees, 917 PhD degrees, and 535 residency/internship or joint residency and higher degree programmes. Practitioners in the USA are now able to qualify in sixteen recognized veterinary specialities. Nearly 5 percent of practices employ veterinarians with diplomate status (*Veterinary practice* **21** (1989): 1). The speciality qualifications are administered by Boards and Colleges: these are listed in Part III. Each provides opportunities for further study and education and organizes examinations and certification programmes. The overall aim is to improve the proficiency and knowledge of members. The American Board of Veterinary Practitioners is a typical organization. It has three areas of certification in companion animal practice, food animal practice and equine practice. To achieve Diplomate status candidates must have completed appropriate internship and residency programmes or have a minimum of six years' experience in a suitable environment, show evidence of following a satisfactory course of postgraduate continuing education and show the ability to write quality manuscripts suitable for publication. Candidates must take an examination and all diplomates must recertify by passing the examination every 10 years. In 1988 forty-five candidates took the examination. Many Canadian veterinarians have become diplomates of the American speciality organizations and postgraduate education is well-established at the universities: about 20 percent of the profession undergo further training to receive MSc, MVSc, PhD or DVSc (Doctor of Veterinary Science) degrees. The latter is through a graduate programme involving both training and research in a speciality.

The university veterinary degree courses in Britain and the training involved are described in the RCVS's booklet *A career as a veterinary surgeon* (RCVS, 1988). It also outlines the possibilites for postgraduate training, giving details on the awards and grants which are available. Apart from the RCVS's booklet Donald (1985) describes the careers available as a veterinary surgeon. A comprehensive guide to degree courses in the UK with a discussion of the entry requirements, course content and character and career paths is available in a careers research and advisory guide (Darke, 1988). It is more difficult to obtain a place to study veterinary medicine than any other subject and only students with the highest educational standards are accepted. The universities advise candidates to obtain some experience of work with a veterinary surgeon prior to beginning the undergraduate course. There are currently six veterinary schools at Bristol, Cambridge, Edinburgh, Glasgow, Liverpool and London and there are about four applicants for each place. The courses last for five or six years and some of the vacation work is spent in a working environment in order to gain specific types of experience. Graduates receive a Bachelor's degree and this entitles them to apply to become a member of the RCVS. An interesting perspective on work in the profession is given in the annual employment survey of new graduates which is published in the *Veterinary record* (most recent: **122** (1988): 316–21).

Postgraduate education is available at the universities and many graduates embark on research for higher degrees. In addition many veterinary graduates undergo postgraduate training in aspects of veterinary science, animal science and production via MSc and Diploma courses. Veterinarians in practice may develop specialist interests in particular fields of veterinary medicine. The RCVS has played an important role in fostering the development of these skills and now awards Certificates or Diplomas in a variety of disciplines such as Veterinary Ophthalmology, Veterinary Radiology, in the health and production of farm animals, and in aspects of equine and small animal medicine and surgery. The Certificates are awarded by examination. The Diplomas are awarded after examination and by satisfying the examining board of extensive practical experience in the area of interest, supplemented by short courses and private study.

The highest qualification in the UK is the Diploma of Fellowship of the Royal College of Veterinary Surgeons. This is usually awarded either for a thesis, in a similar manner to obtaining a PhD, or by examination. Candidates must have been members of the College or have held a registrable degree for at least five years. An FRCVS can also be granted for meritorious contributions to learning. Candidates must be eminent in their field, have held an MRCVS or a registrable degree for over twenty years and have advanced the cause of veterinary science. In 1987 there were 387 Fellows.

References

Allen, K. M. *The human–animal bond: an annotated bibliography*. Metuchen, New Jersey: Scarecrow Press, 1985. 246pp.

Association of Veterinarians in Industry. *AVI careers handbook*. Edited by D. Walker and K. C. Sellers. London: RCVS, 1985. 64pp.

Bergler, R. *Man and dog: the psychology of a relationship*. Oxford: Blackwell, 1986. 188pp.

Boland, C. J. and Morris, R. S. 'Demographic profile of the veterinary profession in New Zealand, 1985'. *New Zealand veterinary journal* **36** (1988): 128–32.

Clutton-Brock, J. *A natural history of domesticated animals*. Cambridge: CUP, 1987. 208pp.

Companion animals in society: report of a working party Council for Science and Society. Oxford: OUP, 1988. 78pp.

Crawford, J. D. *The preveterinary planning guide*. PO Box 34631, Bethesda, Maryland 20817, USA: Betz Publishing, 1987. 200pp.

Darke, P. G. G. *Degree course guide 1988/89. Veterinary science in UK universities polytechnics and colleges*. Hobsons Publishing, Bateman Street, Cambridge CB2 1LZ: CRAC Learning Materials. (Updated biennially; most recent ed. 1988.)

De Wailly, P. 'Charles Vial de Saint-Bel. Père de la médecine vétérinaire en Angleterre et fondateur du Collège Vétérinaire de Londres (1792)'. *Bulletin de l'Academie Vétérinaire de France* **58** (1985): 213–22.

Donald, V. *Careers in veterinary surgery*. London: Kogan Page, 1985. 111pp. (Kogan Page Careers Series.)

Duncan, J. C. *Careers in veterinary medicine*. New York: Rosen Pub. Group, 1988. 129pp.

Dyce, K. M. and Merlen, R. H. A. 'Carlo Ruini and *L'Anatomia del Cavallo*'. *British veterinary journal* **109** (1953): 385–90.

Ford, C. M. 'Aleen Cust – first woman veterinary surgeon in Britain – early influences'. *Veterinary history* **3** (1985): 131–7.

Giamattei, V. M. and Anderson, J. G. *Training programs and careers in animal health technology and veterinary nursing in North America*. Napa, California: Dillon-Tyler, 1985. 164pp.

Karasszon, D. *A concise history of veterinary medicine*. Akadémiai Kiado: Budapest, 1988. 458pp.

Katcher, A. H. and Beck, A. M. (eds) *New perspectives on our lives with companion animals*. Philadelphia: University of Pennsylvania Press, 1983. 588pp.

King, N. B. on behalf of the AVMA Council on Research. 'Contributions and needs of animal health and disease research'. *American journal of veterinary research* **42** (1981): 1093–108.

Lee, M. P. and Lee, R. S. *Opportunities in animal and pet care careers*. Lincolnswood, Illinois: VGM Career Horizons, 1984. 150pp.

Manpower Services Commission. *Work with animals*. Moorfoot, Sheffield S1 4PR: Careers and Occupational Information Centre, 1986. 24pp. ('Working in' Series, no. 84.)

Manpower Services Commission. *Work with animals* and *Animal welfare*. Sheffield: Careers and Occupational Information Centre, 1984. Each 4pp. (Job Outlines Series, nos 92 and 90.)

Rehkemper, U. *Die Welt-Gesellschaft für Buiatrik*. Tierärztliche Hochschule Hannover: Inaugural Dissertation, 1985. 108pp.

Royal College of Veterinary Surgeons. *A career as a veterinary surgeon*. 5th ed. London: the College, 1988. 49pp.

RCVS. *Veterinary nursing: a guide for persons wishing to train as veterinary nurses*. Revised edition. London: the College, 1988. 137pp.

RCVS. *Guide to professional conduct*. London: the College, 1987. 84pp.

Sawyer, M. J. *Veterinary medical school admission requirements in the United States and Canada*. Bethesda: Betz Publishing, 1987. 160pp.

Serpell, J. A. *In the company of animals*. Oxford: Blackwell, 1986. 215pp.

Simmons, M. L. *Career guide to the animal health field: veterinary doctor, veterinary scientist, animal health technologist, laboratory technician*. 2nd ed. Media, Pennsylvania: Harwal Publishing, 1984. 84pp.

Smithcors, J. F. 'Chiron, Apsyrtus & Carlo Ruini'. *Modern veterinary practice* **59** (1978): 433–6

Swope, R. E. *Opportunities in veterinary medicine careers*. Lincolnwood, Illinois: VGM Career Horizons, 1987. 148pp. (VGM Career Books.)

Wise, J. K. 'Employment, starting salaries, and educational endebtedness of 1988 graduates of US veterinary medical colleges'. *Journal of the American Veterinary Medical Association* **193** (1988a): 1317–18.

Wise, J. K. 'Employment of 1988 male and female graduates of US veterinary medical colleges'. *Journal of the American Veterinary Medical Association* **192** (1988b): 1569–70.

Wrathall, A. E. 'Office International des Épizooties (OIE). A forum for international veterinary co-operation'. *State veterinary journal* **40** (1986): (116) 85–95.

Young, H. and Donald, V. *Careers working with animals*. 4th ed. 120 Pentonville Road, London N1 9JN: Kogan Page, 1983. 96pp. (Kogan Page Careers Series.)

2 Veterinary Information: Its Origins and Utilization

The first modern book devoted to an aspect of veterinary medicine, *Anatomia del cavallo, infirmita et suoi rimedii*, was published in 1598, but the veterinary journal was not initiated until 1824 when the *Recueil de médecine vétérinaire* was founded. The first British journals began publication in 1828: *The Farrier and naturalist*, later called *The Hippiatrist*, and *The veterinarian*. The former was only published for three years but the latter was published monthly until 1902. The popularity and demand for the veterinary journal was such that by 1900 there were sixty current periodicals (Houston, 1983) and by 1938 there were 100 titles (Edwards, 1948). Growth in the numbers of journals has continued and in 1984 the Commonwealth Bureau of Animal Health scanned over 1,400 titles. Nowadays accepted knowledge and practices are summarized in textbooks but important research findings and new developments are still best communicated in journals.

It would be difficult to estimate the precise number of veterinary books published each year throughout the world but some indication can be obtained by examining *Veterinary bulletin* and *Index veterinarius*. In 1986 they noted 179 books, of which 133 were in English, 19 in German and 13 in Russian. These services doubtless provide more detailed coverage of books in English than in other languages: some indication of the numbers of books published in other languages is given by Giovannetti and Meissonnier [4], who give information on the numbers of veterinary books on the stock lists of the major publishers.

2.1 JOURNALS

The veterinary journal is the accepted mode of publication for the dissemination of the results of original research. From their outset however they have also been important as an up-to-date, easily accessible means of communication within the profession. The journals with the broadest scope, therefore, are those issued by the national or local associations, such as *Veterinary record*, and those published by veterinary schools, such as *Southwestern veterinarian* and *Cornell veterinarian*. The specialized nature of much veterinary practice has been reflected in the journal literature. Many titles today are, therefore, published by or on behalf of specialist societies. Issues are most commonly monthly, bimonthly or quarterly. The frequency often increases with the titles' success; the *Journal of the American Veterinary Medical Association* appears fortnightly and the *Veterinary record* is the only weekly journal publishing research articles.

The languages in which the literature is published is considered in Chapter 3. The majority of the well-known journals are international in scope and publish almost all their articles in English. Material published in other languages tends to be of local interest. Bilingual countries such as Canada and South Africa publish in both their national languages. Locally produced journals are important for news and topical information about the particular geographic area and for research work which has a direct relevance to the local situation.

2.2 BOOKS

Whereas the journal is used to communicate new ideas and developments, the textbook provides a convenient summary of current knowledge. Most of the standard texts, while primarily written with the student in mind, are equally suitable for practitioners to refer to for revision, practical instructions, or to investigate a speciality with which they are not familiar. As with journals, English is the predominant language of publication but the international market is of such importance that many titles are routinely translated into other languages.

Books are available at all technical levels for the undergraduate, postgraduate and practitioner. Advances in modern printing technology mean that both books and journals are often lavishly illustrated nowadays. A popular form of text is the colour atlas, with photographs of anatomical features, surgical techniques, and clinical and pathological conditions. A majority of veterinarians in the developed countries work in small animal medicine and surgery and because of this there is a very wide range of texts dealing with particular aspects of the medicine and surgery of companion animals. For example one may find books on small animal orthopaedics, canine behaviour, feline trauma management and so on. A special category of materials are the popular discussions on animal health and disease, normally written by veterinarians for the benefit of farmers, stockmen and owners of horses and other companion animals.

2.3 UTILIZATION OF THE LITERATURE

There have been few studies of the habits of veterinarians in information gathering and use.

Ikpaahindi (1985) recently carried out a survey among the staff of the Nigerian Veterinary Research Institute but his findings however are of limited value in assessing the habits of practitioners in developed countries. Of more value is the survey of veterinarians in practice in Indiana which Drake and Woods (1978) carried out prior to establishing a veterinary medical information centre at Purdue University. Respondents were asked to rank various sources consulted in the last two years for critical and non-critical information, critical information being defined as information related to the life or well-being of a patient. Books were the most important sources used (*Table 2.1*). The veterinarians were also asked to indicate the sources most frequently used for new information in six subject areas. Other than for information on equipment and drugs, the most significant sources were books and journals (*Table 2.2*). The mean number of journal subscriptions was 2.5 although 23 percent of the practitioners subscribed to five or more titles.

Another survey, which reinforces the importance of books and journals as information sources, was carried out in the UK recently (Raw, 1987). Five hundred and thirty-seven practices, representing about one-third of all practices, responded to a postal survey on their practice libraries. The main journals taken by the practices are shown in *Table 2.3*. The ranking broadly corresponded to the practitioners' opinion on their relative usefulness. The pre-eminence of the *Veterinary record* was confirmed in a market survey recently carried out on behalf of the BVA (Anon, 1988). Four hundred and one veterinary surgeons were questioned, virtually all of whom (98 percent) said they 'ever read' the *Veterinary record*. The average readership for each of the fifty-one issues was 80 percent and 50 percent kept the *Record* for reference. Although the *Veterinary record* and *Journal of*

Table 2.1 Sources of veterinary information ranked either first or second in importance (percentage of respondents)

	Critical	*Non-critical topics*
Books	71.1	73.4
Other practitioners	34.8	35.4
University clinicians	24	19.5
Journal articles	24	42.8
University diagnostic laboratory	20.1	7.2

Source: Drake and Woods, 1978.

Table 2.2 Ranking of sources of new information

Source	Drugs and biologics	Diseases	Surgical procedures	Preventive medicine	Equipment	Nutrition and management
Journals	2	1	1	1	4	1
Books	7	2	2	2	7	2
National professional meetings	6	4	4	4	6	3
Extension services	10	6	7	5	10	4
Other practitioners	5	3	3	3	5	5
University faculty	3	5	5	7	8	6
Sales representatives	1	9	8	6	1	7
Advertisements received in mail	4	10	9	10	3	8
Advertisements in journals	3	11	—	9	2	9
State veterinarian	11	7	10	8	11	11

Source: Drake and Woods, 1978.

Table 2.3   Main journals taken in veterinary practices in the United Kingdom

Journal	Number and percentage of practices	
	Number	*Percentage*
Veterinary record	526	97.9
Journal of small animal practice	411	76.5
Equine veterinary journal	146	27.1
British veterinary journal	45	8.5
Journal of the American Veterinary Medical Association	25	4.3
Journal of the American Animal Hospital Association	24	4.3
Other journals	90	16.8

Source: Raw, 1987.

small animal practice were the most widely read journals, Raw's survey found that ninety of the practices took over fifty-one different additional journals, indicating the diversity of practitioners' interests.

The number of books in the library of each practice ranged from none to over 500, the most frequent numbers being in the range eleven to thirty. Most of the practices spent between £50 and £100 on books per annum. Practitioners complained about the lack of time to read and to catch up with the literature, so a high regard was held for anything concise and clinically relevant. About half the practices took the *Veterinary annual* and many also subscribed to titles in the *Veterinary clinics of North America* series [71–73] and to titles in the *Current veterinary therapy* series [406, 709, 799, 1643].

The use of journals in an academic environment is very different from that in practice. Veenstra (1987) reports on a journal use study in the Veterinary Medical Library at Auburn University. He presents a table ranking the fifty journals most frequently used which, although representing only 13 percent of all titles used, represents 57 percent of all reported uses. As might be expected the three journals most heavily used were *Journal of the American Veterinary Medical Association*, *American journal of veterinary research* and *Compendium on continuing education*. The *Veterinary record* and *Journal of small animal practice* were ranked fourth and fifth respectively. Surprisingly non-veterinary journals comprised 44 percent of the top fifty journals. These included two of the journals in the top ten titles, *New England journal of medicine* (rank 6) and *Immunology today* (rank 9). Each library is unique and these use patterns cannot be extrapolated too widely; however, it is likely that the requirement for veterinary students, teaching and research staff to use medical journals is common in most academic environments.

The information gathering habits of veterinary students in the United States has been studied recently by Pelzer and Leysen (1988). Students used the library at Iowa State University mainly for referring to coursework and photocopying. There was little use of abstracting and indexing information services and virtually no use of computerized information systems. The authors point out that after graduation most students will work in small practices and have to rely on personally owned books and journals. They highlight the fact that the variety of veterinary practice is such that these may be inappropriate to satisfy information needs. The implication is that students should have greater formal training in information use, and greater exposure to computerized information services.

As we have seen, practitioners read a small number of journals and even in large academic libraries most of the journal use is accounted for by relatively few titles. Apart for Veenstra's study, noted above, another survey carried out at the Danish Veterinary and Agricultural University Library showed that 85 percent of requests for journal articles were satisfied by just 7 percent of the current serials (Hansen, 1981). (The same study indicated that 30 percent of all the requests received by the library were for books.) A variety of workers (cited in Giovannetti and Meissonnier [4]; Cho, 1977; Garfield, 1982; Houston, 1983; Russell *et al.* 1987) have used the technique of citation analysis; that is, examining the references cited in the veterinary literature to determine the major journals. Each of these studies has confirmed that there is a small core list of journals which accounts for most of the citations.

2.3.1 Coping with the Literature

A vast amount of new literature is published each year. The pace at which new publications appear is such that Houston (1983) and Cho (1977) have estimated the half-life of the veterinary literature to be 7.5 and 6.1 years respectively. However by subscribing to or scanning the core journals and by using the services described in Chapter 4, veterinarians may keep up to date. A recent article by White (1988) attempts to reassure those worried by the concept of the 'information explosion' as applied to veterinary medicine.

Research workers, academics and many practitioners develop their own files of reprints or photocopies of articles and other useful literature. Although the practice of requesting reprints from authors is declining, it is still important for workers to make personal contact with experts in the field. Some of the current awareness services are especially useful since they give the authors' addresses and so a direct approach can be made to the authors. Libraries can then be used to supply items not available from the authors themselves.

Stibic's (1980) and Warren's (1981) guides have for many years been the standard texts for professional scientists on methods of coping with the volume of literature. More recently Blood and Brightling (1988) have written on the topic and their book is specifically directed at veterinary practitioners. It takes a wide-ranging view of the storage, handling and retrieval of veterinary information, but is especially concerned with clinical data, and with techniques for handling and using the information required for making a diagnosis. Their work stresses computerized methods of storing and retrieving data. Although the use of computers is becoming increasingly widespread a simple manual system can be quite effective for dealing with published materials. Such systems are cheaper, often simpler to operate, allow one to browse more efficiently and are very flexible in comparison to computerized files. A number of authors have described manual systems for indexing and filing literature (Schindler, 1981; Wolff, 1982; Romatowski, 1987).

Most practices now have computers, however, and the temptation to create computerized records of the literature may prove irresistible. Blood and Brightling discuss some of the systems but new software is continually becoming available. There are two regularly updated guides, which cover specialized software for libraries and information services, as well as more well-known 'business' database packages (Dyer and Gunson, 1988; Kimberley, 1987). Once stored on a personal computer the data can be searched and displayed in many different ways and may be exported to word processing programs when compiling bibliographies and writing articles etc. A further advantage of computerized systems is that data may be 'downloaded' direct from online databases and automatically added to local databases on personal computers. Approval from the copyright holder is required. Many of the database producers have taken this development one stage further and now supply the data on floppy disc. BIOSIS and the Institute for Scientific Information both now have complete packages allowing users to compile and manage their own databases.

2.4 LITERARY STYLE

The style and presentation of the veterinary literature follow the same principles as medical and scientific writing. There are no guides to scientific writing especially published for veterinary authors. Those preparing materials for publication will therefore find general texts covering the art of scientific writing appropriate to their needs. Examples are the books by Day (1988), and Huth (1987), whose work is especially written for medical authors. A useful and inexpensive guide to effective writing for agricultural advisory staff has been published by MAFF (1981). A more advanced and detailed reference work is the *CBE style manual* (1983).

Most journals have their own house style and authors preparing manuscripts must conform to these to have their contributions accepted. Many journals now conform to a uniform set of requirements established by the International Committee of Medical Journal Editors (*see Annals of internal medicine* **108** (1988): 258–65). Apart from this and the general style manuals noted above there are a number of British and international standards which give recommendations for the preparation of theses, research reports and quote methods for citing publications by bibliographic references. A complete discussion of the latter topic has been written by Gray (1982) especially for veterinary authors.

The standard texts on biometrics and medical statistics can be used when analysing experimental and clinical data but Sard [1782] has written a simple introduction to the application of statistical methods in veterinary practice. Epidemiology texts also discuss handling data in some detail.

2.5 VETERINARY LIBRARIES

Specialist veterinary libraries or collections are few in number and most are in veterinary schools or run by national organizations. The situation in Britain, which is described below, is typical of many other countries.

2.5.1 Veterinary Libraries in Britain

Universities and colleges with departments of agriculture, animal science or animal production will have materials on animal health and veterinary science in their libraries. Similarly the libraries of medical schools, and other academic institutes serving zoologists and parasitologists, will have stock on veterinary public health, zoonoses and comparative parasitology. This is exemplified by Roy's (1984) survey of medical schools in the United States which found that their libraries had an average of 171 books on veterinary medicine. However the best collections are in the libraries of the veterinary schools. Apart from these, the major veterinary libraries are in government departments and research institutes. The Royal College of Veterinary Surgeons has a large collection, especially of clinical material, and is the library most likely to be used by veterinarians in practice.

Veterinary Schools

There are currently six undergraduate veterinary schools. The departments of most of these are divided between the main university campuses and field stations, where much of the clinical training and research is performed. The library services may also be divided and this can create difficulties of integration. Usually library staff specifically responsible for the subject field will serve the users, who will include undergraduates, postgraduates and teaching staff. The largest library is that of the Royal Veterinary College. The history of the library, which was founded in 1791, has been described by Catton (1965 and 1982). It has over 30,000 volumes and its historical collection comprises 2,000 volumes. Pre-clinical and historical material is at the main campus while the core veterinary materials are located at the College's field station.

Government Libraries

The largest libraries are those of the British Library. Its Science Reference and

Information Service is in London and materials on veterinary science are held at the Aldwych branch. This is a reference library only. The British Library Document Supply Centre is at Boston Spa and is the major lending library within the UK. Other than the British Library, the most important government libraries are those of MAFF, principally that at the Central Veterinary Laboratory, and those of the laboratories of the AFRC-funded Institute for Animal Health. Details of the major government libraries, their stock and availability to the public are provided in a comprehensive guide (Adkins, 1988).

Royal College of Veterinary Surgeons

The RCVS has one of the most comprehensive veterinary libraries in Britain. The library, which was founded in 1843, now houses the College archives and its historical collection is extensive. Current holdings include 25,000 monographs, over 2,500 having been published prior to 1850, and 245 current periodicals. Catalogues to the older stock have been published [1320, 1321]. The library currently receives about 240 current periodicals. Readers are from all spheres of veterinary practice, so coverage is of every aspect of the subject field, and from elementary to research level. As members of the College are scattered all over Britain, and may also be working overseas, there is an extensive postal enquiry and loan service. A recent survey has shown that the library has been used by over fifty percent of veterinary practices whereas university libraries had been used by 16 percent (Raw, 1987). The library provides a full range of services to members, including carrying out literature searches, preparing reading lists, checking references, answering bibliographical and biographical queries and so on.

2.5.2 Libraries in Other Countries

In the United States there are more veterinary schools than in Britain and therefore more libraries. The section devoted to information sources in the AVMA's *Directory* has a detailed list of the libraries in the veterinary schools of North America and Croft *et al.* (1986) provides details of their organization, stock size and staffing. The best national collections are those of the National Agricultural Library and of the National Library of Medicine, both of which have extensive collections of veterinary materials. The catalogues of both libraries are available online.

The (American) Medical Libraries Association has a Veterinary Medical Libraries Section, established in 1974, to link persons interested in the field and to contribute to the management of veterinary collections. It meets each year at the annual meeting of the Medical Library Association. The Chair of the Section is currently Sue Loubiere (School of Veterinary Medicine Library, Louisiana State University [1840]). The *Bulletin of the Medical Library Association* publishes articles on veterinary topics occasionally and the Veterinary Medical Libraries Section has its own newsletter, *Highlights & news notes*. Another important publication by the Veterinary Medical Libraries Section is *Veterinary serials: a union list of serials held in veterinary collections in Canada, Europe and the USA* (2nd ed., 1987–88). The Chair of its Union List Committee has reported on the prices of veterinary journals over recent years (Anderson, 1988).

Unfortunately there are no similar groupings of veterinary libraries in Britain or Europe, although many British libraries will be members of ASLIB's Biosciences Group. In most countries information staff will be members of the relevant professional organizations. In Britain these are the Library Association and Institute of Information Scientists. Staff in industry are likely to be members of the Association of Information Officers in the Pharmaceutical Industry (AIOPI), which discusses veterinary matters occasionally.

Some of the larger veterinary libraries play an important role in providing documentation services. The ILCA, for example, has prepared microfiche editions of the original agricultural literature from a variety of African countries. It also provides current awareness services to African national research programmes including access to online systems, a document delivery service and the reproduction and circulation of contents pages of journals. A number of the major libraries prepare national bibliographies of veterinary literature. For example, the library of the Veterinary University of Budapest publishes an annual bibliography of Hungarian literature. Similarly the library at the Escola Superior de Medicina Veterinaria in Lisbon publishes a *Bibliografía veterinaria Portuguesa* and has published catalogues of its historical collection. A project is underway at the Universidad Nacional Autónoma de México in developing BIVE (Banco de Información en Medicina Veterinaria y Zootecnia). This is an information bank of the veterinary literature and audiovisual materials produced in Latin America. Almost 5,000 items per year will be added to the database (Sametz de Walerstein, 1986). A unique collaborative scheme is co-ordinated at the library of the University of Montreal (Jetté, 1984). The TELUM database is compiled with the assistance of over sixty veterinary libraries and documentation centres throughout the world. The main input is derived from over thirty North American libraries who provide information on their new accessions. The TELUM database consists of three files: SERUP has information on new serials and on changes to existing titles; MONO gives information on new monographs; and DOC covers literature recently published on veterinary documentation. The TELUM database can be accessed by collaborating libraries online.

Unfortunately there is no worldwide listing of veterinary collections but a list of selected libraries is given in Part III. The various guides to organizations listed in Chapter 3 often include some details of their library resources. Most of the larger libraries and many individuals have joined the International Association of Agricultural Librarians and Documentalists (Secretary: Drs Jan van der Burg, PO Box 4, 6700 AA Wageningen, The Netherlands. Telex: 45015 BIHWG NL). The IAALD have published a useful primer for agricultural libraries (Lendvay, 1980) which has been translated into several languages. Youssef [11] has written another basic guide for non-professional librarians. Apart from these veterinary librarians will find textbooks on the principles and practice of medical librarianship to be of value (e.g. Darling, 1982–88; Matthews and Picken, 1979). The *Quarterly bulletin of the IAALD* includes useful articles and news items on agricultural information and an occasional listing of *Professional literature*. A recent issue gave a list of IAALD members (**XXXIII** (1988): 13–45). The IAALD published a guide to agricultural libraries (Boalch, 1960) a new edition of which is likely to appear during 1989 (under the editorship of Carol Boast). Poland (1988) has compiled another recent guide to biological and medical science libraries which gives good coverage of libraries in developing countries. The CTA have sponsored the publication of guides to information sources in both EEC and ACP (African, Pacific and Caribbean) countries [191].

2.6 CLASSIFICATION SCHEMES AND SUBJECT HEADINGS USED IN LIBRARIES

Most libraries have different physical kinds of materials in separate collections. Thus journals will be shelved separately from books, and there may be collections of conferences, annual reports, audiovisual materials etc. When using a library it is advisable to study the general layout of the stock on the maps and guides available. One should also use the professional skills and knowledge of the librarian to the full. A librarian's function is to exploit and promote the use of information rather than merely being a curator. Librarians will always provide assistance to readers and may be able to simplify the search for specific information.

All libraries will have a catalogue. This is a record of the stock and its function is to direct readers to items of interest using the classification scheme employed in the library. The stock is usually organized according to the class marks given in the classification scheme. The class marks normally consist of an alphanumeric sequence. The catalogue may be on cards, in printed lists, on microfiche, or be available online, and it will normally provide access to the stock via authors, titles and subjects.

Many libraries have developed their own classification schemes but there are five schemes likely to be encountered. The Dewey Classification is used in most public and college libraries. Scientific libraries often use the Universal Decimal Classification which is based on Dewey and can express complex topics by combinations of class marks. The Library of Congress scheme is frequently used in university libraries. In the United States the National Library of Medicine and National Agricultural Library classifications may be used as many of the academic libraries serving veterinary students and staff are based in medical schools or faculties of agriculture.

The major benefits to a library of using the well-known schemes such as Dewey or the Library of Congress are that the schemes are revised frequently, are able to incorporate developments in the subject fields and possess detailed subject indexes and guides. A further advantage is that new books often include the class marks in the cataloguing-in-publication (CIP) data which they include. In addition, libraries can obtain detailed cataloguing records, which may include classification details, from online cataloguing systems. Small libraries may find however that they can create an adequate subject classification using simplifications of these schemes or standard subject heading lists such as the Commonwealth Bureau of Animal Health's *Controlled vocabulary* [161]. A disadvantage of using the larger schemes is that related materials likely to be of interest to veterinarians can be quite widely separated. For example, texts on the physiology of the mammalian eye may be shelved well away from those on both medical and on veterinary ophthalmology. Similarly items on the husbandry of animals may be widely separated from general veterinary works, and from those on the diseases of particular species.

No library is self-sufficient and most libraries make use of a variety of local, regional and international systems for interlibrary loan and document supply. For example, Hansen (1981) has shown that 55 percent of the requests received by the Danish Veterinary and Agricultural Library could be satisfied from stock, 74 percent within Denmark, 86 percent in Scandinavia and most of the rest via the AGLINET network. Only 1 percent required the use of commercial document delivery services. The problem of document delivery is probably greatest in the developing countries.

The British Library Document Supply Centre (BLDSC) was originally set up to cater for British needs for interlibrary lending and document supply but it is now important internationally. Other countries have developed similar national interlending schemes. In 1987/8 the BLDSC received 3,229,812 requests, 767,554 of which came from overseas. Only 7 percent of requests were unsatisfied. Apart from their own stock BLDSC use the resources of a large number of back-up libraries to supply older or more obscure materials. The other major international network is AGLINET, the formation of which was prompted by the IAALD. AGLINET now comprises twenty-seven agricultural libraries who co-operate to provide interlibrary loans and document delivery services. The co-ordinator is Carole Joling (Chief Librarian, David Lubin Memorial Library, FAO [1784]). FAO publish the *AGLINET union list of serials* and this has a list of the national AGLINET libraries.

Although the cheapest and most convenient way to obtain the literature is through the use of established library services it is now possible to order copies of documents though a variety of online systems. Most database producers operate document supply services. CAB International can supply copies of almost all the items abstracted in its journals.

References

Adkins, R. T. (ed.) *Guide to government department and other libraries 1988.* 28th ed. London: The British Library, Science Reference and Information Service, 1988. 100pp.
Anderson, D. C. 'Journals for academic veterinary libraries: price increases,

1977, 1986, and 1987; page costs, 1977 and 1986'. *Serials librarian* **14** (1988): (1/2) 81–8.

Anon 'The profession and its publications'. *Veterinary record* **123** (1988): 189.

Blood, D. C. and Brightling, P. *Veterinary information management*. London: Baillière Tindall, 1988. 177pp.

Boalch, D. H. (ed.) *World directory of agricultural libraries and documentation centres*. Harpenden: IAALD, 1960. 280pp.

Catton, R. 'The historical collection in the library of the Royal Veterinary College'. *Veterinary record* **77** (1965): 503–6.

Catton, R. 'The early history of the library of the Royal Veterinary College'. *Veterinary history* **2** (1982): 91–9.

CBE style manual: a guide for authors, editors and publishers in the biological sciences. 5th ed. Bethesda: Council of Biology Editors, 1983. 324pp.

Cho, Y-J. 'Citation characteristics of periodical literature in veterinary science'. *American journal of veterinary research* **38** (1977): 131–3.

Croft, V. F., Jumonville, J. A., Loubiere, S. and Sessions, R. 'Veterinary school libraries in the US and Canada, 1983–84'. *Highlights and news notes. Veterinary Medical Libraries Section. Medical Library Association* **18** (1986): 1–15.

Darling, L. (ed.) *Handbook of medical library practice*. 4th ed. Chicago: Medical Library Association, 1982–88. 3 vols.

Day, R. A. *How to write and publish a scientific paper*. 3rd ed. Phoenix: Oryx Press, 1988. 211pp.

Drake, M. A. and Woods, L. A. 'An information service for practicing veterinarians'. *Bulletin of the Medical Library Association* **66** (1978): 437–40.

Dyer, H. and Gunson, A. *A directory of library and information retrieval software for microcomputers*. 3rd ed. Aldershot: Gower, 1988. 75pp.

Edwards, J. T. 'The veterinary press: its evolution and present trends I'. *Veterinary record* **60** (1948): 498–502.

Garfield, E. 'Journal citation studies. 35. Veterinary journals: what they cite and vice versa'. *Current contents* **3** (29 March 1982): 5–13.

Gray, D. E. *Bibliographical references in veterinary scientific publications*. 2nd ed. Alnwick: MAFF, 1982. 34pp. (MAFF Booklet 2397.)

Hansen, I. B. 'Use of the Danish Veterinary Agricultural Library by direct library users and users of an online documentation service'. *Quarterly bulletin of the IAALD* **26** (1981): 89–96.

Houston, W. 'The application of bibliometrics to veterinary science primary literature'. *Quarterly bulletin of the IAALD* **28** (1983): 6–13.

Huth, E. J. *Medical style and format: an international manual for authors, editors and publishers*. Philadelphia: ISI Press, 1987. 355pp.

Ikpaahindi, L. 'Information gathering methods of Nigerian veterinary scientists'. *Library and information science research* **7** (1985): 145–57.

Jetté, J. P. 'The TELUM database on the sources of information in veterinary medicine'. *Quarterly bulletin of the IAALD* **29** (1984): 57–60.

Kimberley, R. (ed.) and Rowley, J. (Introduction) *Text retrieval: a directory of software*. 2nd ed. Aldershot: Gower, 1987. Loose-leaf with annual updates.

Lendvay, O. *Primer for agricultural libraries*. 2nd ed. Wageningen: Centre for Agricultural Publishing and Documentation (PUDOC) (for IAALD), 1980. 91pp.

Matthews, D. and Picken, F. M. *Medical librarianship*. London: Clive Bingley, 1979. 173pp. (Outlines of Modern Librarianship 12.)

Ministry of Agriculture, Fisheries and Food. *Effective writing in advisory work*. By G. Cherry and N. Harvey. London: MAFF, 1981. 101pp. (MAFF Reference Book 379.)

Pelzer, N. L. and Leysen, J. M. 'Library use and information-seeking behavior of veterinary medical students'. *Bulletin of the Medical Library Association* **76** (1988): 328–33.

Poland, U. H. (ed.) *World directory of biological and medical science libraries*. Munich: K. G. Saur, 1988. 203pp. (IFLA Publications 42.)

Raw, M. E. 'Survey of libraries in veterinary practice'. *Veterinary record* **121** (1987): 129–31.

Romatowski, J. 'An indexed filing system for journal articles'. *Modern veterinary practice* **68** (1987): 39–42.

Roy, D. E. 'The selection process for veterinary books in the general medical school library'. *Bulletin of the Medical Library Association* **72** (1984): 314–15.

Russell, J. M., Mendoza, M. and Martinez, G. 'Patterns of literature citation by undergraduate students and researchers in the veterinary field'. *Scientometrics* **12** (1987): 73–80.

Sametz de Walerstein, L. 'Development of an information system for the veterinary medicine and animal husbandry schools of Latin America and the Caribbean'. *Quarterly bulletin of the IAALD* **31** (1986): 67–77.

Schindler, R. L. 'A reference file for small animal practices'. *Veterinary medicine and small animal clinician* **76** (1981): 982.

Stibic, V. *Personal documentation for professionals: means and methods*. Amsterdam: North-Holland Publishing, 1980. 214pp.

Veenstra, R. J. 'A one-year journal use study in a veterinary medical library'. *Journal of the American Veterinary Medical Association* **190** (1987): 623–6.

Warren, K. S. (ed.) *Coping with the biomedical literature: a primer for the scientist and clinician*. New York: Praeger, 1981. 233pp.

White, M. E. 'Let's stop loose talk about the "information explosion" '. *Canadian veterinary journal* **29** (1988): 619–20. (*See also* **29** (1988): 965 for correspondence.)

Wolff, A. 'A simple library index system for veterinarians'. *Veterinary medicine and small animal clinician* **77** (1982): 524.

3 Who, What, Where?

Finding out about individuals, organizations, companies and products can be difficult and sometimes almost impossible. Where they exist printed directories are invaluable although they quickly become out of date. Directories which cover the specialities are described in Part II, and only general sources are discussed here.

Where no suitable directory exists then the best way to find information can be to scan the national veterinary journals. Periodicals, such as the *Veterinary record* and the *Australian veterinary journal*, publish a diverse range of material in their news, information and advertisement sections. This can identify societies, which may be advertising forthcoming meetings, manufacturers of particular products, suppliers of services and so on. The national veterinary association will usually provide specific information on request, advise on the existence of specialist groups, and help in identifying individuals with particular expertise and knowledge. Veterinary schools and their libraries can help in this way too. A vast amount of information is in people's heads, much of it not available in any printed form, and one route to this is to contact experts in the field via the libraries, associations and societies listed in Part III.

3.1 GENERAL DIRECTORIES

Unlike some professions, veterinary medicine has few general directories. The nearest equivalents are the membership directories of the national associations and the drug directories and vade mecums both frequently have general reference sections. These sometimes give legislative and organizational information, addresses of government departments, veterinary schools, local veterinary groups and speciality organizations, and details of breed and animal welfare societies. Almost all the drug compendia contain information about only one country; typical examples are the French *Dictionnaire des médicaments vétérinaires* [236] and the British Henston veterinary vade mecums [258, 259]. These directories are produced commercially, although in some cases may be distributed free to practising veterinarians, the production costs having been met by advertising fees.

3.2 DIRECTORIES OF INDIVIDUALS

Veterinary medicine is a closed profession, and registration is a prerequisite to being allowed to practise. Most countries therefore have some kind of published list of registered veterinarians.

For any country, the most comprehensive list of veterinary qualified personnel will be that held by the national or state registration body. In some countries details of registered veterinarians are given in general directories that list medical professionals such as dentists, doctors and pharmacists. In countries where there are many veterinarians, a directory solely devoted to these may be issued. In Britain, for example, veterinary surgeons must register with the Royal College of Veterinary Surgeons (RCVS) in order to practise and the *Registers and directory* [206] is published in accordance with the Veterinary Surgeons Act. The *Registers* includes alphabetical lists of veterinarians giving names, qualifications and the dates they were awarded, and addresses, which may be home addresses rather than those of their practices. Telephone numbers are given for most of the people listed. There are separate lists of veterinary surgeons on the general list, including those who hold EEC veterinary qualifications, and of those holding degrees from recognized Commonwealth universities. There are also geographical listings arranged by town and details of those holding official appointments both in the UK and overseas. There is a list of Fellows of the College. The first list of members of the RCVS after the grant of the Royal Charter was published in 1848 so the series of *Registers* which follows is useful for retrospective searching. As its name implies the *Registers and directory* also contains other information on veterinary medicine in Britain. It gives details of some societies and comprehensive coverage of the activities of the College. A table gives the numbers on the registers since 1935, but since retired veterinarians and those practising abroad can still be registered, it does not indicate the exact number of veterinarians practising in Britain. Also included is a brief history of the profession in Britain.

In Australia, Canada and America the registering bodies are at state level. Each state keeps records of practitioners within their area and in some cases these may be published. For example, the licensing bodies in New York and Texas publish lists.

Most of the national veterinary associations publish lists of members. Since membership of these associations is optional, the lists are less complete than those produced by the registration bodies. The American Veterinary Medical Association's *Directory*, however, is one of the most comprehensive and is particularly useful because of its extensive reference section. Apart from full details of the association's activities and structure it also reproduces AVMA professional policy statements and guidelines, the principles of veterinary medical ethics, digests of veterinary practice acts, gives information on the accreditation status of North American schools, and provides current and historic information about the profession. There are details on many government agencies, veterinary groups and organizations concerned with the health and welfare of animals. The *Directory* lists AVMA member veterinarians alphabetically and geographically and gives some indication of the individual's professional training, current employment and professional activities. Some of the US state veterinary associations publish lists of their members, often as supplements to their journals.

Not all national associations publish lists of members, and none is as complete as that of the AVMA, but where they exist they are an invaluable source of information. Details of individual lists are given in Part II. Sometimes, instead of a separate publication, such lists and amendments to them are published in the association's journal. The national association will usually supply details of member veterinarians on application when this information is not readily available in a printed list.

Specialist societies and professional associations can be invaluable sources of information. They usually publish lists of members, albeit sometimes infrequently, and these identify experts in the field. Such membership directories can range from a simple typewritten list to a comprehensive directory; the *Directory of diplomates* of the American College of Veterinary Surgeons is an excellent example of the latter type. It provides a great deal of personal information about the College's members. Their home and office addresses are given, and there are details of their education and clinical and research interests. There are also photographs of each of the diplomates!

There are a number of who's who-type directories of scientists which contain information on eminent veterinarians. The most recent, and the one with the best international coverage, is the *Agricultural & veterinary sciences international who's who* [188]. CAB International are in the process of compiling a similar international directory. More general biographical directories covering specific geographical regions are *Who's who in science in Europe* [192] and *American men and women of science* [208].

Although directories will be the first resource used, much information about people can be surmised from their contributions to the literature. For example, the best way to check the current address of a research worker, is to check one of their recent publications. An examination of an individual's publications gives insights into sources of funding, career history and professional interests.

3.3 ORGANIZATIONS AND INSTITUTIONS

Specialist veterinary societies are often listed in the relevant national directories. The AVMA *Directory* [211] has a list of national veterinary associations in the United States and gives a contact point. State veterinary associations, and associations in the major market areas, are also listed. The AVMA's *Media guide to veterinary sources and information*, and the Animal Health Institute's similar free guide (*Media resource book*) [212], give contacts in companies, organizations and societies in the USA.

Unfortunately there is no central listing of veterinary associations in Britain, although details of the secretaries of many veterinary groups are published annually in *Veterinary practice* (last **20** (1988) 18 July: 10–12). This *Keyguide* attempts to alleviate the problem of identifying specialist societies in Britain by providing a detailed list of the British groups in Part III. The list in *Veterinary practice* includes the various regional divisions of the BVA, so details of these are not repeated. In Britain many of the officials of the societies are honorary officers and there may be frequent changes in the contact points and their addresses. The details of the officers given in the list of organizations in Part III are therefore subject to change. The appropriate speciality or a general journal should be scanned for the most current information. Up-to-date details of the BVA's Divisions can be obtained from the Association's External Affairs section.

Details of specialist societies in Australia may be found in the Australian Veterinary Association's *Yearbook*. A few Australian societies that publish materials of international interest are listed in Part III.

Part III gives details of the most important European and world veterinary groups. Many international organizations and societies have national representatives in each country in which they have members or in which there are national member societies. Details of these can normally be obtained from the national veterinary association. The AVMA's *Directory*, which is published annually, contains contact points, albeit of the North American representatives, for many international organizations and so can be used to update the information given in Part III. Two other world guides to international organizations are useful to keep up to date with changes: *World guide to scientific associations and societies* (4th ed., 1984) and *Yearbook of international organizations* (annual). Both are published by K. G. Saur.

There are many other organizations which, while not exclusively concerned with veterinary medicine, are related to the subject field, for example in agriculture, animal production and animal welfare. Most of the American bodies are listed in the AVMA's *Directory*. Further details on these and on other non-profit organizations in the United States can be found in the *Encyclopedia of associations* (Detroit: Gale Research Company, 23rd ed., 1988), which is available online. Contacts for British agricultural and farming groups were given in the Royal Agricultural Society's *Reference book and buyers' guide*. This was issued annually and, although it has now ceased publication, details on these groups can still be obtained via the RASE [2263]. Details of British specialist organizations, such as breed rescue societies and other animal welfare groups relevant to small animal practice, are given in the *The Henston veterinary vade mecum (small animals)* [259]. Two other important reference works which are likely to be available in most public libraries and useful for information about organizations in Britain are: *Trade associations and professional bodies of the United Kingdom* (Oxford: Pergamon, 9th ed., 1988) and the *Directory of British associations* (Beckenham: CBD Research, 9th ed., 1988). Only those bodies of major importance and particularly useful as sources of veterinary information are therefore listed in Part III.

There are nearly 400 veterinary schools in the world. These are usually attached to general universities which are listed by the standard reference guides *World of learning* and *Commonwealth universities yearbook*. The World Health Organization published a *World directory of veterinary schools* in 1975 [193]. Although rather out of date it is still of interest since it describes the nature of veterinary education in each country. The World Veterinary Association has produced a more recent list of veterinary schools and faculties, although it concentrates on establishments within WVA member countries. This list originally appeared in the WVA *Bulletin* during the course of 1987 and amendments and additions will be noted in future issues. Individual academic institutions produce calendars and prospectuses giving information on staff, facilities and courses. Certain schools issue annual reports and lists of publications and dissertations produced by students and staff.

The *World of learning* contains information on some research institutes but there is a specialist directory, *Agricultural research centres* [187], to organizations which conduct or finance research and development programmes. The publishers of *Agricultural research centres* also produce regional guides to research laboratories in both Europe and the Pacific [189]. The WVA Secretariat is working on a directory of veterinary research institutes. This will appear in the WVA's *Bulletin*, together with lists of national veterinary associations, veterinary journals and a compilation of information on the organization of veterinary services in different countries.

3.4 RESEARCH

Payne and Payne (1986) examined the articles appearing in *Veterinary bulletin* over a single year in each of the last three decades. This data was used to assess the proportion of the world literature coming from different countries and the intensity of work in each subject area.

Overall ninety-one countries were represented in the survey although the majority published less than 1 percent of the world output. The countries contributing most of the literature are given in *Table 3.1*. Almost a third of the literature comes from countries in the European Community and, together with the United States, these countries produce almost 60 percent of the literature. The survey also indicated the proportion of the literature devoted to various subjects.

Table 3.1   Percentage of the world output from various countries

Year	USA	UK	FRG	Fr	USSR	Eastern Bloc	Australia	Japan
1966	23.8	13.3	8.5	3.2	7.3	19.8	4.9	2.3
1975	24.6	13.7	7.0	3.6	6.0	16.6	4.1	3.5
1985	26.9	10.4	6.4	4.5	3.6	12.1	4.7	4.6

Table 3.2   Percentage of the world output devoted to various subjects

Year	Bacteriology	Virology	Immunology	Pathology	Pharmacology
1966	20.3	17.7	2.4	6.4	3.3
1975	16.8	15.0	2.5	8.6	6.1
1985	23.3	15.3	3.2	9.0	6.0

Bacteriology and virology are by far the most frequent areas of study (*Table 3.2*). Work on parasitology, and on nutritional, metabolic and reproductive disorders was shown to have declined over recent years.

In most countries, research is almost exclusively carried out by the veterinary schools and by government institutes. *Table 3.3* gives the relative shares of the output from different types of organization in the UK; this pattern would doubtless be repeated for other countries.

In Britain, as in most countries, it is the staff and students of the veterinary schools who are numerically the largest body of research workers, their research being carried out in addition to their teaching and clinical work. In most cases finance ultimately comes from government sources, as the universities are funded by the Department of Education and Science. There is no central directive on which areas of veterinary medicine or which research projects should be supported. Some funding is provided by a variety of outside sources and these may include animal health companies, private bequests and animal welfare and other charitable foundations. The Wellcome Trust is an important source of finance for research and teaching activities in Britain. During 1984–6 the Trustees allocated £2.9 million to support research in veterinary medicine. Details of projects currently receiving financial help are given in the Trust's biennial report [2303].

Outside the schools most research activity is funded by the Ministry of Agriculture, Fisheries and Food through its Agricultural Research Service. MAFF has a Priorities Board for Research and Development in Agriculture and

Table 3.3   Numbers of publications from various sources in the UK

Year	University	AFRC	MAFF	DHSS	Industry	Animal Health Trust	Others
1966	207	142	81	61	64	9	37
1975	325	239	152	53	53	20	51
1985	250	188	153	49	49	21	69

Food. This takes a strategic view of UK research and development. The board carries out four-yearly reviews on all aspects of research conducted by the Agriculture Departments and by the Agricultural and Food Research Council (AFRC). The AFRC finances research at its own Institute for Animal Health, which has several research laboratories, and at several other research institutes working on animal physiology and animal production. The AFRC also funds postgraduate studentships at the schools and in other university departments and operates a system linking researchers working in academic institutes with those in its laboratories. The State Veterinary Service of MAFF undertakes research, mainly at the Central Veterinary Laboratories at Weybridge. Research is also carried out at the nineteen regional Veterinary Investigation Centres, although their main tasks are disease investigation and the provision of a diagnostic advisory and consultancy service. Most research in Scotland is funded by the Department of Agriculture and Fisheries for Scotland.

Much research is also carried out by the Animal Health Trust [2092] and is described in the Trust's *Annual report*. The Trust is a charitable institution and works on animal diseases, their diagnosis, cure and prevention. The Trust's overall policy is to co-ordinate clinical investigation with research.

The animal health industry conducts its own research, but much of this remains confidential, at least until a product is launched. The industry is very tightly regulated by drug registration authorities. Although companies submit data to these bodies, in most countries this is completely confidential and not publicly available. There are extensive pre-launch clinical trials and post-launch monitoring and surveillance. These are usually carried out in co-operation with academic workers or with the assistance of the larger practices and veterinary hospitals. Veterinary surgeons in practice make significant contributions by evaluating new techniques, treatments and procedures in a clinical environment and by documenting case reports.

Research in other countries basically follows the pattern outlined for the United Kingdom. In the United States for example, most animal health research is also government funded, in this case by the United States Department of Agriculture (USDA). Major Federal research programmes are carried out by the USDA's

Agricultural Research Service which has a large number of research facilities. Research at state level is supported by the Cooperative State Research Service (CSRS) which funds research at colleges and schools of veterinary medicine, in the State Agriculture Experiment Stations, the land-grant universities and other co-operating institutions. All CSRS funded projects are evaluated to ensure the highest quality of research and prevent duplication of effort.

International organizations such as FAO and WHO also finance and carry out veterinary research. There are several international laboratories backed by these and other organizations funding agricultural development. The International Laboratory for Research on Animal Diseases [1787] is the best known of these laboratories. Most of the national and international research institutes produce regular, usually annual, reports on their activities. ILRAD, for example, produces *ILRAD reports* which has brief articles on research underway at the laboratory and *ILRAD publications* lists newly published material written by its staff.

3.4.1 Research Directories

It is inevitable that information in directories dates very quickly and this is especially so for information on current research. Several sources are discussed here but it is also advisable to search the literature for recent publications. Such a search will highlight the specialists in the field and indicate the main research laboratories.

There are two international systems, CARIS and AGREP, recording data on research in progress, but most of projects covered by each relate to agricultural and not to veterinary research. CARIS (Current Agricultural Research Information System) is co-ordinated by the FAO and began in 1973. It operates as a decentralized network of eighty-three national, regional and international centres inputting to a central database which has details of over 3,000 research projects in developing countries. The database may be searched online by these centres, a list of which is available from FAO. Some of the input centres publish directories covering the research underway in their region. AGREP is an attempt to create a similar directory of research in progress in Europe. A printed version is published occasionally as the *AGREP: permanent inventory of agricultural research projects in the European Communities* [274]. The data is available online. On DATACENTRALEN the database is updated quarterly.

Current research in Britain (CRIB) [277] is the national register of current research being carried out in universities, polytechnics, colleges and other institutions within the United Kingdom. The first edition in 1985 replaced *Research in British universities, polytechnics and colleges*. The biological sciences volume of CRIB lists research underway in the UK veterinary schools and in other institutions concerned with animal health. There is a name index to researchers, a keyword index to specific projects and a study area index giving access to projects within general areas of study.

Veterinarians rarely write their research up in the form of reports, preferring instead to publish in journals. However, reports of US government sponsored research and some non-US technical reports are available in the NTIS database. Although these are records of completed research many of the documents indicate future research plans. Information on ongoing publicly funded research projects in the USA is available in the FEDERAL RESEARCH IN PROGRESS database. Research projects funded by the USDA and carried out by the USDA or co-operating state institutions are described in the CRIS/USDA database (Current Research Information System) and an annual directory is published as the *Inventory of agricultural research*.

In Australia, the Commonwealth Scientific Industrial Research Organisation (CSIRO) maintains a database of CSIRO-sponsored research projects and publishes this annually as the *Directory of CSIRO research programs*. A similar inventory is maintained in Canada [281].

Accounts of research results, often with an indication of the future directions to be followed, are a feature of the annual reports of most organizations carrying out research. Good examples in Britain are those of the Institute for Animal Health [2192], Animal Health Trust [2092] and that of the State Veterinary Service [207].

There are several directories to sources of funds for research. Details on the sources available in the UK and Commonwealth are given in the RCVS's careers booklet (see *Chapter 1*). The *Grants register* [280] gives details of research and travel grants available in the USA, the Commonwealth and the UK. The *Foundation grants index* [279] and the *Directory of research grants* [278] are important source of information about funding programmes in the United States.

3.5 THE ANIMAL HEALTH INDUSTRY

Many types of companies make products for use with or on animals. The pet food and pet supplies industry is the most visible in the developed countries and there are many companies involved in supplying feeds for farm animals. It is however the manufacturers of veterinary drugs that are the largest users and producers of veterinary information.

Table 3.4 shows the leading companies based on 1987 sales worldwide. The industry is a fragmented one and the leading company, Hoffmann-La Roche, only had about 7 percent of the total market. Coopers was the only company in the top twenty solely concerned with animal health and its acquisition by International Minerals and Chemical Corporation in 1989 created the second largest animal health and nutrition group. Although some products, such as Merck's ivermectin/avermectin range, have turnovers in the range of hundreds of millions of dollars worldwide, most have relatively small sales. In Britain, for example, there are nearly 3,000 licensed products and the average turnover is only about £40,000.

Most of the research carried out by animal health companies is performed by relatively few international companies. The leading companies spend an average of 10 percent of their income from animal health and nutrition sales on research and development. In Britain for example the market for animal health products in 1986 was estimated at £130 million; approximately £20 million was spent in research and development, but almost all of this was spent by the three leading companies.

The stages in the development of a new veterinary therapeutic agent are indicated in *Figure 3.1*. The development of a new product may cost between 1.7 and 3.5 million dollars and can last up to seven or eight years. Information is generated at each point in the development process and staff in the companies have need for an enormous range of information in the course of their work. The industry operates under very stringent requirements for the testing and registration of its products. Veterinary therapeutics used in meat and dairy animals require detailed residue studies. Most veterinary medicines are used in a variety of species, and extensive efficacy, toxicity and metabolic studies must be performed in each species. All the data generated during each product's development is kept secure and most companies have departments responsible for its storage and retrieval, normally staffed by information specialists. A detailed discussion of the handling and use of this type of information is not appropriate here but it is worth noting that companies have much unpublished data on their products. They may release this to bona fide researchers, and it will be available to their own staff to deal with customer enquiries or in discussions with the regulatory authorities or with collaborators.

Most of the drug compendia give addresses for companies active in local markets. An international compilation of addresses for animal health companies is the '*Animal health international*' directory [214]. There is a more recent Animal Pharm publication, the *International animal health directory* [218], which gives addresses for 2,409 animal health companies, 161 veterinary regulatory bodies and 140 veterinary institutions.

In the majority of countries the animal health companies have formed trade associations. These are important channels for communication within the industry. In the United States there is the Animal Health Institute [2090] and in the United Kingdom the National Office of Animal Health [2240]. There are also international trade associations such as FEDESA [2167] which is a European organization formed from nine national animal health organizations and twenty-two animal health manufacturers. A world organization, COMISA [2152], has also been created, especially to provide a single voice to liaise with regulatory and intergovernmental groups. In some cases there are trade associations for companies active in specialist markets; examples are FEFANA [2165] and FEFAC [2169], which represent companies engaged in the feed additives and feedstuffs markets in Europe.

Commercial and business news about the industry is reported in *Animal pharm* [322]. This includes a miscellany of news stories about companies, products,

Company	Animal health/ nutrition sales ($m.)	Increase from 1986 (%)	Total group sales ($m.)	Contribution from animal products (%)
Hoffmann-La Roche	720	27	6,072	11.9
Rhone-Poulenc	544	23	10,566	5.1
Pfizer	480	8	4,920	9.8
BASF	452	28	25,629	1.8
Merck Sharp & Dohme	403	23	5,061	8.0
Bayer	360	28	23,658	1.5
Coopers	355	39	355	100
Hoechst	350	19	23,539	1.5
Eli Lilly	341	10	3,644	9.4
SmithKline Beckman	300	20	4,329	6.9
Solvay	250	26	6,761	3.7
Degussa	235	28	7,467	3.1
IMC	221	40	1,883	11.7
American Cyaramid	206	−1	4,166	4.9
Upjohn	170	13	2,521	6.7
Beecham	167	14	4,817	3.5
Ciba-Geigy	161	28	12,422	1.3
Takeda	138	6	4,419	3.1
Monsanto	127	48	7,639	1.7
Sanofi	126	24	2,376	5.3

Table 3.4   Major animal health and nutrition companies

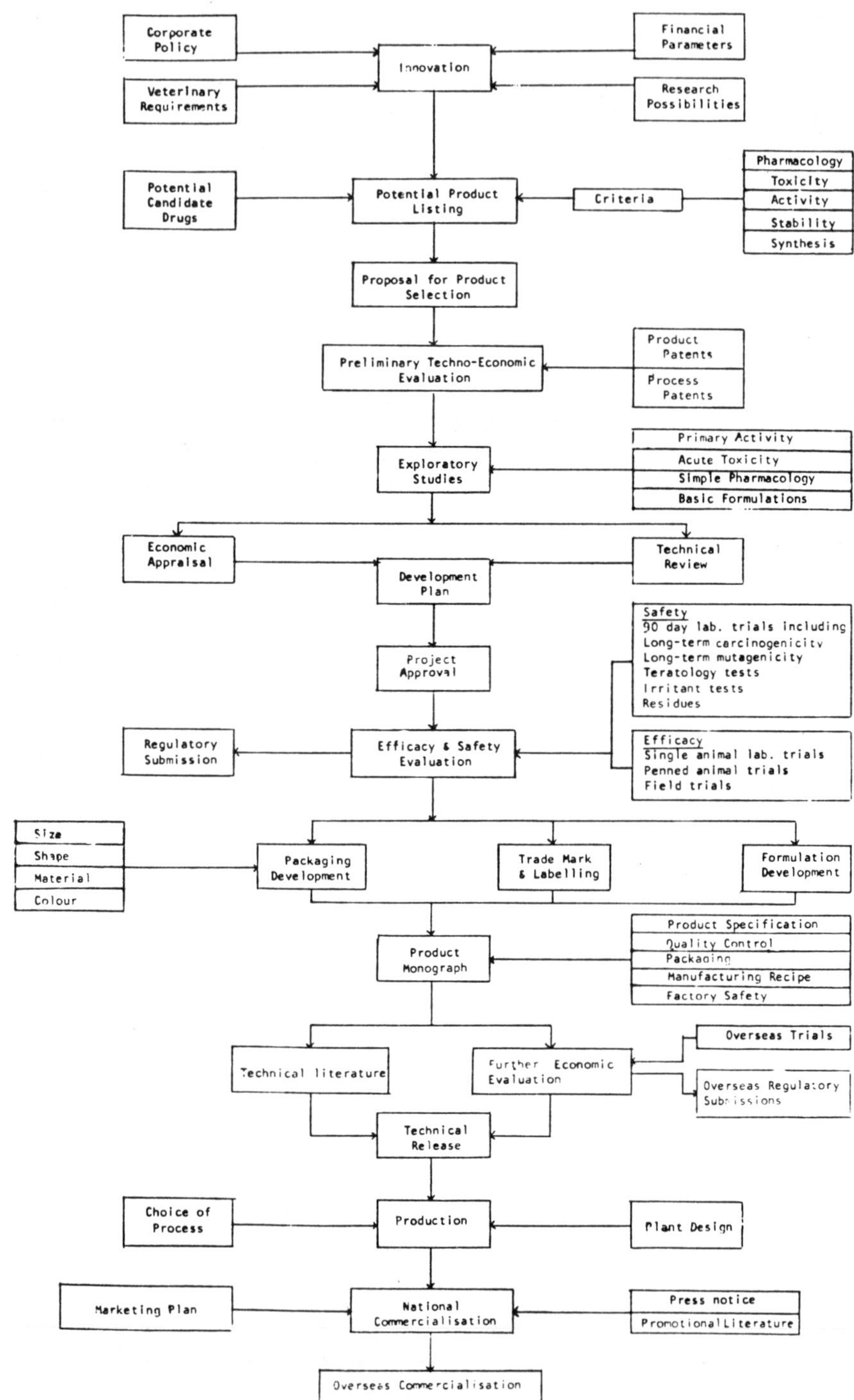

Figure 3.1   Product development path for a new veterinary drug.
(Reproduced by courtesy of Information Research Limited).

business sectors, legislation and related matters. More detailed information about companies can be found in their annual reports which are invaluable for providing overviews of current interests and future plans. An examination of the research publications of the staff of a company will show their interests but is obviously unlikely to disclose many trade secrets! Instead an analysis may be made of a company's patents; this can indicate its research and development projects and give an insight into likely product introductions. When formal annual reports are not issued then company accounts give basic data on the financial health of the concern. There are many online sources of financial information. Data about British and American companies is the most easy to acquire; information about companies based in other countries, especially those based outside Europe, is often difficult to obtain. Dun & Bradstreet is the best-known service with an international coverage. Often however the way to obtain information is simply to make a direct approach to the company itself.

Companies active in the animal health and nutrition sector have parents in the pharmaceutical and agrochemical industries. For this reason background information about the activities of the general chemical and pharmaceutical industry is important. The major sources are online databases including IMSBASE, PHARMACEUTICAL NEWS INDEX, PROMT and CHEMICAL INDUSTRY NOTES (CIN) and the various biotechnology and pharmaceutical news services such as AGRIBUSINESS USA, PHARMAPROJECTS, BIOBUSINESS and CURRENT BIOTECHNOLOGY ABSTRACTS. The animal health industry occasionally figures in the national and international press and executives within the industry may wish to follow general business trends and new stories relevant to agriculture. Online services providing access to news databases can be useful in following this form of information. PROFILE INFORMATION and Reuters TEXTLINE both give access to UK and international news and are typical of these systems. All of these services also include some information on animal health companies, but the online version of *Animal pharm*, PHIND, is the best single source of news and commercial information.

Information on the market size for products, and performance data for their own company and for competitors within the market, is vital to executives within the industry. An inexpensive source of factual data about the market worldwide is published annually by PJB Publications: *Animal health facts and figures* [316]. This gives an overview of the world market for animal health products, discusses the market in each of the major geographic areas and reviews individual companies' performances. A comprehensive business and market information service is provided by Vivash Jones Consultants [318]. County NatWest Securities produce a service similar in scope which includes a newsletter and general market surveys [301]. There are several market research organizations such as Frost & Sullivan which prepare extensive reports analysing and forecasting markets for particular animal health sectors. Each report usually supplies a vast amount of quantitative and qualitative information. Similar, but more general surveys of the markets and the technology likely to be employed in sectors of the animal health business, are prepared by PJB Publications, the publishers of *Animal pharm*. Their reports are much cheaper than Frost & Sullivan's and this reflects the degree of research employed in their preparation and the anticipated volume of sales.

The quantitative sales data and company performance figures used in these reports can be determined from the companies themselves and from a variety of other sources. *Sales exchanges* are usually co-ordinated by the national trade industry association. In a sales exchange companies submit details of their sales to an independent body who compile a detailed report on the overall market and of companies' activities within it. Sales exchanges cover all distribution routes and the figures quoted are at manufacturers' selling price. The level of data reported varies between territories however, and not all companies will be members of the trade association and so some may be excluded. *Audits* provide precise measurements of the market for veterinary medicines by recording transactions at the point of sale. Audits cover all products and packs but do not necessarily cover all distribution routes. Audits can be expensive to purchase. The most important producer is IMS [309]. MILPRO [314] also produce an audit for the UK and there are several companies that prepare audits covering France, Denmark, Sweden and a number of other countries. Finally, in *multi-client studies*, a market research company does the field work and desk research and then sells the final report to recoup costs, sometimes only beginning the work when sufficient purchasers have been identified. Multi-client studies use a sampling procedure and extrapolate from sample data to provide an overall assessment of the national market. Details of the most important of all these services are given in Part II. None of them can ever provide an exact measurement of the precise market because of the variety of distribution channels for veterinary products.

Multi-client studies sometimes include information on farmers and veterinarians' assessments and opinions about products. Another cheap form of market research is the use of omnibus studies. In these a representative sample of farmers or veterinarians are interviewed using questions submitted by the companies willing to share the interview costs. Produce Studies, for example, run an omnibus study covering farmers in the UK.

Most companies engaged in product development will also carry out extensive *ad hoc* market research studies. Market research is a complete field in itself. Market research professionals in the animal health industry may be members of BAMRA (British Agricultural Market Research Association) but the Market Research Society (175 Oxford Street, London W1R 1TA. Tel. 01–439 2585) is the professional association for market research organizations and personnel within Britain. The MRS publish jointly with the British Overseas Trade Board (BOTB) an *International directory of market research organisations* (London, 8th ed., 1987). An international guide to publicly available market research reports is *Marketsearch* (London: Arlington Management Publications/BOTB, annual with mid-year supplement).

Reference

Payne, J. M. and Payne, S. 'Changes in world veterinary output of publications'. *British veterinary journal* **142** (1986): 301–6.

4 Keeping Up to Date with Current Information

4.1 INTRODUCTION

A vast amount of new information relevant to the science and practice of veterinary medicine becomes available each year. Most of this is technical information relating to the new techniques, equipment and drugs which are developed and introduced. Established ideas and methods are constantly being refined and re-evaluated and this too results in changes in practice. However, veterinarians are not only interested in technical matters; because they are business people they need to be informed in areas such as management, health and safety, employment practice and taxation.

Workers in the profession need to make systematic efforts at keeping up to date and every practitioner will have devised a range of techniques for achieving this. The degree of effort expended will vary greatly depending on the needs and interests of the individual. Membership of relevant professional organizations and attendance at their national or local meetings is important; so too is attendance at appropriate continuing education events. Most practitioners will read several journals and newsletters. Veterinary practices usually have a library containing modern textbooks for the various specialities.

Research workers and teaching staff put most effort into remaining informed on new developments. They may scan or read large numbers of periodicals, have individual current awareness services designed for them and search the abstracting services systematically for relevant materials. Many of these abstracting and indexing services are likely only to be used extensively by teachers, students and researchers; practitioners will rely on more appropriate publications. The discussion here is primarily concerned with those of most importance in alerting people to newly published literature; some other services are covered further in Chapter 5.

4.2 INDEX VETERINARIUS AND VETERINARY BULLETIN

Index veterinarius [33] and *Veterinary bulletin* [27] are the main bibliographical tools. They serve dual functions for both current awareness and retrospective searching and are described in some detail because of their importance in finding new and historical material. Both journals are produced by the CAB International Bureau of Animal Health. Previously located at the Central Veterinary Laboratories the Bureau has now moved to CAB International's headquarters at Wallingford and has been expanded to include animal and human physiology, entomology and mycology. The two publications are intimately related and through both the Bureau attempts to document all the significant world literature on veterinary medicine. Subjects allied to veterinary medicine, and likely to be of value to those with an interest in animal health, are covered. All of the items appearing in the two publications from 1972 can be searched online in the CAB ABSTRACTS database.

Index veterinarius (1933–) is a classified title-only listing and has the broadest coverage. It now appears monthly, although prior to 1972, it was quarterly. Each issue contains about 1,600 citations with about 20,000 published in total each year (*Table 4.1*). There are separate subject and author indexes in each issue and the whole is cumulated annually. A sample page from *Index veterinarius* is shown in *Figure 4.1*. Each item may appear under a number of subject headings in the subject index. Each entry gives the full bibliographic details about the item and, where it has been selected for abstracting in *Veterinary bulletin*, then the abstract number is quoted. The types of materials noted in *Index veterinarius* but not abstracted in *Veterinary bulletin* are materials from marginal fields of veterinary medicine, such as history and jurisprudence, minor contributions to the literature such as case reports, correspondence, news items etc., literature written for students or farmers, chapters in books, repetitive literature or that from other fields of the biological sciences. *Index veterinarius* also includes details of all items cited in *Animal disease occurrence*. Within *Index veterinarius* each bibliographic reference is also listed in the author index under the name of the first author, to whom coauthors are referred. In the monthly issues almost all the citations in the author index and in the subject index include the author's address and give the original title for non-English documents, if written in roman script, as well as an English translation. Until recent years this information was only given in the annual cumulations in the main entry in the author index.

The subject headings used in *Index veterinarius* are listed in the Commonwealth Bureau of Animal Health *Controlled vocabulary* [161]. For 1989 these headings conform to descriptors listed in the *CAB thesaurus* [159]. A familiarity with the

955 [En, 13 ref.] Coll. Vet. Med., State Univ., Columbus, OH 43210, USA.

PROTEIN BIOSYNTHESIS
Influence of the gut microflora on protein synthesis in tissues and in the whole body of chicks. MURAMATSU, T.; TAKASU, O.; FURUSE, M.; TASAKI, I.; OKUMURA, J. *Biochemical Journal* (1987) **246** (2) 475-479 [En, 27 ref.]

PROTEIN METABOLISM
[Endogenous urea in the intestinal tract and its importance in nitrogen metabolism in ruminants.] VÁRADY, J.; FEJEŠ, J. Endogenna mocovina v crevnom trakte a jej vyznam v metabolizme dusika u prezuvavcov. *Veterinární Medicína* (1987) **32** (4) 195-200 [Sk, ru, en, de, 15 ref.] Ustav fyziol. Hospodarskych zvierat SAV, Dukelskych hrdinov 1/B, 040 01 Kosice, Czechoslovakia. *Abst.* **8080**
[Renal retention of urea in sheep.] LENG, L.; SZANYIOVÁ, M. Renalna retencia mocoviny u oviec. *Veterinární Medicína* (1987) **32** (4) 201-208 [Sk, ru, en, de, 28 ref.] Ustav fyziol. hospodarskych zvierat SAV, Dukelskych hrdinov 1/B, 040 01 Kosice, Czechoslovakia. *Abst.* **8088**

PROTOZOOLOGY
[Comparative medical protozoology. Vol. II. Myxozoa, Microsporidia, Ascetospora, Apicomplexa. 1. Coccidioses (sensu lato).] EUZÉBY, J. Protozoologie médicale comparée. Vol. II. Myxozoa—Microspora—Ascetospora Apicomplexa, 1: Coccidioses (Sensu lato). Lyon, France; Marcel Mérieux (1987) 475pp. ISBN 2-901773-47-8 [Fr] *Abst.* **8216**

PSEUDOMONAS
[Review of virulence characteristics of Pseudomonas and studies on enterotoxin formation.] FEHLHABER, K.; SCHEIBNER, G. Übersicht über Virulenzmerkmale bei Pseudomonaden und Untersuchungen zur Enterotoxinbildung. *Monatshefte für Veterinärmedizin* (1987) **42** (15) 549-552 [De, ru, en, 34 ref.]
[Studies on Pseudomonas strains using skin tests and keratoconjunctival strains.] SCHEIBNER, G.; FEHLHABER, K.; BARTELT, E. Untersuchungen an Pseudomonas-Stämmen im Hauttest und Keratokonjunktivaltest. *Monatshefte für Veterinärmedizin* (1987) **42** (15) 552-554 [De, ru, en, 6 ref.]

PSITTACIFORMES
[Vitamin deficiency in a one-year old hyacinth macaw (*Anodorhyncus hyacinthinus*).] HOCHLEITHNER, M.; TIPOLD, A.; LECHNER, C. Vitaminmangel bei einem einjährigen Hyazinth-Ara (*Anodorhynchus hyacinthinus*). *Wiener Tierärztliche Monatsschrift* (1987) **74** (5) 186-188 [De, en, 6 ref.]
Outbreak of psittacosis associated with a cockatiel. BUTTERY, R. B.; WREGHITT, T. G. [Correspondence]. *Lancet* (1987) **2** (8561) 742-743 [En, 1 ref.]

PUERPERAL DISORDERS
[Microbial aetiology of the mastitis-metraitis-agalactiae syndrome among sows kept intensively.] KORUDZHIISKI, N.; BOXHKOVA, G.; GULUBINOV, G. V.; DZHUROVA, I.; GEORGIEV, S.; DICHEV, R. *Veterinarnomeditsinski Nauki* (1987) **24** (5) 11-15 [Bg, en, ru, 13 ref.] Tsentralen Veterinarnomed. Inst., Sofia, Bulgaria. *Abst.* **7981**
Types and incidence of aerobic bacteria in different puerperal conditions in bovines. AMBROSE, J. D.; PATTABIRAMAN, S. R.; VENKATESAN, R. A. *Cheiron* (1986) **15** (5) 176-179 [En, 8 ref., 2 tab.] Dep. Obstetrics & Gynaecol., Vet. Coll. Madras-600 007, India. *Abst.* **7973**
[Effectiveness of various treatments in the late puerperium.] BÖHME, H.; BETHGE, B.; VINZELBERG, D. Untersuchungen zur Effektivität von Behandlungsvarianten im Spätpuerperium. *Tierhygiene-Information* (1986) **18** (Sonderheft 54) 171-180 [De] Bezirksinst. Veterinarwesen, Haferbreiter Weg 132-135, DDR-3500 Stendal, German Democratic Republic. *Abst.* **7979**

PULMONARY ADENOMATOSIS
Experimental coinduction of type D retrovirus-associated pulmonary carcinoma and lentivirus-associated lymphoid interstitial pneumonia in lambs. DEMARTINI, J. C.; ROSADIO, R. H.; SHARP, J. M.; RUSSELL, H. I.; LAIRMORE, M. D. *JNCI (Journal of the National Cancer Institute)* (1987) **79** (1) 167-177 [En, 36 ref., 13 fig.] Dep. Path., Coll. Vet. Med. Biomed. Sci., State Univ., Fort Collins, CO 80523, USA. *Abst.* **7924**

PYRETHRINS
[Insecticidal treatment for pig houses in the presence of pigs.] LEKANOVA, L. SH.; KERBABAEV, E. B.; KUZNETSOV, V. D.; LEKANOV, V. N.; TIKHOMIROV, S. M. *Veterinariya, Moscow, USSR* (1987) No. 7, 28-29 [Ru] Vsesoyuznyi Institut Veterinarnoi Entomologii, USSR. *Abst.* **7805**
[Ear tags impregnated with insecticide [fenvalerate] used to prevent summer mastitis of cows in Norway.] RØN, I. Oremerker med insektmiddel til bruk mot sommermastitt hos sinkyr og kviger i Norge. *Norsk Veterinaertidsskrift* (1987) **99** (6) 443-447 [No, en, 6 ref.] Norske Melkeprodusenters Landsforbund, Postboks 9066 Vaterland, 0134 Oslo 1, Norway. *Abst.* **7581**
[Tolerance of "Wellcare" permethrin emulsion by horses, particularly its effect on erythrocytes and locomotion.] ANDRESEN, U.; PAVEL, G. Untersuchungen zur Verträglichkeit von Wellcare Emulsion für Pferde unter besonderer Berücksichtigung des roten Blutbildes und der Lokomotion. *Deutsche Tierärztliche Wochenschrift* (1987) **94** (7) 385-391 [De, en, 20 ref.] Bahnhofstrasse 15, D-2243 Albersdorf, German Federal Republic. *Abst.* **7993**

PYRIMIDINES
Urinary orotic acid excretion in hyperammonaemic sheep. MOTYL, T.; ORZECHOWSKI, A.; PIERZYNOWSKI, S. *Journal of Veterinary Medicine, A* (1987) **34** (7) 522-528 [En, 31 ref.] Dep. Anim. Physiol., Agric. Univ., Nowoursynowska 166, 02-766 Warsaw, Poland. *Abst.* **7952**

PYRROLIZIDINE ALKALOIDS
Pyrrolizidine alkaloid poisoning of sheep in New South Wales. SEAMAN, J. T. *Australian Veterinary Journal* (1987) **64** (6) 164-167 [En, 27 ref.] Agric. Res. Vet. Centre, Forest Rd, Orange, NSW 2800, Australia. *Abst.* **8006**
Metabolism and toxicity of anacrotine, a pyrrolizidine alkaloid, in rats. MATTOCKS, A. R.; DRIVER, H. E. *Chemico-Biological Interactions* (1987) **63** (1) 91-104 [En, 17 ref.]

PYTHIUM
***Pythium destruens* sp.nov., an agent of equine pythiosis.** SHIPTON, W. A. *Journal of Medical and Veterinary Mycology* (1987) **25** (3) 137-151 [En, 26 ref.] Bot. Dep., James Cook Univ., Townsville, Qld. 4811, Australia. *Abst.* **7766**

QUAIL
Keeping quail. A guide to domestic and commercial management. THEAR, K. Saffron Walden, Essex CB11 3SP, UK; Broad Leys Publishing Co. (1987) 96pp. ISBN 0-906137-15-2 [En, £3.95]

QUERCUS
Determination of total phenolics in acorns from different species of oak trees in conjunction with acorn poisoning in cattle. BASDEN, K. W.; DALVI, R. R. *Veterinary and Human Toxicology* (1987) **29** (4) 305-306 [En, 12 ref.] Toxicol. Lab., Sch. Vet. Med., Univ., Tuskegee, AL 36088, USA. *Abst.* **8004**

RABBIT
Optimising the use of rabbits for antisera production—a moral approach. I. An animal technician's approach. WILLS, J. E.; THORNTON, S.; GARDINER, D. J. *Animal Technology* (1987) **38** (2) 99-120 [En, 2 ref.]
Normal development of behaviour in rabbits. HEM, A.; SANNES, E.; NAFSTAD, I. *Zeitschrift für Versuchstierkunde* (1987) **29** (5/6) 257-264 [En, de, 8 ref., 4 fig., 3 tab.]

RABBIT DISEASES
Gastric ulcerations in rabbits: a histomorphological study. GEORGE, K. C.; SOMVANSHI, R. *Indian Journal of Animal Sciences* (1987) **57** (5) 416-420 [En, 9 ref., 4 fig., 2 tab.] Indian Vet. Res. Inst., Izatnagar, Uttar Pradesh 243 122, India. *Abst.* **7903**
Pathogenesis of Pasteurella multocida in experimentally infected rabbits. SOKKAR, S. M.; MOHAMED, M. A.; FETAIH, H. *Archiv für Experimentelle Veterinärmedizin* (1987) **41** (4) 516-521 [En, de, ru, 23 ref., 5 fig., 2 tab.] Fac. Vet. Med., Cairo Univ., Egypt. *Abst.* **7539**
[Intestinal diseases of rabbits.] SAMOGGIA, G. Le enteropatie. *Rivista di Coniglicoltura* (1987) **24** (8) 12-15 [It]

Figure 4.1   Part of the subject index of *Index veterinarius*.
(Reproduced by courtesy of CAB International).

controlled vocabulary/thesaurus is vital for efficient searching. English names are used for diseases and for domestic animals but Latin or scientific names are used for pathogens, zoo animals and wildlife. English spelling is used. The index headings can be quite specific, and are often phrases, such as *Anthelmintics for sheep*, *Immunity to protozoa* or *Synthetic prostaglandins*. Because of this, and since there are relatively few cross references in the main body of the subject index, some initiative is required to determine all the relevant headings under which to search for relevant literature. The subject headings have altered over the years. A complete search may be very time consuming. This is because of the large number of headings which may need to be checked, and because prior to 1972, *Index veterinarius* appeared quarterly without an annual cumulative edition.

Veterinary bulletin (1931-) is a companion to *Index veterinarius* and provides abstracts for all major items of veterinary literature. About six review articles are also published each year. *Veterinary bulletin* is monthly, each issue contains about 750 abstracts, so there are abstracts for about 45 percent of the items in *Index veterinarius*. Each abstract is published in one of twenty-six main sections (*Figure 4.2*) and there are cross references to abstracts on related topics printed in other sections. Subject and author indexes are in each monthly issue and cumulated versions of the indexes are published annually.

Most of the main headings are subdivided which makes it easy to scan issues for relevant material. For example the Virology and Viral Diseases section may have abstracts under headings for specific viral diseases such as Foot and mouth disease, Aujeszky's disease and Rabies, for families of viruses such as Poxvirus infections and Influenza viruses, and for viral diseases in particular animals, such as Viruses of cattle and Viruses of swine. These section headings can be searched online and offer a useful additional retrieval point.

On 1986, 87 percent of the items included in the two services were journal articles and a list of the serial publications contributing to the database in 1988 has been published [81]. Coverage is wider than the periodical literature however, and books, conference proceedings, theses, annual reports and most other forms of literature are included. Patents are not covered. *Figure 4.4* shows that almost three-quarters of the literature included is in English, with German in second place. An

Table 4.1   Number of items published in *Veterinary bulletin*, *Index veterinarius*, *Small animal abstracts* and *Animal disease occurrence*

	1988	*1987*	*1986*
Veterinary bulletin	8,059	8,224	9,001
Index veterinarius	18,865	17,337	20,491
Small animal abstracts	2,033	1,547	1,745
Animal disease occurrence	1,276	1,035	1,022

Vol. 57   No. 3   March 1987   Abstracts 1162–1794

Veterinary Bulletin

CONTENTS

Review Article: Ovine squamous cell carcinoma. By P. W. Daniels and R. H. Johnson   153

	Page		Page
Bacteriology and Bacterial Diseases	169	Haematology	233
Virology and Viral Diseases	183	Anatomy	234
Mycoses and Mycotoxicoses	193	Hygiene	235
Protozoology and Protozoal Diseases	195	Zootechny	236
Arthropod Parasites	198	Radiations and Radioisotopes	237
Helminth Parasites	200	Food Inspection	237
Regional and General Pathology	205	Techniques and Apparatus	239
Neoplasms and Leukosis	211	Surgery	240
Nutritional and Metabolic Disorders	213	Veterinary Services and Education	242
Reproductive Disorders	214	Reports	242
Toxicology	215	Books	242
Immunology	218	Conferences	244
Pharmacology and Therapeutics	221	AUTHOR INDEX	(1)
Physiology and Biochemistry	227	SUBJECT INDEX	(7)

Figure 4.2   Contents page of an issue of *Veterinary bulletin*.
(Reproduced by courtesy of CAB International).

analysis of the 1973 volume of *Index veterinarius* showed 68 percent of items were from the veterinary literature, 18 percent from medical, 8 percent from agricultural and 6 percent from general science literature (*Veterinary bulletin* **44** (1974): abstract no. 5836).

4.3 VETERINARY UPDATE

Veterinary update: clinical abstract service [28] provides abstracts of clinical papers appearing in about seventy English language periodicals. There are three editions intended for practitioners dealing with horses, food animals and small animals respectively. Each abstract is presented in a form for easy scanning; thus each item has a short title, a one line summary and an abstract giving the pertinent facts concerning types of animals involved, diagnosis, treatment and clinical results. Typical items are shown in *Figure 4.5*. There are annotated indexes in each issue and cumulative six-monthly indexes.

Selected abstracts from the three editions of *Veterinary update* appear in a variety

A new, accurate, sensitive capillary gas chromatographic assay for methylmalonic acid (MMA), tested on blood plasma and urine of lambs deficient in vitamin B_{12}, confirmed previous reports that urinary MMA was negatively correlated with vitamin B_{12} and/or cobalt status. It was important to express urinary MMA value as a function of creatinine concentration. The best correlation coefficient between urinary and plasma MMA in lambs was 0.87. Cobalt adequate lambs had plasma MMA values of less than 5 μmol/l, urinary MMA less than 120 μmol/l, and urinary MMA/creatinine values of less than 0.022 μmol MMA/mmol of urinary creatinine. Plasma MMA appeared to rise above 5 μmol/l only in lambs with vitamin B_{12} values less than 250 pg/ml. However, 38% of lambs with plasma vitamin B_{12} below 250 pg/ml had plasma MMA values below 5 μmol/l. Flock status is best assessed with a small group of lambs.

Other animals

939 SCOTT, D. W.; SHEFFY, B. E. **Dermatosis in dogs caused by vitamin E deficiency.** *Companion Animal Practice* (1987) **1** (4) 42-46 [En, 17 ref.] Coll. Vet. Med., Cornell Univ., Ithaca, NY 14853, USA.

Twelve Beagles on a vitamin E deficient diet developed signs of skin disease within 2-4 months. First there was defective keratinization (seborrhoea sicca), then inflammation (erythroderma) and a tendency to develop secondary pyoderma. Histological changes in skin biopsy samples are described. All signs disappeared 8-10 weeks after the dogs had been placed on a vitamin E adequate diet. It is pointed out that none of the signs is diagnostic.

REPRODUCTIVE DISORDERS

Horse

See also abst. 762

940 CLOUTIER, P.; GUAY, P.; KING, W. A.; BEAUREGARD; M. **[Ovarian hypoplasia in a mare.]** Hypoplasie ovarienne chez une jument. *Médecin Vétérinaire du Québec* (1987) **17** (3) 137-138 [Fr, en, 8 ref.] Fac. Méd. Vét., Univ. Montréal, CP 5000, St-Hyacinthe, Que. J2S 7C6, Canada.

The XO syndrome was diagnosed in an infertile 4-year-old Standardbred with ovarian hypoplasia. One sex chromosome was absent.

Cattle

See also abst. 937

941 KASSAM, A.; BONDURANT, R. H.; BASU, S.; KINDAHL, H.; STABENFELDT, G. H. **Clinical and endocrine responses to embryonic and fetal death induced by manual rupture of the amniotic vesicle during early pregnancy in cows.** *Journal of the American Veterinary Medical Association* (1987) **191** (4) 417-420 [En, 10 ref.] Dr. R.H. BonDurant, Sch. Vet. Med., Univ., Davis, CA 95616, USA.

Pregnancy was terminated in 4 cows by manual rupture of the amniotic vesicle on day 41 (n = 1) and day 46 (n = 3) after insemination. The cows were killed 36 days after vesicle rupture, by which time only one had come into oestrus. Luteal activity, monitored daily by plasma progesterone assay, was still evident in 2 cows 35 days after fetal death; in the remaining 2 cows, regression of the corpus luteum (CL) was achieved at 28 and 32 days, respectively. Uterine release of prostaglandin $F2\alpha$ ($PGF2\alpha$) was monitored by a plasma sampling schedule; specimens were obtained every 4 hours. There were no appreciable releases of $PGF2\alpha$ associated with fetal death. The first appreciable $PGF2\alpha$ release in episodic form was seen only in conjunction with CL regression. In all cows, a palpable membrane slip was evident for 18 days after rupture of the amniotic vesicle, although at that time, uterine resilience was diminished in the 2 cows in which the CL subsequently regressed. After 18 days, the uterus was noticeably oedematous and fluid-filled in all cows; in 1 of the cows with a regressed CL, the uterus had returned to

prepregnancy size and tone by day 33. The 2 cows with intact CL post mortem had varying amounts of flocculent material in the uterine lumen, but the 2 cows with regressed CL had none.

942 HÖPFNER, H. W. **[Intrauterine treatment of endometritis in cows with a glucose drug combination.]** Untersuchungen zur intrauterinen Behandlung der Endometritis des Rindes mit einer Glukose-Arzneimittelkombination. *Monatshefte für Veterinärmedizin* (1987) **42** (15) 535-539 [De, ru, en, 13 ref.] Staatl. Tierärztliche Gemeinschaftspraxis, Halberstädter Strasse 4, DDR-3237 Schwanebeck, German Democratic Republic.

A glucose-electrolyte-vitamin combination (7.6 g of glucose, 47.6 ml of isotonic electrolyte solution, 240 000 IU of vitamin A/100 ml) were compared with Lugosol and Solupront by intra-uterine infusion in 50 cows with endometritis of differing severity. The glucose combination, was effective, with results equal to those recorded with the two other standard preparations. The following year, the entire herd, consisting of 1400 cows, was put under a therapeutic régime for endometritis using preparations free from antibiotics and sulfonamides, with good results.

943 WOUDA, W.; ELGERSMA, A. **[Fatal ovarian bleeding in two donor cows after embryo transplantation.]** Fatale ovariële bloeding bij twee donorkoeien na embryotransplantatie. *Tijdschrift voor Diergeneeskunde* (1987) **112** (20) 1177-1179 [Nl, 2 fig.] Gezondheidsdienst voor Dieren, PO Box° 361, 9200 AJ Drachten, Netherlands.

One 6-year-old cow was found dead 12 hours after, and another cow of the same age died a few hours after ova had been recovered by uterine irrigation under spinal anaesthesia. Haemorrhage occurred from ruptures 1.5-2 cm long in the ovaries, caused apparently by manipulation of the uterus during irrigation.

Sheep and goat

944 GIMBO, A.; ZANGHI, A.; GIANNETTO, S. **Ram testicular hypoplasia. Anatomical and histopathological observations.** *Schweizer Archiv für Tierheilkunde* (1987) **129** (9) 481-491 [En, de, fr, it, 19 ref.] Fac. Vet. Med., Univ., Via S. Cecilia 30, I-98 100 Messina, Italy.

A histological study of the bilateral condition in young crossbred rams (Bergamasco/Pinzirita) from one farm is described. The occurrence of fetal Sertoli cells indicated a development disorder.

945 MATEJKA, M.; CRIBIU, E. P.; RICORDEAU, G.; CHAFFAUX, S. **[Frequency of freemartinism in Romanov ewes.]** Fréquence du freemartinisme chez des agnelles Romanov. *Recueil de Médecine Vétérinaire* (1987) **163** (6/7) 635-638 [Fr, en, es, 11 ref.] INRA Centre Rech., 78350 Jouy-en-Josas, France.

Cytogenetic analysis of peripheral lymphocyte cultures from 125 Romanov ewes born as twins to a male are reported. Of 6 animals diagnosed with a sex chromosomal chimerism (54,XX/54,XY), 5 are freemartin and infertile and one is normal and fertile. The frequency of freemartinism in this breed is between 0.8 and 1.9% and half of infertile ewes are confirmed as freemartins.

Swine

See also abst. 1006

Other animals

946 ROBINSON, R. **Genetic defects in cats.** *Companion Animal Practice* (1987) **1** (3) 10-14 [En, 66 ref.] St. Stephens Rd Nursery, Ealing, London, W13 8HB, UK.

A list of some 40 defects with established modes of inheritance and about 20 suspected of genetic aetiologies.

Figure 4.3   Part of typical page from *Veterinary bulletin*. (Reproduced by courtesy of CAB International).

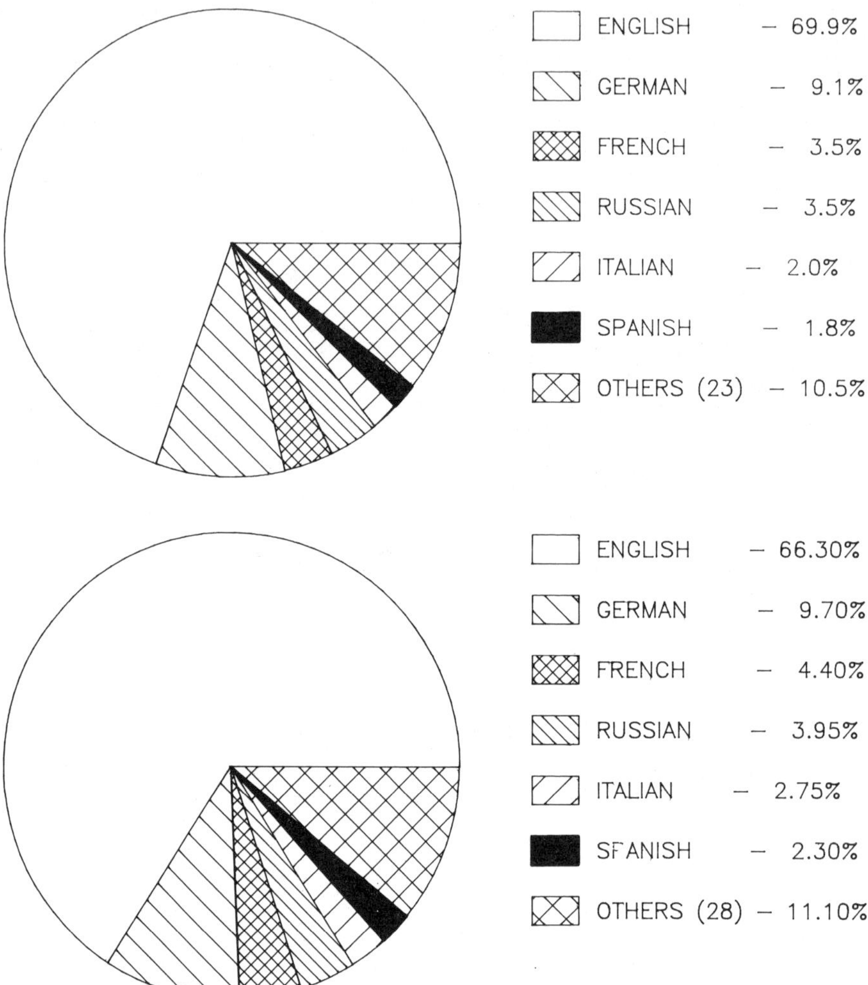

Figure 4.4   *Veterinary bulletin* (upper figure) and *Index veterinarius* (lower figure): language coverage 1986.

of other forms. The same publishers also issue *Modern veterinary practice* [22], each issue of which now consists of a selection of about fifty abstracts considered to be of greatest interest. Veterinary surgeons in Britain have access to the majority of the abstracts in *Veterinary update* since most are published in *Clinical insight* [103] in their *Clinical literature digest* section. The only items excluded are those relating to clinical situations which would not be encountered by a veterinary surgeon practising in Britain or Europe. Similar arrangements to republish materials from *Veterinary update* have been established with the Post-Graduate Committee in Veterinary Science of the University of Sydney [2258] who publish them as *Article summaries*

GLOMERULONEPHRITIS AND HEPATITIS FOLLOWING IMMUNOTHERAPY

Signs of hepatitis resolved after cessation of immunotherapy.

A 10-yr-old 30-kg spayed mixed-breed with partial anorexia, vomiting, progressive lethargy and polyuria/polydipsia for 1 wk had been given repeated IV injections of killed <u>Corynebacterium parvum</u> vaccine (Wellcome) for 10 mo as adjuvant immunotherapy after a cutaneous melanoma was excised. The dog had exhibited minor side effects of <u>C parvum</u> treatment (vomiting, anorexia) 4-6 hr after injection.

The dog was jaundiced, depressed, and had a palpable abdominal mass caudoventral to the right costal arch, but no visible recurrence of the melanoma. Lab findings included elevated BUN, creatinine, total bilirubin and inorganic phosphorus, with high serum lactic dehydrogenase, alanine transaminase and alkaline phosphatase values. Acidosis was evident and prothrombin and activated partial thromboplastin times prolonged. On radiographs, a mass craniomedial to the right kidney originated from the liver.

Treatment included lactated Ringer's solution IV and ampicillin IV at 25 mg/kg TID. Because progressive hypoalbuminemia resulted in facial and cervical edema, and coagulation times were progressively prolonged, the dog was given fresh frozen plasma from A-negative donors IV at 2000 ml/day on days 4-6. Tissue sections taken during laparotomy revealed cirrhosis and chronic active hepatitis and proliferative glomerulonephritis. The dog improved clinically with supportive care and was healthy 1 yr later.

> C.E. Leifer et al. Animal Medical Center, New York, New York. **Proliferative glomerulonephritis and chronic active hepatitis with cirrhosis associated with Corynebacterium parvum immunotherapy in a dog.** JAVMA 190:78-80, 1987.

EFFICACY OF OXFENDAZOLE AGAINST <u>TOXOCARA</u> IN PUPS

Oxfendazole was effective against adult <u>Toxocara</u> in pups.

In 4 unweaned Greyhound pups 30 days old, oxfendazole (Synanthic DC: Syntex) PO at 10 mg/kg SID for 3 consecutive days reduced the adult <u>Toxocara canis</u> burden 98.5%, compared with 4 untreated littermates at necropsy on day 40. When 10 pups were similarly treated, beginning at 5 days of age, overall efficacy on day 21 compared with 10 littermates was 75.8%, indicating oxfendazole was ineffective against larvae in early stages of development. The pups readily accepted the oxfendazole, and no side effects were observed.

> D.E. Jacobs et al. Royal Vet Coll, Hatfield, England. **Evaluation of the efficacy of oxfendazole against larval and adult <u>Toxocara canis</u> in unweaned dogs.** J Small Anim Pract 27:783-786, 1986.

Figure 4.5   Typical entries from *Veterinary update*.
(Reproduced by courtesy of American Veterinary Publications).

[14] and with a publisher in Japan, Chikusan Shuppan Sha, who publish *Companion animal practice*.

4.4 QUARTERLY INDEX AND SMALL ANIMAL ABSTRACTS

There are two abstracting services that cover the literature relevant to small animal practitioners.

The *Quarterly index* [770] is a thorough and remarkably cheap compilation of the literature appearing in some of the core veterinary journals. With the exception of the *Journal of small animal practice* all of these are North American periodicals. The *Veterinary record* is not included. Each issue of the index includes abstracts of every article, case report, letter, abstract or correction likely to be of interest to a practitioner dealing with small animals or exotic pets. Reviews of new books are also noted. These items are arranged and numbered sequentially according to the journal issue in which they appear. This makes it easy to scan particular journal issues for items of interest. *Quarterly index* is published quarterly and there are author and subject indexes which are cumulative during the course of the year. The final issue of each year is a cumulation giving a single volume reference work for the whole year. A typical page from the *Quarterly index* is shown in *Figure 4.6*. The abstracts can be lengthy and are clinically oriented. The database may be searched online on VETERINARY NETWORK. In 1987 the *Quarterly index* included 2,172 items.

Whereas the *Quarterly index* provides very detailed coverage of the North American literature, the world's literature on small animals, particularly that on cats and dogs, is best covered by *Small animal abstracts* [771]. The numbers of items appearing in *Small animal abstracts* in recent years are shown in *Table 4.1*. In 1987, of the 1,547 abstracts published 957 were also published in *Veterinary bulletin*. Of the remaining 590 items, 557 were noted as titles-only in *Index veterinarius*, although abstracts for all of the 590 items were published in one or more of the CAB International abstracts journals.

4.5 OTHER CAB INTERNATIONAL JOURNALS

Small animal abstracts is one of several specialist journals produced by CAB International from their database. Other 'species-oriented' abstracting journals which will be of interest to veterinarians are *Pig news and information* [619] and *Poultry abstracts* [1035]. CAB International publish a number of other main abstracting journals, some of which have been published for some considerable time, which are of value to workers in particular fields. Some are concerned with animal science and production: *Animal breeding abstracts* [1636], *Dairy science abstracts* [417] and *Nutrition abstracts and reviews* [1411]. Others deal with some of the

**JOURNAL OF THE AMERICAN VETERINARY
MEDICAL ASSOCIATION
Volume 191, Number 1   July 1, 1987**

JVMA.198--Recommends reanalysis of data
          -Comments and reply on the article,
"Factors affecting prerace dehydration and performance of racing Greyhounds" in JAVMA, Dec 15,
1986, pp 1572-1574 (86-JVMA.510 in the *Quarterly
Index*).
          A statistical error in the article is pointed out and
reanalysis of the data made.
<<J Am Vet Med Assoc, Vol 191, No 1 (Jul 1'87) pages
4 Letter 0 refs

JVMA.199--Career pathways
          -Comments on the "sad fact that a DVM
degree closes doors to many interesting opportunities".
<<J Am Vet Med Assoc, Vol 191, No 1 (Jul 1'87) pages
4-5 Letter 0 refs

**JVMA.200--Prefers veterinary technician to animal
technician**
<<J Am Vet Med Assoc, Vol 191, No 1 (Jul 1'87) pages
5-6 Letter 0 refs

**JVMA.201--Regression of canine transmissible venereal
sarcoma**
-Discussion of canine transmissible venereal sarcoma.
Viable tumor cells can be transplanted into other dogs
and even other Canidae. The tumor will progressively
grow for 2-4 months, then in adults it will regress.
Whereas in immunosuppressed dogs and neonates, it will
metastasize. Tumors in adults are smaller, and re-
gressing tumors contain more lymphocytes (especially T
cells) and have spindle-shaped cells instead of the
round cells seen in progressively growing tumors.
Serum antibodies have been seen in dogs with the
tumors. Lymphokines may be helpful when used with
conventional chemotherapy in eliminating residual
tumors.
<<J Am Vet Med Assoc, Vol 191, No 1 (Jul 1'87) pages
6 Letter 0 refs

JVMA.202--The bond of being a veterinarian
          <<J Am Vet Med Assoc, Vol 191, No 1 (Jul
1'87) pages 26-28 Reflections 0 refs
Dr. John B. Herrick
Iowa

JVMA.203--Continuation of coverage provisions
          -Coverage of the spouse after death or
divorce and coverage after termination of membership
or employment are discussed.
<<J Am Vet Med Assoc, Vol 191, No 1 (Jul 1'87) pages
31 Insurance Note 0 refs
Dwight Porter
Professional Society Insurance Service, Chicago, Il
60604

**JVMA.204--Malpractice insurance--some legal considera-
tions**
-Things to know about the nature and extent of
malpractice insurance coverage.

<<J Am Vet Med Assoc, Vol 191, No 1 (Jul 1'87) pages
32-33 Legal Brief 0 refs
Harold W. Hannah, LLB
Texico, IL 62889

**JVMA.205--Cardiopulmonary and behavioral effects of
fentanyl-droperidol in cats**
-Evaluation of the cardiopulmonary and behavioral
effects of fentanyl-droperidol in 12 healthy cats.
          Experimental design. The narcotic fentanyl (0.4
mg/ml) and the butyrophenone tranquilizer droperidol
(20 mg/ml) combination (Innovar Vet: Pitman Moore)
was given the 12 cats at 1 ml/9 kg BW SC. Arterial
blood pressure, heart rate, arterial pH, PaCO2, PaO2,
rectal temperature, and respiration were measured
prior to and at 30, 60, 90, and 120 minutes following
injection. Behavior was also monitored.
          Results. Respiratory rate was significantly de-
creased and heart rate significantly increased throughout the study compared to baseline values. Body
temperature was significantly decreased at 90 minutes
postinjection. No other significant changes were seen
although blood pressure did decrease.
          By 20-30 minutes postinjection, 8 cats were tranquil
and often laterally recumbent and 4 showed signs of
euphoria (eg., kneading, purring, friendliness). By 30-
45 minutes postinjection, these 4 cats were also
tranquil and often laterally recumbent. All were
responsive to loud noises, particularly the first 60
minutes postinjection. One cat experienced respiratory
difficulty and a marked decrease in PaO2, was
extremely sensitive to noise, and would become very
agitated.
<<J Am Vet Med Assoc, Vol 191, No 1 (Jul 1'87) pages
59-61 Original Study 19 refs
[1]J. L. Grandy, DVM; R. B. Heath, DVM, MSc
[1]Dept of Clin Sci, College of Vet Med & Biomed Sci,
Colorado State Univ, Fort Collins, CO 80523

JVMA.206--Ivermectin toxicosis in a dog
          -Case report of a 2.5 year old male Old
English sheepdog-type.
          History. The dog was given ivermectin at 150 ug/kg
PO (7 ml of Sheep Ivomec: Merck Sharp & Dohme) for
suspected endoparasitism. Within 2 hours it began to
exhibit progressive neurologic signs beginning with
hindlimb ataxia.
          Clinicopathologic findings on admission 20 hours
later included stupor, difficulty in arousing, fever,
dyspnea, hypersalivation, bilateral absence of the
menace response, mitotic but light responsive pupils,
ventromedial to ventrolateral strabismus. The rest of
the neurologic exam, CBC, serum biochemistries,
urinalysis, CSF analysis, blood gas and acid base values
were normal.
          Treatment was supportive, consisting of dexa-
methasone and fluid therapy.
          Marked sinus arrhythmia and bradycardia de-
veloped 8 hours after admission and were responsive to
atropine and glycopyrrolate administration. The dog
was ataxic, walked aimlessly, and had periods of deep
sleep after 48 hours, but was eating and drinking. On
release (after 8 days) hindlimb ataxia and episodes of
abnormal behavior were still present. The dog gradually
improved and was normal when reexamined 2 months
later.
          There are 2 previous reports of ivermectin causing

Figure 4.6   Typical page from *Quarterly index*.
(Reproduced by permission of Veterinary Interface).

veterinary specialities: *Helminthological abstracts* [1476], *Protozoological abstracts* [1590], *Review of applied entomology* [1478] and *Review of medical and veterinary mycology* [1396]. All of the items published in these journals since 1973 are included in the CAB ABSTRACTS database.

4.6 VETDOC

VETDOC provides access to literature on the research, development and use of all kinds of veterinary pharmaceuticals. Most of the subscribers to the service are animal health companies. VETDOC [26] only covers the journal literature, but it publishes about 4,000 abstracts each year, which are mostly of articles in the core veterinary journals (Gibb, 1988). The service is prompt in publishing detailed abstracts which contain much factual information on the experimental methods and results reported, often making recourse to the original article unnecessary. A typical abstract is shown in *Figure 4.7*. This is taken from the basic printed product, the *VETDOC abstracts journal*, which is issued twenty times a year.

VETDOC began in 1968 and subscribers, as well as receiving the printed journal, can also search the data online on ORBIT SEARCH SERVICE. The database is divided into two files, the earlier covering the period 1968 to 1982. Unfortunately only brief abstracts are available online in the most recent file, and there are none at all in the closed file, so the full abstracts are only available from the printed abstracts journal or its microfilm version. The indexing of the database is thesaurus controlled. Since 1983 it has also been highly structured, so very precise searches can be carried out simply. Because of the interests of its users VETDOC pays special attention to indexing chemical compounds. A comparison of its performance to that of CAB INTERNATIONAL has shown VETDOC to be particularly useful for retrieving data on trade or brand-named products (Oakes, 1986). A search of the current file is shown in *Figure 4.8*.

VETDOC is produced by Derwent Publications who also compile the related PESTDOC and RINGDOC. The former covers the journal and conference literature on insecticides and other pesticides; RINGDOC deals with the journal literature on human pharmaceuticals. Both services can be useful to those engaged in veterinary research.

4.7 CONTENTS LISTS AND CURRENT AWARENESS SERVICES

Current contents [41] is the best-known service. It appears weekly in several editions, veterinary journals being included in the *Agriculture, biology and environmental sciences* title. The *Life sciences* and *Clinical practice* editions may be of value to those wishing to follow developments in bioscience and medical research. Each issue of *Current contents* reproduces the tables of contents of recently published journals. The

Z S   **86-60360**
Investigating Ivermectin Toxicity in Collies.
Vet.Med. (80, No. 6, 33, 36-40, 1985)
/Merck-USA/ Pulliam J D; Seward R L; Henry R T; Steinberg S
A/ Rahway, N.J.; Perkasie; Philadelphia, Pa., USA

In an investigation of ivermectin toxicity in Collie dogs 3 doses of the drug were tested orally. 3/4 Dogs in each of the groups treated with the 2 higher doses were adversely affected, 1/4 showing serious signs. Toxic symptoms included ataxia, depression, tremors, recumbency, mydriasis, excessive salivation, shallow respiration with panting, and incoordination. Ivermectin tissue assays showed high concentrations of ivermectin in the CNS systems. The degree of response to ivermectin did not seem to be related to Collie eye anomaly.

Equal numbers of male and female rough-coated Collies were obtained, half of which had Collie eye anomaly. The ages ranged from 7 mth to 9 yr and 8 mth. The 4 treatment groups were: group 1 untreated controls; group 2 ivermectin 0.1% p.o. solution at 50 ug/kg; group 3 ivermectin 0.3% p.o. solution at 200 ug/kg; group 4 ivermectin 0.3% p.o. solution at 600 ug/kg. Each group contained 1 male and 1 female affected with Collie eye anomaly, and 1 male and 1 female free of the condition.
2 Dogs given 200 ug/kg and 2 dogs given 600 ug/kg showed signs of toxicity. 4 Hr after treatment, 1 dog from group 4, a 19-mth-old female unaffected by the eye anomaly, had progressive postural difficulty. Although muscle strength and strong reflexes persisted, the dog became less aware of stimuli. Excessive salivation and panting were observed. 28 Hr post-treatment, the animal was euthanized. A 7-yr-old male with the eye anomaly showed ataxia, staggering, hypermetria, incoordination, hypersalivation and increased diaphragmatic respiration. At 51 hr, the animal died. Mild neurologic effects were seen in other dogs from groups 3 and 4. Pathologic changes included mild pulmonary congestion and mild to moderate multifocal hemorrhages in the cerebellum and brain-stem, but these were considered artifacts following death or euthanasia. 4 Tab. 15 Ref. (CLW)
Merck Sharp & Dohme Research Laboratories, Merck & Company Incorporated, P.O. Box 2000, Rahway, New Jersey 07065, U.S.A.

Figure 4.7   Item from the *VETDOC abstracts journal*.
(Reproduced by courtesy of Derwent Publications Limited).

Institute of Scientific Information prides itself on the promptness of its products and subscribers may well be aware of items from *Current contents* before the journals themselves have arrived in Britain. Each issue has author and title word indexes and these are cumulated. Authors' addresses are listed in the index. There is a triannual cumulative journal index allowing one to locate every journal issue published in *Current contents* during a four month period. The data are now available online in CURRENT CONTENTS ONLINE and can be obtained on disc.
All the larger abstracting and indexing services are now produced using

```
YOU ARE NOW CONNECTED TO THE VETDOC UNIFIED DATABASE.
COVERS 1983 THRU 87-63201 (8710)
SEE ALSO VETDOC (1968-1982)

SS 1 /C?
USER:
ivermectin/st link dog

PROG:
SS 1 PSTG (18)

SS 2 /C?
USER:
1 and collie:

PROG:
SS 2 PSTG (7)
print ti 1-7

-1-
TI  - The Safety and Efficacy of Ivermectin in Heartworm Prevention.

-2-
TI  - Clinical Observations in Collies given Ivermectin Orally.

-3-
TI  - Response to Physostigmine Administration in Collie Dogs
        Exhibiting Ivermectin Toxicosis.

-4-
TI  - Intoxication of a Collie with Ivermectin. (Ger.).

-5-
TI  - Adverse Reaction to Ivermectin in a Rough-Coated Collie.

-6-
TI  - Investigating Ivermectin Toxicity in Collies.

-7-
TI  - Ivermectin in the Dog.
```

Figure 4.8   Online search of the most recent VETDOC file for information on adverse effects of ivermectins in dogs. Eighteen items are identified and the search is narrowed to papers on collies. The titles of the seven references are printed and the fourth is printed in full.
(Reproduced by courtesy of Derwent Publications Limited and ORBIT SEARCH SERVICE).

```
SS 2 /C?
USER:
print all 4-4


-4-
AN  - 87-60341 T Z S M V E
PN  - (G)
AU  - Berninghaus H
LO  - Werl, Ger.
JN  - PRTIAV; Prakt.Tierarzt (67, No. 7, 575-77, 1986)
TI  - Intoxication of a Collie with Ivermectin. (Ger.).
AB  - The fatal poisoning of a collie with ivermectin is reported.  A
      4-yr-old male collie was given an unknown dose of Ivomec
      (ivermectin) s.c. to control endo- and ectoparasites.  2 Days
      later the animal's respiratory rate had increased slightly, its
      pupils were dilated, its reflexes were diminished, slight ataxia
      was apparent, and the dog kept going over on its hind quarters.
      It received amoxicillin i.v., vitamin B complex, Crataegus, and
      infusions of electrolyte and mannitol solutions.  The symptoms
      worsened and cortisone infusions were given.  Despite the use of
      the antidotes RO15/1788 (Hoffmann-La Roche) at 0.08 and 0.04
      mg/kg i.v., and picrotoxin at 1 mg/min in isotonic dextrose
      solution and when the animal was in a coma at 8 mg, the outcome
      was fatal
CT  - DOG/FT; EXITUS/FT; CASE-HISTORY/FT; IN-VIVO/FT; SMALL-ANIMAL/FT
LT  - *01* IVERMECTIN/ST; IVERMECTIN/TR; IVOMEC/ST; IVOMEC/TR;
      NEMATODIASIS/TR; INFESTATION,ECTOPARASITE/TR; INTOXICATION/ST;
      S.C./FT; INJECTION/FT; ANTHELMINTICS/FT; IVERMECTI/RN; ST/FT;
      TR/FT
LT  - *02* FLUMAZEPIL/TR; ROCHE/FT; INTOXICATION/TR;
      BENZODIAZEPINE-ANTAGONIST/FT; I.V./FT; INJECTION/FT;
      BENZODIAZEPINE-ANTAGONISTS/FT; FLUMAZEPI/RN; TR/FT
LT  - *03* AMOXICILLIN/TR; INTOXICATION/TR; I.V./FT; INJECTION/FT;
      ANTIBIOTIC/FT; ANTIBIOTICS/FT; AMOXICILL/RN; TR/FT
LT  - *04* B-COMPLEX/TR; INTOXICATION/TR; VITAMINS-B/FT; B-COMPLEX/RN;
      TR/FT
LT  - *05* MANNITOL/TR; INTOXICATION/TR; DIURETIC/FT; DIURETICS/FT;
      LAXATIVES/FT; MANNITOL/RN; TR/FT
LT  - *06* CORTISONE/TR; INTOXICATION/TR; CORTICOSTEROID/FT;
      CORTICOSTEROIDS/FT; CORTISONE/RN; TR/FT
LT  - *07* PICROTOXIN/TR; INTOXICATION/TR; ANALEPTIC/FT; ANALEPTICS/FT;
      PICROTOXI/RN; TR/FT
```

Figure 4.8 *cont'd*

```
SS 2 /C?
USER:
STOP Y

PROG:
TERMINAL SESSION FINISHED 02/15/88  4:25 A.M.  (EASTERN TIME)
ELAPSED TIME ON VETDOC UDB: 0.05 HRS.
ELAPSED TIME THIS TERMINAL SESSION: 0.06 HOURS.
ORBIT SEARCH SESSION COMPLETED.  THANKS FOR USING ORBIT!
```

Figure 4.8 *cont'd*

computerized techniques. The availability of these data in machine-readable form means that the publishers can produce bulletins of current information in specific subject areas in a form appropriate for individual researchers. These usually appear fortnightly or monthly and provide abstracts of relevant literature.

Few of these titles are concerned exclusively with veterinary topics – a notable exception being the *Mastitis literature survey* produced by CAB International. Most of the bulletins available are only of minor interest to veterinarians in practice. AGDEX Information Services, for example, produce several monthly bulletins containing references and brief abstracts of material from the UK agricultural sources [37]. Most of the other services available are likely to be of most value for those carrying out research and working in the fields of biochemistry, physiology and pharmacology. Typical titles in the BIOSIS/CAS Selects series, produced by BIOSIS/Chemical Abstracts Service, for example, are: *Antiviral agents*, *Immuno-chemical methods* and *Monoclonal antibodies*. BIOSIS also publish the *Bioresearch today* and *BIOSIS standard profiles* series derived from the BIOSIS database and Chemical Abstracts Service publish the *CAS selects* and *CAS BioTech updates* series, both compiled solely from *Chemical abstracts*.

A number of the abstracting and indexing services also offer users the ability to specify their own subject interests; a 'profile' can be designed for computer searching of the literature, and subscribers can receive individually tailored current awareness bulletins. Those with direct access to online systems can develop profiles for themselves and these can easily be modified in the light of changing interests.

4.8 INFORMATION ON NEW BOOKS

Evaluative reviews of books are included in many journals but unfortunately these reviews may only appear some time after the book has been published. *Index veterinarius* and *Veterinary bulletin* also note new books and in 1986 and 1987 these services noted 179 and 140 books respectively. The abstracts which *Veterinary bulletin* publishes are intended to indicate the books contents and the expected level of the readership rather than being critical reviews.

The most up-to-date information about new books is available from the publishers themselves who are obviously keen to inform potential purchasers about new works. Occasionally publishers have inserts included in journals or arrange for mailshots to be sent to members of societies. Advertisements for new books are sometimes placed in journals. Publishers produce detailed catalogues and stock lists, but these may be of limited value since, for the larger publishers at least, few of the titles may be relevant to veterinary medicine. Many publishers now compile specialist catalogues. One may be devoted to titles in veterinary science or there may be catalogues covering the broader topics of animal sciences or agriculture which may contain details of veterinary works. A useful feature of publishers' catalogues is that they frequently include announcements of forthcoming titles. Most publishers are happy to add potential purchasers on to their mailing lists: addresses for the more important publishers are given in Part III.

Booksellers are also important sources of information about new books because they often produce comprehensive catalogues of new titles and editions. The most important in Britain are Heffers, Kimptons Medical Bookshop and H. K. Lewis. The Veterinary Book Guild in the United States issue a useful catalogue which lists major works from several publishers. Similarly a number of other foreign booksellers produce detailed catalogues of veterinary titles. That of the Librairie Zoothèque gives a thorough list of French works; those of Nicholás Moya and Librería Agrícola are useful for details of books in Spanish. Addresses for these booksellers are given in Part III.

A good source of up-to-date information on new books available in Britain is the British Council's *British book news* [38]. This is especially useful to those outside the UK since in many countries the magazine is available via a controlled free circulation system. The British Council also administers the ELBS (English Language Book Society) scheme. This makes low-priced editions of many standard textbooks available to students in almost ninety developing countries. A complete catalogue of the books available can be obtained from the Council.

4.9 TRADE LITERATURE

Veterinarians in practice receive large amounts of unsolicited material. Manufacturers of veterinary equipment, supplies and drugs often send out mailshots advertising their products to practitioners. Much of this is of limited value since it is largely produced as a marketing exercise and so may include only brief technical information and may not give full price data. None the less advertising and promotional items like this can be of interest, especially to others working in the animal health industry. Unfortunately this type of material is often difficult to obtain. By its very nature it tends to be fugitive and ephemeral, and is rarely collected and organized systematically. The most easily accessible is the advertising which forms a large component of many journals, although in many libraries advertisements are removed from journals prior to binding. Some promotional materials are included as loose inserts to journals, but these are not usually kept by libraries.

Most companies produce catalogues of their products although even these might not be widely available. These sometimes contain full technical information or may simply duplicate data given on packaging. In most countries it is mandatory for companies to prepare and distribute information on their products and many of the directories of veterinary drugs reproduce these data [214–273]. Detailed technical information about particular products can be supplied by companies' technical services departments.

Of special note are the various controlled-circulation magazines and journals. These are basically funded by advertising and so could be considered a form of trade literature. They are sent free to practitioners, the titles have a large readership, and they undoubtedly serve a useful role in keeping practitioners up to date in professional matters. In the UK *Veterinary practice* and *Veterinary times* have a newspaper format, and *Clinical insight* contains more formal, well illustrated articles with a relevance to clinical practice.

4.10 CONFERENCES AND CONTINUING EDUCATION EVENTS

Veterinarians are gregarious people and the subject field is one in which it is useful to exchange practical information. As a result a large number of specialist societies have been formed. Each of these, plus the national and international associations, hold regular symposia, conferences and meetings of varying degrees of formality. Many of the specialist associations meet at the annual conferences of the national veterinary associations. In the United States for example many of the speciality groups meet at the AVMA's annual meeting or prior to or at the AAHA's annual conference.

Where there are printed proceedings from meetings these will usually be noted in *Index veterinarius* and *Veterinary bulletin*. The form of proceedings varies greatly however and often all that is available are photocopies of abstracts of the papers or of the authors' manuscripts. These may only be available at the meeting itself. Where more formal printed proceedings are produced this is noted under the entry for the sponsoring organization in Part III. Sometimes abstracts, or the full text of the papers presented at meetings, are published in the journal of the sponsoring organization. The BVA for example publishes a brochure which has abstracts for the papers presented at the annual congress. This is distributed as a supplement to *Veterinary record*.

Most events are open to non-members of the societies and are advertised widely in journals and newsletters. The national veterinary journals usually include calendars of the major forthcoming meetings. The *Veterinary record*, for example, provides news of forthcoming events in its diary section and British regional and other veterinary associations advertise in the journal's classified columns. More general agricultural events held in the UK are noted in the *Farm diary* [331] and in the RASE's *National calendar of events* [332]. Similarly *Feedstuffs* [327] includes a full list of agricultural events in the United States. Conferences on specialist topics will be advertised in the relevant journals. One notable list, covering parasitology, appears in each issue of the *International journal for parasitology*. A calendar of events of international interest is published in the *Bulletin of the World Veterinary Association* [326]. Another comprehensive international list appears in the *Journal of the American Veterinary Medical Association* [329]. This journal also publishes a list of events occurring in the USA, including details on meetings of the state veterinary associations. The American Veterinary Exhibitors Association compile a calendar of the coming year's veterinary and related meetings and non-members may subscribe to this convention schedule. The American Veterinary Distributors Association publish a similar listing.

The most prestigious conference is the World Veterinary Congress. The first was held in Hamburg in 1863 and the event is now held every four years, recent ones being in Moscow 1979, Perth 1983 and Montreal 1987. The Montreal congress was attended by 5,439 people from eighty-four countries. Almost half of those attending were veterinarians. Over 700 papers and 350 posters were presented. The next congress, the twenty-fourth, will be in Rio de Janeiro in 1991. Many of the larger congresses have commercial and trade exhibitions. New products are often launched at the congresses and the exhibitions are a good source of trade literature. At the last World Veterinary Congress 1,400 staff were involved in the exhibition and there were 225 exhibition stands.

4.10.1 Continuing Education

The pace of new developments in veterinary medicine is very great. Even recent graduates find that refresher courses, in which the newer techniques and developments are discussed and demonstrated, are important in keeping them up to date. These meetings are known as continuing education or continuing professional development (CPD) events. The national associations play an active role in encouraging veterinarians to participate in these events because they are important in maintaining high standards of veterinary care. The BVA and RCVS work together in promoting continuing professional development throughout the UK and in publicizing information on forthcoming events [330]. A list of continuing education events in the United States is published in the *Journal of the American Veterinary Medical Association* quarterly.

These events are organized by a variety of bodies. The veterinary schools are very active in continuing education programmes; most of the specialist associations organize courses for their members; in the United States the state veterinary associations may sponsor the courses. There are a variety of other organizations which may offer courses in particular areas, for example the Hunterian Institute at the Royal College of Surgeons of England offers a variety of animal care courses for veterinarians, other scientists and technicians, working with laboratory animals. Many of the events receive commercial sponsorship. In the UK the BSAVA/C-Vet courses are perhaps the best known; there is a comprehensive range of courses for veterinary surgeons and also a programme of courses for veterinary nurses.

The course notes distributed at events held in Britain and the United States are normally available only to participants. However the presentations made at courses organized by the Post-Graduate Committee in Veterinary Science of the University of Sydney [66] and those of the Foundation for Continuing Education of the New Zealand Veterinary Association [63] are published.

References

Gibb, M. 'Letter to the editor'. *Journal of veterinary pharmacology and therapeutics.* **11** (1988): 227–9.

Oakes, S. C. *A comparative study of CAB and VETDOC, two commercial databases in the veterinary information field.* The City University, Department of Information Science: M.Sc. Dissertation, 1985. 209pp.

5 Finding Out About the Literature

All information has a cost. Even that freely given by colleagues has a price: the time spent discussing and, where necessary, documenting the problem and its solution. Often, however, one's colleagues and acquaintances cannot provide the information required. It is then appropriate to make a systematic attempt to identify appropriate information sources using formal bibliographic aids. This chapter is concerned with these information tools, which will usually only be available in the larger libraries.

5.1 GUIDES TO THE LITERATURE AND BIBLIOGRAPHIES

This work is merely the latest in a series of guides to the veterinary literature. These provide an overview of the various information sources and identify the most appropriate for particular enquiries. The earlier guides are still valuable; each is cumulative, and builds upon the knowledge documented in the previous titles. Indeed, the field is so wide-ranging, and so many veterinary titles have by now been published, that it would be impossible to compile a complete bibliography. The works listed in Part II, therefore, are a selection of the most important and the most recent titles. The other guides can be consulted for earlier publications. If one cannot identify a suitable source of information using these guides then one would use computerized information systems, perform extensive searches through printed abstracting and indexing journals, or use more general bibliographies.

Kerker and Murphy's *Comparative and veterinary medicine: a guide to the resource literature* [5] was the most complete guide when first published. Apart from key veterinary works it includes many of the medical and life sciences publications relevant to veterinary science. It is now very out of date but two guides to the literature of agriculture have been published subsequently and each contains sections on both the animal and veterinary sciences [2, 6]. D. E. Gray's chapter in *Information sources in agriculture and food science* [6] is a concise survey and he has compiled a more recent and very extensive bibliography of veterinary books [53]. Developments in veterinary science are closely linked to advances in human medicine and veterinary researchers make use of information and techniques in the basic life sciences. For these reasons guides to sources of information in the life [10] and medical [7] sciences can be useful.

Apart from these detailed subject bibliographies those looking for information can use the more general lists of books which are available. A variety of titles are listed in Part II [43–59], at least some of these will be available in any library of a reasonable size. Some of these bibliographies are commercially produced, such as *Books in print* [46] although most countries produce national bibliographies, like the *British national bibliography* [49] which attempts to list all new books and serials. Some of the bibliographies compiled by veterinary libraries have been discussed in Chapter 2 but the catalogues of other major libraries, such of those of the Science Reference and Information Service [47] and the British Library Document Supply Centre, can also be useful. The *Catalogue of Lewis's medical, scientific and technical lending library* [50] covers books acquired by the library up to 1972 and there have been regular supplements.

A number of specialist subject bibliographies are also available covering particular aspects of veterinary science. CAB International have compiled many bibliographies from their database and titles are available in a number of areas of veterinary medicine, including general medical topics, mycology, protozoology, parasitology and therapeutics. A particularly well known item is the anuual *Mastitis literature survey* [418]. CAB International also publish a number of annotated bibliographies, such as Dubey and Towle's *Toxoplasmosis in sheep* [544], which also include reviews of the literature.

5.2 REVIEWS

Review papers collate and summarize the new information presented in the literature. They bridge the gap between the original publication of research as journal articles and the more formal presentation of current knowledge given in textbooks. Reviews often deal with topics in great depth and they usually contain extensive bibliographies. Authors of review articles usually evaluate the literature, so reviews supplement the information available in textbooks by listing both the more important and recent publications. Reviews are particularly appropriate to those needing information in unfamiliar fields or wishing to update their knowledge in a subject. They are especially popular with practitioners because they provide an excellent way of keeping up to date. They provide an invaluable service in relating advances reported in the research literature to everyday problems and practice. Articles written for practitioners are usually concise and often exceptionally well illustrated.

There are two major annual review series. *Advances in veterinary science and comparative medicine* [60] contains exhaustive reviews, suitable for those carrying out research, with the subjects covered in considerable depth. The articles in the *Veterinary annual* [70], in contrast, are intended for the veterinary surgeon in practice. When the *Veterinary annual* began it attempted to review all the significant literature appearing in the previous year; the size of the literature is so great that such a task would be impossible nowadays. Each issue now has about forty brief articles. These tend to be on topics of current importance to practitioners in Britain, but the *Veterinary annual* has international appeal.

Most journals include review articles occasionally but such is the popularity and demand for reviews that several journals now consist of them exclusively. In particular there are several journals which are intended to assist practitioners in continuing education. *In practice* [64] is well known in the UK and there are several US periodicals. Common features of these journals are self-assessment tests and quizzes so that readers can check their knowledge. The *Compendium on continuing education for the practicing veterinarian* [62] can be used with a formal continuing education programme at the University of Pennsylvania School of Veterinary Medicine. Several review series and journals are published for practitioners interested in specific groups of animals. The *Veterinary clinics of North America* [71–73] are well known, and apart from the edition dealing with small animals, there are now series dealing with equines and food animals. The format of the *Veterinary clinics* is for each volume to be devoted to reviews on aspects of a single topic. There are now two other titles devoted to small animal practice: *Advances in small animal practice* [773], which is annual, and *Contemporary issues in small animal practice* [774].

Unfortunately neither *Veterinary bulletin* nor *Index veterinarius* index reviews as a separate group of items in their printed indexes. Reviews are therefore best identified by searching online.

5.3 ABSTRACTING AND INDEXING SERVICES

Most of the services described in Chapter 4 in relation to current awareness can be used for retrospective searching. *Veterinary bulletin* and *Index veterinarius* however are the major tools for retrospective searching. There are two other services which cover the world veterinary literature and have not been mentioned so far: *Referativnyi zhurnal. Veterinariya*, published in Russian, and *Agroselekt. Reihe 4. Veterinärmedizin*, published in German. Both are of most interest internationally for their coverage of literature from Eastern Europe and Russia. *Veterinary bulletin* began publication in 1931. Prior to this the only abstracting service was in

German, *Jahresbericht Veterinärmedizin*. This, and its predecessor, give retrospective coverage back to 1881.

The remarkably comprehensive coverage of the veterinary literature by the current abstracting services is exemplified by Gray's study (1974). He took a 20 percent sample of 1,350 references quoted by authors in *Advances in veterinary sciences and comparative medicine*, 1,000 in *Annales de recherches vétérinaires* and 1,000 in *Deutsche tierärztliche Wochenschrift* and checked *Veterinary bulletin, Landwirtschaftliches Zentralblatt. Abteilung 4: Veterinärmedizin* and *Biological abstracts* to see if the references could be found in these abstract journals. Of the sample 99.3 percent were included in one or more of the abstract journals.

All of the major abstracting services covering the biosciences literature have veterinary sections. *Biological abstracts* and its sister publication *Biological abstracts/ RRM (reports, reviews, meetings)* provide comprehensive coverage of the basic research literature in biology and biomedicine. These two services are the principal source for information on biochemistry, immunology, physiology and the other preclinical sciences. *Zoological record* [35] indexes the world's zoological literature. Its coverage of the veterinary literature is slight but it can be useful for retrieving information on taxonomy, parasitology, zoogeography and other aspects of the biology of animals, particularly of wild animals and invertebrates. Although it has now ceased publication, the *Index-catalogue of medical and veterinary zoology* [1477] is an invaluable source of information on animal parasites.

The principal services indexing the world's agricultural literature have sections devoted to veterinary medicine and animal husbandry. The *Bibliography of agriculture* [30] is compiled by the National Agricultural Library and is available online as AGRICOLA. *Agrindex* [29] is the printed product of AGRIS (International System for Agricultural Sciences and Technology). AGRIS is co-ordinated by staff at the FAO in Rome but its operations are a co-operative venture of 128 national and 18 regional and international centres. It gives good coverage of non-conventional documents, publications from non-western European countries and it includes most FAO documents. AGRIS became operational in 1975 and the online file is available on several on-line systems and via a number of national AGRIS centres. AGROVOC [167] is used to index items.

The most important printed services documenting medical literature are *Index medicus* [32] and *Excerpta medica* [20]. *Index medicus* covers most of the core veterinary journals and is available in all but the smallest medical libraries. *Excerpta medica* excludes most veterinary literature but is still of interest. It is published in sections each devoted to a medical speciality. It is therefore a suitable aid for those wishing to search in specific areas of medicine. Veterinary scientists working in the areas of drug development and chemotherapy will also find *Chemical abstracts* invaluable. About one third of *Chemical abstracts* is devoted to life science related material and it has strong coverage of the literature of biochemistry, pharmacology, molecular biology, pharmacy and pharmaceutical technology.

A unique form of searching is provided by the *Science citation index* [34] in which it is possible to search by references cited by authors. This technique is particularly useful when there are key papers in the field which are likely to be cited by new workers and when following developments in methodology.

5.4 COMPUTERIZED INFORMATION RETRIEVAL SYSTEMS

Computers are used in many aspects of veterinary practice. They have had a traditional role as interfaces to laboratory and diagnostic equipment for the collection and analysis of data; they may also be used to maintain databases of epidemiological data; sophisticated packages are now available for controlling records about patients or clients, and managing the practice or animal hospital. A variety of systems are now available for controlling the health, production and management of farm animals.

The application of computers in a clinical setting is most advanced in the developed countries. A questionnaire survey of veterinary practices in the UK, carried out in 1986, showed that 62 percent of the practices possessed a computer. The same report analyses the market for computers in veterinary practice and reviews existing software (Cook and Cook, 1986). The use of computers is most widespread in the United States and the American Veterinary Computer Society holds annual symposia and produce a newsletter, which until recently was published in *Modern veterinary practice*. The Post-Graduate Committee in Veterinary Science of the University of Sydney issue *Computer software market*, a news-sheet on new software products. Developments in the range of software which is available occur very quickly. The larger and more established companies now market their products very efficiently, primarily by advertising in professional journals and by representation at trade exhibitions.

A recent issue of the *Canadian veterinary journal* (**29** (1988): (3)) was devoted to the use of computers in veterinary practice and gives an overview of current applications. It includes descriptions of two services, PROVIDES and CONSULTANT, which may be of particular interest to clinicians since they provide computer-assisted diagnoses. Both services were developed at Cornell University. They suggest diagnoses and possible approaches to treatment using clinical signs input by the clinician. Relevant literature references are provided by both systems. PROVIDES deals with small animals only and uses the articles in *Quarterly index* to create its knowledge base. PROVIDES is marketed in the United States by Animed Computer Systems. CONSULTANT is more general in scope and is updated with literature received in the Flower Veterinary Library at Cornell, older references being deleted from the database. CONSULTANT is available online via Cornell University's computing facility and a document ordering system is part of the service. White (1987) has published an analysis of the journals contributing to CONSULTANT.

5.4.1 Online Information Systems

Online searching involves searching databases on a remote computer using the telephone network as a telecommunications route. All that is required is a personal computer, appropriate communications software and a modem or acoustic coupler to connect the personal computer to the online network via the telephone system. One also requires contracts with each of the online host systems. The user must be familiar with both the databases themselves and the particular command languages used. Some of the electronic news services offer links to these online information services. For example, COMPUSERVE and the VETERINARY COMPUTERISED INFORMATION SYSTEM can be used as gateways to other services. Any particular database may be available on several online systems. Normally one only needs a contract with the online host, although some databases, like VETDOC, are only available to subscribers.

A database can be any collection of data held in machine readable form. Some contain factual data: these databases are known as databanks. Examples are MINE (Microbial Culture Information Network) which provides data on micro-organisms and cell lines in culture collections, RTECS (Registry of Toxic Effects of Chemical Substances) which contains toxicology data, and the MERCK INDEX which is a chemical dictionary/encyclopaedia. Most databases, however, are concerned with bibliographic data; that is, they contain the full text or summaries of printed materials. There are several guides to the range of databases available and some of the guides themselves are available online. The most complete index to the databases and the online systems is the Cuadra/Elsevier *Directory of online databases*. It gives details on over 3,400 databases and over 500 online services. Hall's work (1986) gives more detailed descriptions of 250 of the major databases. His book also includes a full bibliography of online searching. The same publishers have prepared a series of guides to the databases in different subject areas. The titles currently available include: *Business and company databases*, *Medical databases*, *Patents and trademarks databases* and *Management and marketing databases*.

There are many benefits from searching the data online. One pays only for the information one uses but has access to a wide variety of sources. The major advantage is that there is much greater flexibility in searching the data online than when using the hard copy versions. An online record from CAB ABSTRACTS is shown in *Figure 5.1*. This record could only have been found in *Index veterinarius* by the eight subject headings listed as descriptors, or through the author indexes. Only three of the descriptors are used as main entries in the subject index to *Veterinary bulletin*, although in this case one could find the item by scanning the sections in *Veterinary bulletin* in which the item appeared or is noted. By contrast, in the online database almost every piece of data is searchable. Moreover the searching process is conversational and one can modify the scope of the search easily. An important advantage of online systems is that the clerical effort of the search is reduced. Items from the databases may be printed easily and sorted by

```
0525417  OV057-00134; OI055-00001
   Tickborne fever: efficacy and effects on pharmacokinetics of some
chemotherapeutic agents in the goat.
   Comparative veterinary pharmacology, toxicology and therapy [edited by
A.S.J.P.A.M. van Miert and others]. Proceedings of the 3rd Congress of the
European Association for Veterinary Pharmacology and Toxicology.
   Anika, S. M.;   Nouws, J. F. M.;   Vree, T. B.;   Duin, C. T. M. van;
Nieuwenuijs, J.;   Miert, A. S. J. P. A. M. van  (Van Duin, C. T. M.;
Van Miert, A. S. J. P. A. M.)
   Dr. C. Van Duin, Fac. Diergeneeskunde, PO Box 80.176, 3508 TD Utrecht,
Netherlands.
   Lancaster, UK; MTP Press
   1986.  415-426  (21 ref.)
   Language: English
   Document Type: UP  (Unnumbered Part)
   Status: NEW
   Subfile: OV  (Veterinary Bulletin); OI  (Index Veterinarius)
Experimental  tickborne  fever  in  dwarf  goats has an acute character:
fever,  dullness,  anorexia,  tachycardia,  a moderate inhibition of rumen
contractions,  leukopenia  and  a  decreased  serum  alkaline  phosphatase
activity. Goats receiving oxytetracycline, chloramphenicol or trimethoprim
(plus sulphonamides) showed improvement, whereas ampicillin and spirâmycin
were  ineffective.  Changes  in  drug metabolism were observed in infected
goats  treated  with  chloramphenicol  or  sulphadimidine; the elimination
half-life values of these drugs and of oxytetracycline were prolonged. The
pharmacokinetics  of  ampicillin, spiramycin and sulphamethylphenazole did
not  show  marked differences between healthy and tickborne fever-infected
animals.

Descriptors:  goat  diseases; experimental infection; ehrlichia; tickborne
     fever;  drug  therapy;  chloramphenicol;  ehrlichia  phagocytophila;
     trimethoprim
Section Heading Codes:  OVB63; OI
Section  Headings:    BACTERIOLOGY AND BACTERIAL DISEASES (FROM 1976. SEE
     ALSO OV01000 TO OV02536) - RICKETTSIALES  (SC=OVB60);   (SC=OI)
```

Figure 5.1   Typical record from the CAB ABSTRACTS database.
(Reproduced by permission of CAB International).

date, author, journal etc. An important limitation of online searching however is
that most databases are only available from the late 1960s onwards. MEDLINE is
exceptional in that one can search back to 1964. Prior to this one must carry out
searches of the hard copy printed abstracting and indexing journals.

The costs of online searching have three components: the connect time charge of the online host, the telecommunications charges and the cost of displaying results. Aslib have published a straightforward guide to setting up an online information retrieval service (Turpie, 1987). A particularly useful work to those new to online searching is Armstrong and Large's (1988) guide to developing search strategies. It includes chapters on searching databases in various subject areas including agriculture, biological sciences and health sciences.

Introductions to the equipment and techniques used in searching the literature of veterinary medicine online have been provided by Self (1986), Nielsen (1985) and MacNeil (1986). By far the most important database is CAB ABSTRACTS although many searchers, particularly in the United States, use MEDLINE as the main source. MEDLINE is cheaper than CAB ABSTRACTS and most of the core veterinary journals are included. A further reason for the popularity of MEDLINE is that much of the searching is carried out by staff in joint medical/veterinary libraries where MEDLINE is the most familiar database.

The performance of the various online databases in providing veterinary information was last evaluated in the early 1970s (Brodauf *et al.*, 1977). These authors used ninety test questions submitted by veterinarians in the European Community. The results have little relevance nowadays since the systems which are available online have changed so radically. Most printed abstracting and indexing services of interest to the veterinarian are now available as online databases but CAB ABSTRACTS is the most complete service. CAB AB-STRACTS is available on seven online systems: BRS, CAN/OLE, DIALOG, DIMDI, ESA-IRS, JICST and TSUKUBA DAIGAKU (in Japan only). The database includes *Veterinary bulletin* and *Index veterinarius* from 1972; the other CAB abstracts journals are included from 1973. A reference manual for the database is available (1988). On both DIMDI and BRS/Colleague the CAB ABSTRACTS database is available in several smaller subfiles: one of these is devoted to veterinary science and parasitology. Other online databases which are particularly useful are MEDLINE, VETDOC (for literature on veterinary drugs), BIOSIS (for basic biosciences information) and the various *Chemical abstracts* databases which are available (for pharmacology, physiology and biochemistry). TOX-LINE and RTECS are the primary sources of toxicology data.

Apart from the main bibliographic databases such as CAB ABSTRACTS, MEDLINE, TOXLINE and BIOSIS, which cover the scientific and technical literature, there are a wide variety of different types of online databases. Details of the stock of the Danish Veterinary and Agricultural Library are available online in the DJVB database on DATACENTRALEN. The American farming press is covered in AGRIBUSINESS USA and AGDEX gives similar coverage of the British agricultural and government publications. AGDEX gives good coverage of grey and non-conventional literature. SIGLE (System for Information of Grey Literature in Europe) has no printed equivalent. It covers grey literature such as reports, conferences, theses etc. There are several databases giving information on culture collections. MiCIS gives data on collections in the UK. MINE gives data on European microbial collections. MINE is a collaborative venture sponsored by the EC Biotechnology Action Programme. AGNET, run by the University of Nebraska, gives access to online agribusiness and farm management information, for example state and international animal import regulations from the USDA-APHIS. It also provides electronic mail and a bulletin board facility. The VETERINARY COMPUTERISED INFORMATION SYSTEM provides subscribers with a range of information services. It gives links to databases on DIALOG and to various electronic information systems such as online files from the USDA and FDA. The main service is the VETERINARY STOCK*FINDER. This has information on 15,000 animal health products derived from manufacturer's and distributor's literature. Users may order products online. A similar computerized stock list is being developed in the UK – each product in the Register of Veterinary Products has a unique barcode number and veterinary surgeons will order products using these numbers by reading stock details directly and sending the details to the wholesaler online without manual intervention.

There are two services which although not generally available online use computerized files of information and are of particular interest to North American veterinarians: VSDB (Veterinary Services Data Bank) [2362] and FARAD [2346] (Food Animal Residue Avoidance Databank). VSDB is a collection of literature on diseases and pests considered to be a threat to animal health in the United States. Over 65,000 articles have been collected; information on these is stored in a computer database and full texts of articles are kept on microfilm. The database is used to compile bibliographies, current awareness services and special reports on exotic diseases. FARAD (Sundlof, 1986) is a compilation of information on chemicals used in animals in the United States with data on regulatory, pharmaceutic and pharmacokinetic aspects. The pharmacokinetic data can be used to estimate residue depletion times for xenobiotics in livestock, indicating withdrawal times in cases of emergency due to overdosage, non-label use etc.

5.4.2 Optical Disc Technology

This technology is becoming increasingly widespread. It is changing rapidly and includes several techniques for recording information in either digital or analogue forms on a variety of types of disc. The most relevant to published information are Compact Disc (CD-ROM) systems. CD-ROM stands for Compact Disc-Read Only Memory. A CD-ROM disc is a metal disc with information written into its surface in digital form by laser. The disc is coated in plastic and is extremely durable. The data are read by laser using either a special reader/player linked to a microcomputer or a specially adapted microcomputer as a workstation.

A single disc can store approximately 550 megabytes of information. This is equivalent to more than 250,000 A4 pages or 1,500 floppy discs. This means that information products such as directories, dictionaries and abstracting and indexing services can now be distributed cheaply on disc. The retrieval software used on CD-ROM systems has the same capabilities as the online retrieval systems but users do not have any telecommunications problems. This makes them particularly attractive to users in the developing world. A further advantage is that purchasers or subscribers to the products can use the data as often as they wish without paying additional access fees. Because there are no charges for online connect time nor for printing records or for telecommunications costs, CD-ROM systems are attractive to users who would frequently use the same databases online. The pricing of CD-ROMs encourages use and this make them particularly attractive for end-user searching. The principal disadvantage is lack of currency since CD-ROMs are updated less frequently than the equivalent online version of the databases. Conversely for hard-copy printed directories the CD-ROM version will be more up to date than the original, which may only be published infrequently.

Initially printed reference works such as dictionaries, encyclopaedias, chemical directories seemed to be the most popular products, but many producers of bibliographic databases now make their databases available in this form. Of particular interest from a veterinary standpoint is that CAB International have prepared a CD-ROM containing a portion of their database. This has been tested in several countries but as yet is not available for sale. Both AGRICOLA and MEDLINE (Bruce, 1988) are available and ISI are marketing a CD-ROM version of the *Science citation index*. The CD-ROM versions of these databases may not be exactly equivalent to the online forms. Moreover the same database may be available as a CD-ROM product from a variety of suppliers and these may offer different features and ways of searching.

The products in CD-ROM format are listed in several directories, examples being *CD-ROMs in print 1988–89* (Emard, 1988) and *The CD-ROM directory, 1989* (Cormack, 1988). These directories give full information on the companies producing and selling the products and list books, journals, conferences and exhibitions relevant to the CD-ROM industry. There are several newsletters and journals covering CD-ROM technology and its applications in library and information work. These include *CD-ROM librarian* and *The laserdisk professional*.

References

Armstrong, C. J. and Large, J. A. (eds) *Manual of online search strategies*. Aldershot: Gower, 1988. 831pp.

Brodauf, H., Hoffman, W. D. and Klawiter-Pommer, J. H. T. *Searching the veterinary literature retrospectively: a comparative study of results from 10 data bases covering the period January 1972 to December 1974*. Oxford: Oxford Microform Publications (for the Commission of the European Communities), 1977. 56pp + 4 microfiche. (EUR 5886.). Summary report in *Veterinary record* **101** (1977): 461–3.

Bruce, N. J. 'Introducing new library technology to veterinarians in small group instruction'. *Journal of veterinary medical education* **15** (1988): 46–8.

CAB ABSTRACTS online manual. Wallingford: CAB International, 1988. Looseleaf with supplements.

Cook, R. and Cook, A. *Computing in veterinary practice in the UK.* 1 Pondwicks Close, St. Albans AL1 1DG, England: the Authors, 1986. 130pp.

Cormack, E. (ed.) *The CD-ROM directory, 1989.* 3rd ed. 22 Peter's Lane, London EC1 6DS, England: TFPL Publishing, 1988. 283pp.

Cuadra/Elsevier *Directory of online databases.* PO Box 1672, Grand Central Station, New York 10163: Cuadra/Elsevier. Annual (two main issues plus two updates per year).

Emard, J-P. (ed.) *CD-ROMs in print 1988–89.* London: Meckler, 1988. 164pp.

Gray, D. E. *Survey of the existing position in veterinary information and the relationship of veterinary information to AGRIS.* Rome: FAO, 1974, 37pp. (FAO/AGRIS 14.)

Hall, J. L. *Online bibliographic databases: a directory and sourcebook.* 4th ed. London: Aslib, 1986. 509pp.

MacNeil, K. 'Online medical databases'. *Modern veterinary practice* **67** (1986): 68–72.

Nielsen, J. N. 'Searching the veterinary literature via computer'. *Journal of the American Veterinary Medical Association* **186** (1985): 1058–61.

Self, D. A. 'Searching the literature of veterinary science'. *Medical reference services quarterly* **4** (1986): 17–28.

Sundlof, S. F., Craigmill, A. C. and Riviere, J. E. 'Food Animal Residue Avoidance Databank (FARAD): a pharmacokinetic-based information service'. *Journal of veterinary pharmacology and therapeutics* **9** (1986): 237–45.

Turpie, G. *Going online 1988.* London: Aslib, 1987. 89pp.

White, M. E. 'An analysis of journal citation frequency in the CONSULTANT data base for computer-assisted diagnosis'. *Journal of the American Veterinary Medical Association* **190** (1987): 1098–101.

6 The Literature of Veterinary Medicine

6.1 ORIGINAL CONTRIBUTIONS

6.1.1 Serials

Almost all original research is published as articles in journals, since this ensures that findings are communicated to a wide audience without delay. The most general journals are those produced by the national associations. These periodicals publish research reports but, since the majority of the readership is in general practice, include more material of interest to the practising veterinarian. The content of this kind of journal is diverse: editorials, clinical trials, review articles, epidemiological information and case reports, practical hints and reviews and correspondence, as well as scientific and technical papers. The emphasis is on the clinical, rather than the scientific or theoretical aspects of veterinary medicine, since practitioners will be most interested in aspects of research and development that may affect the medical and surgical techniques available to them. Specialized research papers are not excluded, however.

In countries conducting large amounts of veterinary research, then the national associations may produce several journals one of which specializes in publishing accounts of research. Thus the AVMA publish the *Journal of the American Veterinary Medical Association*, which deals with news relevant to the profession and general papers on veterinary developments, while the *American journal of veterinary research* reports on basic research. Similarly in Britain the BVA publish *Veterinary record*, the classic journal for the practitioner, while research papers appear in *Research in veterinary science*. The BVA also publish the *British veterinary journal* which includes longer research papers considered to be of general interest and review articles.

The journals of the national associations are a suitable medium appropriate for the publication of research undertaken in those countries. These journals reflect current research interests and practices or problems in the various countries: often they will be the first choice for many potential authors submitting manuscripts and papers by foreign authors are rarely included. Almost all journals operate a refereeing procedure to control the quality of the contributions and although most national associations produce a journal, the international importance is greater for some than others.

The subject field has grown so large that, as well as the general journals published by the national associations, there are now journals devoted to many of the veterinary specialities, for example *Veterinary microbiology*, *Veterinary parasitology*, and journals devoted to particular species, for example *Avian diseases*, *Equine veterinary journal*, *Journal of fish diseases*. Items published in these advanced-level journals are again subject to a careful refereeing process, and are of high standard. Papers which are published are recognized as significant contributions to veterinary literature. Naturally, both authors and readers are spread worldwide. Many of these periodicals are published by, or on behalf of, a specialist society or association.

A less formal method of exchanging tips on technique, reporting interesting findings and pooling clinical experiences is the *Control & therapies* series published by the Post-Graduate Committee in Veterinary Science of the University of Sydney [2258]. This is monthly and contains about thirty brief items in each issue.

Some animal health companies issue newsletters and journal-type magazines. Some have become well-established as periodicals, an example being Bayer's *Veterinary medical review*. This title and Hoechst's *Blue book for the veterinary profession* (now ceased) mainly publish papers on the company's products. Others, such as Upjohn's *Pro veterinario*, contain more general articles. Other examples are *Kal kan forum*, which has articles for small animal practitioners, *Norden news* and Norden Laboratories' *Bovine veterinary forum*.

Controlled-circulation journals flourish, practitioners in most countries receiving two or three titles. There are also a number of controlled-circulation journals in the area of animal production which contain some veterinary information. Examples are *Poultry international* and *Pig international*. Many farming journals and magazines are available free in this way.

6.1.2 Guides to Serials

A selective list of the important veterinary journals which have general coverage, rather than being devoted to a particular speciality, is given in Part II. The journals which specialize in publishing matter dealing with either particular species or one of the veterinary specialities are noted in the appropriate sections in Part II. Many of these titles are included in the list of journals that has been prepared by the Veterinary Medical Libraries Section of the Medical Library Association [77].

This is intended as a core list of journals deemed essential to a veterinary medical library in the United States or Canada. There are, however, a great many other journals which may contain information of interest to veterinarians and there are a wide variety of sources available to identify current titles.

A variety of other lists and directories to serials are noted in Part II [76–86]. The *List of serials abstracted* [81] by the Commonwealth Bureau of Animal Health is a very complete list but only the titles of the periodicals are given. Descriptive information on the journal's contents and subscription and ordering details are available in *Ulrich's international periodicals directory* [85], with veterinary journals grouped together under a separate subheading. Many of the libraries noted in Part III publish lists of their serials holdings and there are a number of union lists giving the stock of groups of libraries. The union list of veterinary periodicals prepared by the Veterinary Medical Libraries Section of the Medical Library Association (*see* Chapter 2) is a useful guide to the current holdings of some of the important veterinary libraries worldwide.

A German list *Periodika der Veterinärmedizin und ihrer Grenzgebiete* (Berlin: Freie Universität Berlin, Dokumentationstelle für Veterinärmedizin, 1971) is a compilation of the titles covered by three abstracting services, and of the journals taken by three veterinary libraries (Schönherr, 1972). Since the list was published there have been many alterations and additions to the periodicals listed, but it is a source for information on defunct titles and name changes. Other tools for retrospective use are the *World list of scientific periodicals* [86] and the *British union catalogue of periodicals* [78]. Again these are of most use for identifying changes of name and obscure titles.

Several abstracting services compile and publish lists of journals which contribute to their databases. These can be useful to check journal titles and to assess if abstracts are likely to be included in the databases and whether the full texts of articles can be supplied from the publishers. The *CAB serials checklist* [79] is the most useful but similar lists have been compiled for the BIOSIS database [83] and for Chemical Abstracts Service.

6.1.3 Theses

A thesis or dissertation is usually prepared by a student studying for a higher degree and it describes their original research in some depth. The most important findings of these workers will usually be published as one or more scientific articles but the original thesis can still be a valuable source of information. It may be published before more conventional reports of the work and it may describe the research methodology and results in far more detail than would be appropriate in a journal article. In addition the thesis will usually contain a comprehensive review of the subject or, at the very least, a detailed bibliography.

There are, however, several problems in trying to make use of theses. First, they are bulky documents; partly for this reason only a few copies are produced and obtaining one can therefore be difficult. General guides to the availability of theses submitted to different institutions have been prepared by Borchardt and Thawley (1981) and Allen and Deubert (1984). A second problem is that it can be difficult to find out about new theses. Some universities publish lists of theses in their annual reports or provide details for publication in journals but these are of little practical use. Luckily a good alerting and abstracting service for newly published theses is provided by *Veterinary bulletin* and *Index veterinarius*, which index about 700 theses each year. One-third of these are in English; the majority of the rest are inaugural dissertations from the Federal Republic of Germany.

There are also several other services which document recent theses. Items acquired by the British Library are announced in *British reports, translations and theses* [149] and duplicate copies of these are available from the British Library Document Supply Centre (BLDSC). From July 1988 onwards British doctoral theses acquired by the BLDSC are included in DISSERTATION ABSTRACTS ONLINE. Author abstracts are included. However a more complete guide to British theses is the *Index to theses with abstracts* [150], produced by Aslib. About 10,000 theses are included each year and there is a detailed abstract for each item. The abstracts are presented in broad classified order but there are also author and keyword indexes.

European theses are noted in *Dissertation abstracts international. Section C: European abstracts* [148] published by University Microfilms International (UMI). The same publisher also produces a series of titles documenting North American dissertations. Copies of the full texts of most of the theses and dissertations are available from UMI and BLDSC can provide copies on loan.

6.2 REFERENCE BOOKS

Two general encyclopaedias of veterinary medicine were produced in the 1960s. *The international encyclopedia of veterinary medicine* [361] has general articles on a range of topics but there are few references to further work. The *Veterinary encyclopedia* [363] was published in loose-leaf form and the intention was that the work should be regularly updated although in fact only one set of additional material appeared. It seems unlikely that new works of such a general character will be prepared. Veterinary knowledge is increasing at such a rate that it cannot reasonably be contained in one publication and yet remain up to date and valid. Having said this though, Wamberg and Macpherson's work remains popular and is in print in French and German translations. In scientific fields encyclopaedias appear to be being superseded in everyday use by dictionaries.

A number of directories, which could also be considered appropriate for this chapter, are discussed in Chapter 3.

6.2.1 Dictionaries

Until recently the only modern dictionary in everyday use was *Black's veterinary dictionary* [157]. This is essentially a popular work and the profession is fortunate in having two new dictionaries published in 1988. The most complete, with the greatest number of keyterms, is *Baillière's comprehensive veterinary dictionary* [158]. Each entry defines and, where appropriate, explains the terms. A briefer and more compact work intermediate in depth of coverage between these two titles is the *Concise veterinary dictionary* [160].

General medical dictionaries may also be useful. The most comprehensive British title is *Butterworth's medical dictionary* (2nd ed., 1978). There are several popular American texts including *Dorland's illustrated medical dictionary* (27th ed., 1988), *Stedman's medical dictionary* (24th ed., 1982) and *Mosby's medical and nursing dictionary* (2nd ed., 1986).

Apart from straightforward dictionaries there are a number of subject glossaries of note. The *Nomina anatomica veterinaria* [1226] and *Nomina anatomica avium* [1036] provide lists of standard anatomical terminology. The *Systematized nomenclature of veterinary medicine* (SNOVET) [165] provides a nomenclature and coding standard by which to record diseases and treatments. It is intended for use with clinical data but could be used for indexing scientific literature or creating personal filing systems. The *Animal disease thesaurus* [156] is an annually revised listing of terms used by the USDA-APHIS in indexing animal health literature. The terms currently used in the *Animal disease thesaurus* will be incorporated in the next edition of SNOVET which was due in 1988.

There are several other thesauri which cover the veterinary sciences, most having been compiled in order to assist the indexing of databases. Probably the most useful is the *Controlled vocabulary* [161] used to index the Commonwealth Bureau of Animal Health's journals. This replaces the *Veterinary subject headings* [166]. The indexing terms for all the CAB International journals and for the AGRICOLA database are now selected from the *CAB thesaurus* [159].

M. Villemin has produced a French-language dictionary, now in its third edition, the *Dictionnaire des termes vétérinaires et zootechniques* [184]. E. Wiesner and R. Ribbeck's *Worterbuch der Veterinärmedizin* [185] is a German-language work, equivalent to Baillière's dictionary in scope and comprehensiveness.

6.2.2 Miscellaneous Reference Books

A unique single volume reference work, initially prepared for the American veterinarian, but full of information for practitioners in other countries, is *The Merck veterinary manual* [362]. There are sections devoted to all the main fields of practice and there is strong coverage on the diagnosis and treatment of disease. Overall it is the ideal desk reference and a quick source of facts and figures. The index is very detailed.

The other main reference works likely to be used by the practitioner are guides to drugs and therapy. The *Current veterinary therapy* series is well-known and highly regarded and now has titles devoted to large animals, equines, small animals and theriogenology. These are multi-authored works, providing brief articles on clinical problems and approaches to diagnosis and to their medical treatment. Although reflecting practice in the United States the basic background information is valuable, and the therapeutic procedures discussed are usually relevant in most countries. A range of vade mecums have been produced covering the diseases likely to be encountered and the therapy likely to be employed in Australia [1676]. Similar vade mecums covering small and large animals are distributed to veterinarians in Britain. Veterinary surgeons in Britain also receive copies of *Index of veterinary specialities*, *Animal health news and index* and a copy of the *Compendium of data sheets for veterinary products* produced by NOAH. With the exception of the NOAH *Compendium* all these titles classify the drugs according to their therapeutic use. They are therefore useful as guides to products available for particular conditions.

6.3 TEXTBOOKS AND MONOGRAPHS

The scope of veterinary medicine is now so wide that it is not practical to encompass all the aspects of the subject in a single text. There are, however, many detailed and comprehensive monographs dealing with the medicine and surgery of particular groups of animals. Blood and Radostit's *Veterinary medicine* [403] is a classic text dealing with large animal medicine, for example. Leman *et al.*'s *Diseases of swine* [639] is another example of a definitive textbook. Similar comprehensive works are available dealing with all the major species of animals and with most of the veterinary specialities. There is an especially wide range of general texts on small animal medicine and surgery. Most of the larger monographs are multi-authored, with chapters written by experts in the field. A range of titles dealing with each species and each speciality is listed in the appropriate sections in Part II.

Although many publishers issue veterinary works, some have established special reputations. The best-known publishers are Lea & Febiger, Williams & Wilkins and those in the Harcourt Brace Jovanovich Group (Baillière Tindall, W. B. Saunders and Academic Press). Butterworths specialize in publishing technical works on animal physiology and husbandry. In West Germany Paul Parey and Springer-Verlag are important publishers. Some publishers specialize in particular areas; for example J. A. Allen are well-known for their books on veterinary history and on horses. The most important publishers are listed in Part III.

In recent years colour atlases have become popular: they are a useful teaching aid and illustrate many of the conditions encountered by the clinician. Developments in modern printing technology have allowed publishers to produce superb atlases. Most of these are concerned with anatomy, either gross, radiological or microscopic. Wolfe Medical Publications specialize in producing atlases of colour photographs accompanied by a concise explanatory text. Such books can be useful diagnostic aids and important teaching tools.

There are several book series written for the veterinary surgeon in practice. The

Library of Veterinary Practice (Blackwell) and the Veterinary Practitioner Handbook Series (Wright) are well known in the UK. Each volume presents data in a form allowing quick reference, particularly to the information useful to the clinician. The titles are well illustrated and are equally suitable for use by students and practitioners. Many of the volumes in these series deal with a body system in large or small animals, or an aspect of veterinary practice such as nursing, or radiography. These are small sized, pocket guides.

A number of veterinary associations and societies publish works of use to their members. The BSAVA's series of manuals is typical. Manuals have been produced on canine behaviour, exotic pets, psittacine birds and several other topics. A variety of new titles covering neurology, radiology, endocrinology, dentistry and oncology are in preparation. These handbooks are reasonably priced and written specifically for the veterinarian in practice.

Animal health is of interest to farmers and stock breeders and to pet owners and many popular works have been published intended for these groups. A representative sample of these works is included in this guide. The 'TV Vet' Eddie Straiton has written a variety of well-illustrated books dealing with the different species and over half a million copies have been sold around the world. Farming Press produce many works on animal husbandry which contain chapters on animal health and diseases. In the United States, The Interstate Printers and Publishers have many works on animal science, many authored by M. E. Ensminger. Longman publish many agricultural texts and have an extensive list in the Intermediate Tropical Agriculture Series; these books are intended for those in developing countries and deal with the husbandry of animals in the tropics and discuss health in passing. Much of the programmes of preventive veterinary medicine is concerned with factors other than disease, disease often showing itself where management is faulty. Agriculture and animal husbandry books are therefore useful since good husbandry is an essential component of good preventive veterinary medicine. Agricultural texts are also useful to veterinary students since veterinarians need a good understanding of animal husbandry practice.

References

Allen, G. G. and Deubert, K. *Guide to the availability of theses. 2: non-university institutions.* Munich: K. G. Saur, 1984. 124pp. (IFLA Publications 29.)

Borchardt, D. H. and Thawley, J. D. (compilers) *Guide to the availability of theses.* Munich: K. G. Saur, 1981. 443pp. (IFLA Publications 17.)

Schönherr, S. 'Die Periodika der Veterinärmedizin und ihrer Grenzgebiete'. *Tierärztliche Umschau* **27** (1972): 535–8.

7 Sources of Special Information

Veterinarians use conventional documentary materials – books and journals – as their main sources of information. There will be occasions, however, when these are inappropriate or insufficient and a great deal of valuable information appears in other forms: government and intergovernmental publications (including legislation), standards, patents, trade marks, statistical data and audiovisual materials. This chapter reviews the salient features of some of this material.

7.1 GOVERNMENT PUBLICATIONS

Governments are concerned to ensure that the practice of veterinary medicine is efficient because good animal health practices make a significant contribution to improvements in livestock production, and because of the need to protect the health of the consumer of meat products. The degree to which central government involves itself with the practice of veterinary medicine varies from country to country. In many of the developing countries, and in countries which have controlled economies, such as those in Eastern Europe, the majority of veterinarians are employed by the state. In countries where private practice is the norm then the government may do little more than establish a legal and administrative framework governing the profession, with the control of those entitled to practise achieved via a Veterinary Surgeons Act and through a registration system. Even in these countries though, veterinarians in private practice may carry out some work on contract for local or national government.

This is mainly in the fields of meat inspection, other aspects of veterinary public hygiene and in animal welfare.

In countries where the majority of veterinarians are self-employed there is a general concern within government and the profession that supply of veterinarians from the schools should match the demand for their services. Governments in a number of countries have therefore carried out reviews of the profession. The British government, for example, set up a Committee of Enquiry into the Veterinary Profession. This was chaired by Lord Swann and the Committee's report appeared in 1975 (London: HMSO, 1975. Cmnd 6143 and 6143–1). The Committee recommended that there should be regular manpower reviews, the most recent of which concluded that a reduction of 10 per cent in the numbers of students entering the profession was required (MAFF, 1985). Two other major reviews into aspects of veterinary practice in the UK have been carried out recently. The 'Wildy report' (1987) was written by a Working Party of the Agriculture Departments in Great Britain and the AFRC and examined public sector funded research and development in farm animal diseases. The 'Riley report' (1989) made recommendations on the future of veterinary education in the UK and was prepared by a committee established by the University Grants Committee.

In most countries there is a government publisher who will publish most official documents. In Britain this is HMSO, Her Majesty's Stationery Office. HMSO issue a variety of catalogues: the *Daily list* gives details of items under the name of the department or other body issuing them; there is also a *Monthly catalogue, Annual Catalogue* and five-yearly consolidated indexes. HMSO have recently announced the availability of *HMSO in print on microfiche*. This is issued quarterly and lists available HMSO publications. There is no subject index but publications are cross-referenced by title, government department, parliamentary number and author (including Chairmen of Committees). HMSO also produce *Sectional lists*, individual catalogues of current non-parliamentary publications based on divisions of responsibility between government departments. *Sectional list 1* is entitled *Agriculture, forestry, fisheries and food* and contains most of the items likely to be of use to veterinary scientists. The complete HMSO database is available online from 1976 on BLAISE-LINE.

Not all government publications are published by HMSO and many important government documents are neither published nor sold by them. A useful directory to these documents is Chadwyck-Healey's *Catalogue of British official publications not published by HMSO* [39]. Of particular interest are publications from the Ministry of Agriculture, Fisheries and Food. MAFF produce fact-sheets, brochures, posters, leaflets and other publications on animal health intended for farmers, journalists and lay people. These contain basic information and can be useful starting points for the novice. A catalogue of MAFF publications, including ADAS priced publications, is available from MAFF Publications. Many of the unpriced leaflets can be supplied by ADAS advisers at their discretion. An index to the unpriced ADAS publications was prepared by Tom Norton (Chief Librarian at MAFF) in 1987. However it is unlikely to be updated and the best source is now Alnwick itself.

In the United States, most official documents are available through either the US Government Printing Office or the National Technical Information Service. The NTIS is part of the US Department of Commerce and publishes a vast array or reports and other docuemnts each year. The main printed indexes are the *Monthly catalogue of United States government publications* (issued by the US GPO) and *Government reports annual index* (issued by NTIS). Both the US GPO and NTIS databases are available online. As is the case with MAFF and ADAS in Britain, the USDA publish many advisory publications for farmers and the general public. Most are listed in the Animal and Plant Health Inspection Service's catalogue of *Available publications*. At state level the Land-Grant Universities produce many advisory publications. All of these types of material are well covered in the AGRICOLA database. In Britain Microinfo act as agents for NTIS and GPO and can also supply other government and intergovernmental publications such as those of the US National Standards Association, World Bank and International Monetary Fund.

Most Ministries of Agriculture produce annual reports which include reviews of developments in animal health over the year. Sometimes more specialist reports are produced by the government's own veterinary organization. The report of the Chief Veterinary Officer [207], for example, gives a comprehensive survey of the work of the State Veterinary Service in Britain.

7.2 INTERGOVERNMENTAL PUBLICATIONS

The two most important organizations, the Food and Agriculture Organization (FAO) and the World Health Organization (WHO), are both operational organizations of the United Nations (UN). A recent directory [1] describes the databases and information systems of UN organizations active in agriculture and a more general guide to UN databases and services has been published (ACCIS, 1984).

The WHO is primarily concerned with international health matters and public health. Its major publications are described in a *Catalogue of WHO publications 1974–79* and *WHO publications catalogue 1980–85*. These are updated by a biannual catalogue of *New books*. Many of the WHO's reports have a limited distribution however; a typical example is the *Guidelines for the diagnosis, prevention and control of dermatophytoses in man and animals* (WHO/CDS/VPH/86.67). Such documents are best obtained by contacting the agency concerned within WHO as there is no publicly available list of these reports.

The FAO is concerned with the improvement of agricultural production and the more effective use of available food resources. It publishes several thousand documents each year, many of which contain information relevant to animal health and production. These are described in three basic catalogues: *FAO books in print, FAO list of documents* and *FAO documentation – current bibliography*. Only the latter is a priced publication. It lists all new publications and recently completed technical and terminal field reports. It is compiled bimonthly by the FAO's David Lubin Memorial Library which holds copies of over 85,000 FAO documents. Most of these appear in the AGRIS database and can be supplied in microfiche form.

Both the FAO and WHO issue many of their publications in series devoted to particular subjects. The FAO monographs which are likely to be of most value are those in the *Animal Production and Health Papers* series [371] and those in the *Animal Production and Health Series* [372]. Both the FAO and WHO have established systems of working through panels and committees which consist of international groups of experts that provide both bodies with the latest scientific and technical advice. These often review information in the field periodically. A typical example is the FAO's European Commission for the Control of Foot-and-Mouth Disease. This meets annually in Rome and its proceedings are valuable reviews of developments in the control of FMD. Many of the groups of experts are joint FAO/WHO bodies and the committee's reports may be published by both organizations. An important example of the collaborative work of the FAO and WHO is the Codex Alimentarius Commission. This publishes the results of its annual meetings and has set up a specialist Codex Committee on Residues of Veterinary Drugs in Foods. Further examples are the titles in the *FAO Plant Production and Protection Papers* series, which include the *Pesticide residues in food* volumes. These appear annually and provide surveys of residue and toxicology data for the evaluation of the safety, metabolism and environmental impact of pesticides, including veterinary insecticides. The reports of the various WHO Expert Committees and Joint FAO/WHO Expert Committees are published in the *WHO Technical Reports Series* [374]. WHO also publish a monograph series [373].

Both the FAO and WHO have world-wide lists of sales agents. In the UK their publications are available from HMSO which acts as agents for many international organizations. New publications are listed in HMSO daily and monthly catalogues and in a separate *International organizations annual catalogue.* In the United States UNIPUB act as the local sales agent for many international organizations.

The EC publish a lot of material relevant to animal health and agricultural development. The Commission of the European Communities organizes many meetings in its various programmes for the co-ordination of research. The proceedings of these normally appear either as reports in the EUR series [364] or in the *Current Topics in Veterinary Medicine and Animal Science* series [365]. Many of the meetings deal with specific diseases and the proceedings often contain summaries of their incidence and economic significance in European countries and on their diagnosis, treatment and control. Abstracts of scientific reports issued by the Commission are given in *Euroabstracts* which appears monthly. Details also appear in the catalogue of the Office for Official Publications of the CEC which gives bibliographic details of these reports plus other CEC publications.

The Commission has established a specialist organization, operating under the

Lomé Convention, the CTA (Technical Centre for Agricultural and Rural Cooperation) [2283], whose role is to foster collaboration between the EC and African, Caribbean and Pacific (ACP) countries. Its main aims are to provide better access to information, research training and innovation in the spheres of agriculture and rural development. This includes working towards the improvement of animal production and animal care in these regions. As a result of this work it has published several useful documents including guides to sources of information [191].

7.3 LEGISLATION

Amendments to legislation are announced in the catalogues of official publications. Thus in Britain they appear in the HMSO catalogues. A useful annual survey of changes in legislation also appears in the report of the Chief Veterinary Officer [207]. In the United States most of the legislation in force relating to veterinary medicine and the use of animal drugs, feeds and related products is published in the *Code of Federal Regulations* (Title 21). This is reissued annually. Changes in legislation are noted in the *Federal register* which is published on weekdays by the US GPO.

The practice of veterinary medicine is controlled by much legislation apart from the basic Veterinary Surgeons Act. In Britain, for example, veterinarians are affected by legislation such as the Medicines Act 1968 (which is the principal statute governing the licensing, use and supply of medicines), the Health and Safety at Work Act, Pet Animals Act and employment statutes. Articles on legal matters affecting the profession are frequently published in the journals of the national associations. H. W. Hannah has written many articles on legislative matters in the United States and a compilation of these has been published (*Legal briefs from the Journal of the American Veterinary Medical Association*, Schaumberg: AVMA, 1986, 256pp.). Articles on practice management often discuss legal matters.

The national associations play an important role in representing the profession's interests during the formulation of legislation. They are also very active in explaining the implications of legislation to their members. The RCVS produces an excellent guide [1367] covering the position in the UK. The BVA has published a variety of guides to specific areas of legislation and to certain management aspects of veterinary practice.

The Commission of the European Communities [2147] also publishes legislation. Many of its Directives relate to agriculture and animal health and are especially important in regulatory and business matters. The Commission is involved in harmonizing the rules, regulations and working practices of companies throughout Europe and in promoting trade throughout the European Community. Information and notices concerning the Commission's work is published in the C series of the *Official journal of the European Communities*. New legislation is announced in the L series. The S series of the same journal publishes notices of public works contracts, supply contracts and invitations to tender of the European Development Fund. All Community law is available online in the CELEX database. Bibliographical information on the principal Community acts, official publications and documents issued by European institutions and articles relevant to Community affairs are available online in SCAD.

In Britain those in the industry concerned with regulatory matters will be members of the British Institute of Regulatory Affairs (Drayton House, 30 Gordon Street, London WC1H 0AX).

7.4 STANDARDS

The traditional type of industrial standard, that is, a document defining an approved level of quality or test method, is of most relevance to manufacturers of veterinary equipment and supplies. This type of standard is issued by many national standards bodies and also by the International Organization for Standardization. Current British standards are listed in the *BSI standards catalogue* [335] and international standards in the comparable *ISO catalogue* [337]. Work currently underway on proposed new British and ISO standards, and details of newly published standards, is announced in *BSI news*. In America a variety of organizations issue standards: the American Society for Testing and Materials issues an *Annual book* [334] and the American National Standards Institute issues an annual *Catalog of American national standards* [336]. New and revised American standards are listed in *Standards alert*. This is a free publication issued monthly by American Technical Publishers (68a Wilbury Way, Hitchin, Herts SG4 0TP, England: Tel. (0462) 37933).

The national and international pharmacopoeias are used as standards of quality and purity for drugs, biologicals and other articles used in veterinary medicine and pharmacy. In addition, national drug regulatory bodies, and intergovernmental bodies such as the OIE, FAO or WHO, may issue specifications and standards for individual products or their components. An example is the WHO's recent catalogue of the sources of virus strains and antisera of animal viruses (WHO/ZOON/87.164). The proceedings of meetings organized by the International Association for Biological Standardization [369] contain valuable information in the field of biological products.

Certain standards have been developed for practitioners. Examples are the standards for animal hospitals developed by the American Animal Hospital Association and the British Veterinary Hospital Association. National associations have developed codes of professional practice and the national associations and some specialist associations and societies have also developed standards and guidelines for particular operations and procedures.

7.5 PATENTS AND TRADE MARKS

Patents and trade marks are often called 'industrial property'. The terminology indicates that each has a commercial value to the owner and that both are likely to be most widely used by companies. The grant and practical use of both patents and trade marks are governed by complex legal and procedural rules. Eisenschitz (1987) and Williams (1986) have written general guides outlining the salient features of these materials and indicating how they may be exploited. Rimmer (1988) has compiled a thorough guide to the official publications of over fifty patent issuing authorities. Her guide also includes information on utility models, designs and trade marks. Online systems are particularly important in patent and trade mark information and Marchant (1987) has provided a brief but thorough survey of the relevant databases.

7.5.1 Patents

When a patent is granted it gives an inventor a monopoly on the commercial exploitation of their original work within the particular issuing territory. The benefit to society is that, prior to or at the time of grant, the patent is also published – the technology disclosed therein can then be used by others in their research. Also, since a patent has a limited life, the invention can be used freely by others when it expires.

Patents are often considered only to be of importance to inventors, most of whom are engaged in industrial research and development. Nowadays, however, researchers in government and academic institutions are under strong pressure to commercialize their work and need to pay attention to patent protection. There are other reasons for using patents; the most important being the large amount of technical information they contain. Most of this is never reported in the conventional literature, but even when it is, the patent will usually be the first disclosure. Patents can also be used to provide commercial intelligence, to track competitor activity, to preview market developments and to identify licensing opportunities.

Any important invention will be patented in many countries and this is partly the reason why almost a million patents are published each year. About a quarter are in Japanese, and about 15 percent are from the Federal Republic of Germany. There are obvious problems in deciphering complex scientific documents in foreign languages. Fortunately excellent abstracts of almost all significant patents are provided by Derwent Publications' *Chemical patents index* [18]. The first patent to be published on an invention is commonly termed the 'basic' patent and subsequent patents on the same invention are called 'equivalents', the whole collection forming the patent 'family'. Derwent provide an invaluable service in identifying the patents in the family so making it possible to find English language equivalents.

Derwent have been active in the field of patent information since the 1950s and have produced comprehensive services documenting pharmaceutical patents since 1963 and agricultural patents since 1965. They publish two types of abstract for each patent. First an altering abstract, which summarizes the key features of the invention, and later a documentation abstract. The latter is very detailed and contains all the invention's salient features and includes graphics where appropriate (*Figure 7.1*). The Derwent database, WORLD PATENTS INDEX (WPI), is now available on several online systems. Derwent's detailed subject indexing allows the database to be searched in many different ways.

Derwent abstract the patents of thirty-one patent issuing authorities but the most complete database in terms of country coverage is INPADOC. This is produced by the World Intellectual Property Organization and it includes the patents of fifty-five countries and patent authorities. Over 18,000 new records are added weekly and the database now contains over 34 million records. INPADOC is of value when as complete information as possible is needed about the family. In contrast to WPI, INPADOC provides only brief bibliographic data on the patents, in the original language, and there are no abstracts. An important feature is that the database also gives information on changes in the legal status of individual patents for ten of the major issuing authorities. Legal status information for Japan is not given on INPADOC but this is available in the PATOLIS database.

General abstracting and indexing services often cover patents to some degree and the most important of these is *Chemical abstracts*. This includes the basics of all patents relating to chemistry, including pharmaceutical technology. It is the best source for a quick check on the basic patent cover of individual compounds since the file can be searched online using Chemical Abstracts' registry numbers. Some of the standard printed reference works can be useful; the *Merck index* gives the earliest patents for most of the compounds it includes; Slack and Nineham's work covers very old compounds (now out of patent cover) [225].

Collections of patents are usually only available at the larger national libraries but copies can be obtained through normal inter-library document supply schemes or purchased from the patent offices. Derwent operate a patent supply and translation service.

7.5.2 Trade Marks

A trade mark comprises words or figurative elements or a combination of the two. Information on the literature of trade marks is available in a recently published guide (Newton, 1988). Trade marks serve to link a product or service with its producer or supplier. Those of most significance are the brand and trade names used for veterinary products. Individual trade names can be identified using the product directories listed in Part II [214–273]. The status of a particular trade mark in a territory can be checked using the national registry and a number of these registries are now available online. For example, details of all UK trade marks are given in BRITISH TRADE MARKS and US trade marks are

| 85-081135/14 | C03 B07 P33 P42 | ALEX/ 28.10.83 | BC(11-C4) *I* | 0 1 1 |

ALEXANDER A M
*AU 8434-465-A

28.10.83-NZ-205056 *(14.02.85)* A61j-01 B05b-15/06

Holder for veterinary medicament cartridge during admin. - fits onto user's upper arm and holds cartridge replaceably

C85-035308   Holder for a cartridge during admin. with a hand-held device supplied from the cartridge (2) via a flexible tube (4) can be secured to the user's arm to hold the cartridge replaceably. The holder (1) pref. has an outwardly depending protrusion from which a cartridge can be held inverted by a loop on the cartridge base engaging over the protrusion.

There are pref. members which releasably engage the cartridge neck, and lateral parts which engage the user's upper arm on either side, these being of resiliently deformable material with securing straps between the parts.

There is pref. a holster (20) for carrying the device when not in use. One major wall of the cartridge is pref. concave.

ADVANTAGE
Secures the cartridge conveniently out of the way and ameliorates the disadvantages of a variable distance between cartridge and device.

USE
The holder is for a cartridge contg. fluid medicaments. (17pp1358LHDwgNo-1/11).

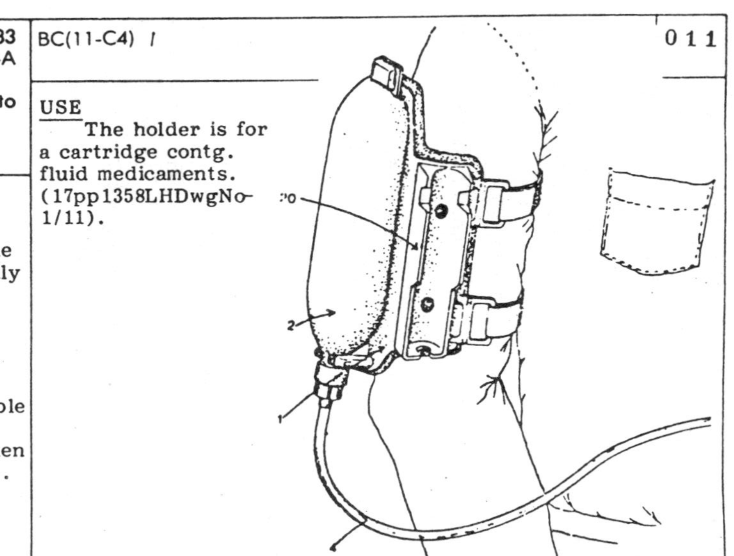

Figure 7.1   Documentation abstract from the *Central patents index*. Relates to Bayer's Armadose worming system, launched in the UK in 1989. The patent was published in 1985.
(Reproduced with permission of Derwent Publications Limited.)

available in two TRADEMARKSCAN databases which cover federal and state marks. The best international collection is the '*Animal health international*' *directory* [214]. This lists over 50,000 product names used for veterinary products in thirty-six countries. Unfortunately it is no longer being kept up to date and there is now no complete collection of animal health trade marks. A relatively new online service is IMSMARQ. This provides access to a variety of national registry files, common law and reference files. It gives access to pharmaceutical trade marks in use in over forty countries. COMPUMARK is a similar computerized service. Most of these online databases can be searched for strings of characters within a mark and some allow phonetic searching and searching for graphics.

An interesting historical collection of emblems and devices is given in Katic's *World atlas* [1324].

7.6 STATISTICAL DATA

A directory of 113 animal health and disease data sources was published in 1982 (Ostroff, 1982). This gave details of online databases which may contain animal health data and of the computerized and manual recording systems used by both international organizations and national veterinary services. The guide needs to be updated. Current developments in animal disease recording systems are often reported at the conferences of the International Society for Veterinary Epidemiology and Economics [2218].

There are several compilations of data on the incidence of animal diseases worldwide produced by the international organizations. The OIE began publishing *World animal health* [296] in 1985. This is now issued in two parts *No. 1: New animal disease outbreaks – statistics* and *No. 2: Animal health status and disease control methods*. The statistics volume gives the disease status of one hundred countries with regard to the sixteen most contagious animal diseases which can cause major economic losses (OIE list A). The second volume presents tables on disease in each country with regard to the diseases on both OIE lists A and B. This gives data on the occurrence, number of outbreaks, number of cases and deaths and on the disease control measures used. The volume also has reports on the animal health situation in about seventy countries. The reports are in English, French or Spanish. The *Animal health yearbook* [285] is another world livestock disease report. Tables present information on over 130 diseases and the species in which they occur in over 170 countries. Data are provided on the prevalence of each disease and an indication is usually given on the method of control practised in each country. Numbers of livestock, human populations and numbers of veterinarians and animal health auxiliary personnel are also given. Each volume has an extensive section on FMD. There is a review of changes in the world epizootiological situation. The numerical data are held in a databank by the Animal Production and Health Division of FAO. Finally, *Animal disease occurrence* [284] is published by CAB International in collaboration with the Commission of the European Communities. It gives abstracts of literature which gives information on the incidence of animal diseases and tabulates information on outbreaks of all notifiable diseases plus other diseases of economic importance.

Most of the national veterinary services keep records on the incidence of animal disease. Some of the services publish these data in a special report and other countries include summaries of the disease situation in their annual reports. Sometimes these data are published in the national veterinary journals. For example, reports compiled by MAFF on the disease situation internationally and in the UK appear in the *Veterinary record* regularly.

Within each country there may be a variety of systems for recording animal health and disease data. One of the largest and best known is the Veterinary Medical Data Program [2298]. This is a collaborative venture among twenty-seven North American veterinary schools. Data on over 4 million case records seen at the member hospitals is coded and input to a database. Data are included on age, breed, sex, diagnosis, length of stay, weight, mortality, treatment, procedures and outcome. The database may be used to follow trends in disease, mortality or treatment. Blood and Brightling (1988) describe the construction and use of veterinary information recording systems like these and discuss their relevance to practitioners.

The FAO Statistics Division maintains important collections of data on livestock and livestock products. These are summarized in the *FAO yearbooks* [291 and 292] but are also available in an FAO database, AGROSTAT. Data on animal populations and livestock production figures are best obtained from national ministries of agriculture, although there are several compilations of data for the UK, Europe and USA [286, 288, 290, 294].

7.7 AUDIOVISUAL MATERIALS

Because of the practical nature of veterinary medicine audiovisual materials are an important tool in both undergraduate training and in continuing education. Videotape has now almost completely taken over from film as the major form of audiovisual material for these purposes. Exhibitions of videos are a common feature of most of the larger conferences; at the last World Veterinary Congress more than 300 videos were on show. The World Veterinary Association has compiled a detailed list of the films and videos available which is revised periodically [339].

There are two video libraries based in the United Kingdom: the Allan White Memorial Video Library [348] and the Unit for Veterinary Continuing Education [352]. The UVCE has the widest range of materials with over 250 audiovisual programmes. Most are for veterinarians but about fifty titles are for veterinary nurse training and for use with lay audiences.

In the United States the AVMA runs a film library which is free to members and covers many topics. Both technical films and films suitable for showing to clients and animal owners are included. Details of the AVMA library are given in the AVMA's *Directory*.

Most academics have extensive collections of slides and photographs which they use in teaching. In recent years some of these collections have formed the basis of a number of published atlases with excellent colour illustrations, especially in the fields of anatomy and parasitology. Animal health companies can also be useful as sources of illustrative materials. Organizations within the state veterinary services usually have extensive collections of slides and photographs which are used in advisory work.

References

ACCIS (Advisory Committee for the Co-ordination of Information Systems). *Directory of United Nations databases and information systems 1985.* New York: United Nations, 1984. 323pp.

Blood, D. C. and Brightling, P. *Veterinary information management.* London: Baillière Tindall, 1988. 177pp.

Eisenschitz, T. S. *Patents, trade marks and designs in information work.* London: Croom Helm, 1987. 236pp.

Marchant, P. *Patents and trademarks databases 1988.* London: Aslib, 1987. 50pp. (Updated annually.)

Ministry of Agriculture, Fisheries and Food. *Manpower review of the veterinary profession in the United Kingdom.* Alnwick: MAFF, 1985. 34pp.

Newton, D. C. *Trade marks: a guide to the literature and directory of lists of trade names.* 2nd ed. London: British Library, 1988. 80pp.

Ostroff, J. (ed.) *International directory of animal health and disease data banks.* Beltsville: National Agricultural Library, 1982. 93pp. (USDA Miscellaneous Publication, no. 1423.)

Rimmer, B. M. *International guide to official industrial property publications.* 2nd ed. London: British Library, 1988. 200pp.

Williams, J. F. *A manager's guide to patents, trademarks and copyright.* London: Kogan Page, 1986. 168pp.

8 Language Problems

Veterinary medicine is now an established profession in most of the world and in many countries professional organizations have existed for over a hundred years. These bodies, the numerous specialist associations which have been formed, and the various educational establishments have usually ensured that literature is available in the local languages. Understandably, they have concentrated on publishing information relevant to local practitioners, although many also publish research journals, of interest to a wider audience.

The veterinary scientist wishing to keep up to date with international developments will, however, need a working knowledge of English. *Figure 4.4* shows that most of the literature considered to be of international importance is now published in English, and it has recently been shown that this proportion is increasing (Payne and Payne, 1986).

Certainly more textbooks and reference works are published in English than in any other language: the importance of this English material is reflected in the high proportion of English-language monograph stock in some of the major veterinary libraries (*Table 8.1*). Nevertheless, monographs covering aspects of veterinary science are now available in most languages. Moreover original works in the local languages are supplemented by English textbooks which are now frequently published in editions in other languages, translations into German, French and Spanish being the most common. For example, Blood and Radostits' *Veterinary medicine* [403] has been translated into French, Spanish, Portuguese, Italian and Japanese. The translation of non-English works is less common, although many works have been translated from German. The importance of translations is illustrated by the 1986–7 catalogue of the French publisher Vigot: of the

Table 8.1   Percentage of monograph stock of some veterinary libraries which is in English

	Percentage
Danish Veterinary and Agricultural University	75
Faculté de Médecine Vétérinaire de l'Université de Liège	50
Institut d'Élevage et de Médecine Vétérinaire des Pays Tropicaux	45
Faculty of Veterinary Medicine – University of Milan	30

Source: Tropical agriculture information sources [191].

thirty-seven items this contains, eleven have been translated from English and five from German.

Many of the publications of the international agencies such as the FAO and WHO are available in several languages. The Office International des Épizooties has a unique role as an international body co-ordinating efforts on disease control. It encourages information flow by publishing all of its monographs in English, French and Spanish.

It is research workers who are most likely to use foreign language materials, mostly journal articles. Unlike in some other disciplines, few veterinary journals are published in cover-to-cover translation. Notable exceptions to this rule are the *Veterinary clinics of North America, Veterinary record* (published in a Dutch edition) and *Deutsche tierärztliche Wochenschrift* (published in a Spanish edition). The OIE is again unique in publishing most of the articles in its journals simultaneously in English, French and Spanish. Animal health companies issue some of their journals and newsletters in several languages; examples are Upjohn's *Pro veterinario* and Bayer's *Veterinary medical review*.

Although English is the preferred language of publication for most research workers, a significant amount of literature appears in other languages. German was particularly important in the first half of the twentieth century. Many German and also French authors now publish in English, the percentages having risen from 2.7 and 1.0 percent in 1966 to 17.7 and 23.4 percent in 1985 (Payne and Payne, 1986). This strategy, which undoubtedly ensures that their contributions are more widely read, is being followed by many of the researchers in Scandinavia, The Netherlands and other Western European countries. Probably the greatest problems therefore remain in exploiting literature written in Russian, other Eastern European languages and Japanese.

The first step when dealing with foreign-language materials is to obtain suitable abstracts. Articles in many non-English journals include abstracts in one or more languages, although the quality and usefulness of author abstracts can vary greatly. The various abstracting services described in Chapters 4 and 5 may provide alternative summaries, although there is an increasing trend for these services to use the authors' abstracts. These resumés, together with a close examination of the tables and diagrams within the text, may provide an adequate indication of the paper's content.

There are few aids available for those wishing to study the text of such articles in more detail. Some veterinary terms will be found in biological, medical or general scientific dictionaries so translating dictionaries in these fields may be useful. Several of the more useful translating dictionaries covering aspects of agriculture and animal husbandry are listed in Part II. Giovannetti and Meissonnier [4] give details of some other works. The only translating dictionaries specifically for the veterinary sciences are R. Mack's two works for Russian and German [178, 179] and two works for Spanish [180, 183]. Roy Mack is now compiling an English–French veterinary dictionary. Other multilingual dictionaries, such as the *Veterinary multilingual thesaurus* [170], may help. This thesaurus defines 4,922 terms in English, German, French and Italian. *Elsevier's lexicon of parasites and diseases in livestock* [174] covers a narrower topic in the same languages plus Spanish and Latin.

If a fuller translation is required, then those working in the larger practices or in academic and research institutions may find that their own colleagues have useful linguistic abilities. Readers near London can also use the services of the British Library. Veterinary materials are held at the Aldwych branch and staff there will give a verbal interpretation of the content of foreign technical publications. Further information is available from the British Library Science Reference and Information Service, Aldwych, 9 Kean Street, London WC2B 4AT, England (Tel. 01–636 1544).

Professional translators can be used when a complete translation is required. Most local Chambers of Commerce, the Institute of Translation and Interpreting (318a Finchley Road, London NW3 5HT, England. Tel. 01–794 9931) and the Translators Association (84 Drayton Gardens, London SW10 9SB, England. Tel. 01–373 6642) can supply lists of translators. A further source is the *Register of translators and translating agencies in the United Kingdom* (Morris and Weston, 1987). In the USA, the American Translators Association (109 Croton Avenue, Ossining, New York 10562. Tel. (914) 941 1500) maintains and publishes a directory of members (*Translation services directory*. 6th ed., 1987). The International Federation of Translators (Secretary General: Dr R. Haeseryn, Helveldstraat 245, B-9100 Saint-Amandsberg/Ghent, Belgium) has most national professional organizations as members.

References

Morris, P. and Weston G. *Register of translators and translating agencies in the United Kingdom*. 58 Wood Lane, Beverley, North Humberside HU17 8BS, England: Merton Press, 1987. 233pp.

Payne, J. M. and Payne, S. 'Changes in world veterinary output of publications'. *British veterinary journal* **142** (1986): 301–6.

PART II

Bibliography

9 General Works

GENERAL SOURCES

General Bibliographical Guides (Chapter 5)

1   **Advisory Committee for the Coordination of Information Systems (ACCIS).** *ACCIS guide to United Nations information sources on food and agriculture.* ACCIS Guides to United Nations Information Sources No. 1. Palais des Nations, 1211 Geneva 10, Switzerland: ACCIS, 1987. 124pp.

2   **Blanchard, J. R.** and **Farrell, L.** (eds) *Guide to sources for agricultural and biological research.* Berkeley: University of California Press, 1981. 735pp.
Chapter D, *Animal sciences* by M. Merala, J. R. Blanchard and J. Kimball (pp. 287–377), contains a section on veterinary medicine.

3   **Bush, E. A. R.** *Agriculture: a bibliographical guide.* London: Macdonald, 1974. 2 vols. 1561pp.
Very dated now but of interest since it includes review articles with extensive reference lists as well as other reference sources.

4   **Giovannetti, J. F.** and **Meissonnier, E.** 'Sources of information in the fields of animal production and animal health. I. Primary information in English, French and Spanish. II. Secondary information, data bases and data banks'. *Revue scientifique et technique de l'OIE* **4** (1985): 751–72 (plus 747–50) and **6** (1987): 27–39 (plus 19–25).

5   **Kerker, A. E.** and **Murphy, H. T.** *Comparative and veterinary medicine: a guide to the resource literature.* Madison: University of Wisconsin Press, 1973. 308pp.

6   **Lilley, G. P.** (ed.) *Information sources in agriculture and food science.* London: Butterworths, 1981. 603pp. (Butterworths Guides to Information Sources.)
Chapters 16, *Veterinary science* by D. E. Gray, (pp. 418–39) and 15, *Animal production* by I. J. Lean and R. C. Campling (pp. 407–17) are particulary relevant. A new edition is in preparation.

7   **Morton, L. T.** and **Godbolt, S.** (eds) *Information sources in the medical sciences.* 3rd ed. London: Butterworths, 1984. 534pp. (Butterworths Guides to Information Sources.)

8   **Stephens, G.** *Guide to the literature of veterinary medicine.* New York: Haworth Press. Forthcoming.

9   *UNIDO guides to information sources.* Vienna International Centre, PO Box 300, A–1400 Vienna, Austria: United Nations Industrial Development Organization.
Guides have been published for the following industries: dairy products manufacturing, meat processing, pharmaceuticals and pesticides.

10   **Wyatt, H. V.** (ed.) *Information sources in the life sciences.* 3rd. ed. London: Butterworths, 1987. 191pp. (Butterworths Guides to Information Sources.)
The previous two editions were published as *Use of the biological literature.*

11   **Youssef, F. I.** *Manual for small veterinary libraries.* Alexandria: FAO, 1972. 65pp. (Near East Animal Health Institutes Handbook, no. 8.)
The list of references and bibliographical works is now outdated but the first part of the work remains a simple guide to library routines and operations for the non-professional librarian.

Abstracting Services (Chapters 4 and 5)

12   *Abstracts of Bulgarian scientific literature. Series B. Animal breeding and veterinary medicine.* 1956–. 125 Lenin Blvd., Block 1, Sofia, Bulgaria: Center for Scientific, Technical and Economic Information. Quarterly.
The equivalent institutes in a number of other Eastern European countries produce annual bibliographies of veterinary and/or agricultural literature.

13   *Agroselekt. Reihe 4. Veterinärmedizin.* 1956–. Berlin, German Democratic Republic: Akademie-Verlag. Monthly.
Formerly *Landwirtschaftliches Zentralblatt. Abteilung 4: Veterinärmedizin.*

14   *Article summaries.* 1988–. Sydney: Post-Graduate Committee in Veterinary Science. Monthly.

About forty to fifty abstracts are issued each month in two editions (*Large animal* and *Small animal*). The abstracts are taken from *Veterinary update: clinical abstract service*.

15 *Biological abstracts*. 1926/27–. 2100 Arch Street, Philadelphia, Pennsylvania 19103: BIOSIS (BioScience Information Service). Fortnightly.

Available online from 1969 with [31] in BIOSIS. The database is also used to compile two other abstract services of interest: *Abstracts of entomology* (1970–) and *Abstracts of mycology* (1967–). Both are published monthly; each contains about 14,000 abstracts and content summaries annually.

16 Cambridge Scientific Abstracts, 7200 Wisconsin Avenue, Bethesda, Maryland 20814.

Publishers of a range of abstracting journals covering the biological sciences. Titles of particular interest are: *Animal behaviour abstracts* (1973–), *Aquatic sciences and fisheries abstracts* (1969–), *ASFA aquaculture abstracts* (1984–), *Entomology abstracts* (1969–), *Immunology abstracts* (1976–), *Microbiology abstracts* (in 3 parts) (1965–), *Toxicology abstracts* (1978–) and *Virology and AIDS abstracts* (1967–).

17 *Chemical abstracts*. 1907–. 2540 Olentangy River Road, Columbus, Ohio 43202: American Chemical Society. Weekly.

Available online from the early 1960s in a variety of forms through STN INTERNATIONAL and several other online systems.

18 *Chemical patents index*. 1963–. Rochdale House, 128 Theobalds Road, London WC1X 8RP, England: Derwent Publications. Weekly.

The AGDOC and FARMDOC sections deal with agricultural and pharmaceutical inventions respectively. Both contain patents relevant to veterinary medicine. The database (WPI) is available on the TELESYSTEMES, DIALOG and ORBIT search services.

19 *Chirurgia veterinaria*. 1964–78. 1–14. Berlin: Paul Parey.

Appeared quarterly and included about 400 abstracts per year on anaesthesia, surgery, ophthalmology and radiography.

20 *Excerpta medica*. 1947–. PO Box 1527, 1000 BM Amsterdam, The Netherlands: Excerpta Medica. Monthly.

Issued in many sections each concerned with a medical speciality. Available online as EMBASE PLUS since 1974.

21 *Jahresbericht Veterinärmedizin*. 1928–1943. Berlin: Springer-Verlag.

Succeeded *Jahresbericht über die Leistungen auf dem Gebiete der Veterinärmedizin* (1881–1927).

22 *Modern veterinary practice*. 1920–. Goleta: American Veterinary Publications. Ten times a year.

Formerly a journal specializing in publishing brief, well illustrated articles for practitioners. From **69** (1988): (4) comprises selected summaries of new literature provided from *Veterinary update: clinical abstract service*. The abstracts are grouped into sections on dogs, cats, horses, cattle, pigs and sheep.

23   *Pascal sigma* and *Pascal thema*. 1973–. Paris: Centre de Documentation Scientifique et Technique. Many sections, each issued ten times per year.
Originally published as *Bulletin signalétique*. Veterinary science is not covered in a separate section but the database, PASCAL, which is available online from 1973 gives good coverage of European bioscience and biomedical literature.

24   *Referativnyi zhurnal. Veterinariya*. 1963–. Baltijskaya ulitsa, 14, 125219 Moscow A–219, USSR: VINITI. Monthly.
Continuation (from 1980) of *Referativnyi zhurnal. Zhivotnovodstvo i veterinariya*.

25   *Tropical veterinary bulletin*. 1912–30. **1–18.** London: Bureau of Hygiene and Tropical Diseases.
Superseded by *Veterinary bulletin*.

26   *VETDOC*. 1968–. London: Derwent Publications. Twenty issues per year.

27   *Veterinary bulletin*. 1931–. Wallingford, Oxfordshire OX10 8DE, England: CAB International. Monthly.

28   *Veterinary update: clinical abstract service*. 1986–. Goleta: American Veterinary Publications. Bimonthly.
Published in three editions: *Equine, Food animal* (cattle, pigs, sheep and goats) and *Small animal* (mainly dogs and cats). The latter appears monthly. There are annotated indexes in each issue and quarterly and six-monthly indexes. A continuation of *Veterinary reference service update*.

Indexing Services (Chapters 4 and 5)

29   *Agrindex*. 1975–. Rome: FAO. Monthly.
Has about 10,000 references per month arranged in broad subject categories. Each issue has a list of the centres participating in AGRIS and of AGLINET libraries.

30   *Bibliography of argiculture*. 1942–. 2214 N. Central Avenue, Encanto, Phoenix, Arizona 85004: Oryx Press. Monthly.
Available online in AGRICOLA from 1970.

31   *Biological abstracts/RRM (reports, reviews, meetings)*. 1967–. Philadelphia: BIOSIS. Fortnightly.

Complements *Biological abstracts*. Covers research reports, conferences, reviews, US patents and books. Until 1980 known as *Bioresearch index*.

32 *Index medicus*. 1879–. Bethesda: National Library of Medicine. Monthly with annual cumulations.
Published in its present form since 1960. Available online back to 1966 as MEDLINE (available from 1964 on DIMDI). About three-quarters of the online records contain author abstracts.

33 *Index veterinarius*. 1933–. Wallingford: CAB International. Monthly with annual cumulation.

34 *Science citation index*. 1945–. 3501 Market Street, Philadelphia, Pennsylvania 19104: Institute for Scientific Information. Bimonthly, annual cumulation.
Each issue comprises: a list of references cited (citation index), an author index which gives details of the items citing them, keyword subject index and a corporate index. Cumulations are published every five and ten years. Available online as SCISEARCH from 1979.

35 *Zoological record*. 1864–. Philadelphia: BIOSIS. Annual.
Consists of twenty-seven sections; one deals with comprehensive zoology, one lists new generic and subgeneric names and the others index the literature on a particular taxonomic group. Available online from 1978 as ZR ONLINE.

Current-awareness Services

36 *Acta veterinaria Japonica*. 1956–. Nihon University, Shimo-uma, Setagaya-ku, Tokyo 154, Japan: Research Institute for Veterinary Science. Quarterly.
Recent issues have been appearing annually and have consisted of a classified list in English of items published in Japanese journals.

37 *AGDEX monthly bulletins*. Edinburgh: AGDEX Information Service.
Titles available include: *Animal nutrition, Animal health, Animal breeding, Dairying, Beef, Pig production, Sheep, Poultry production, Food* (meat products), *Fisheries* and *Equitation*. Prepared from the AGDEX database.

38 *British book news*. 1940–. 65 Davies Street, London W1Y 2AA, England: The British Council. Monthly.
Gives full bibliographic details and details of the contents of forthcoming British books and other news about British publishing.

British national bibliography. (See [49].)

39 *Catalogue of British official publications not published by HMSO*. Cambridge Place,

Cambridge CB2 1NR, England: Chadwyck-Healey, 1980–. Quarterly with annual cumulation.
Available online.

40   *Current advances in* . . . 1984–. Oxford: Pergamon. Monthly.
A series of twelve journals each covering a biological speciality and listing references in broad subject headings. Titles of particular interest are those in *Biochemistry, Immunology, Microbiology* and *Pharmacology and toxicology*. Available online in CABS.

41   *Current contents*. 1958–. Philadelphia: Institute for Scientific Information. Weekly.
Available online as CURRENT CONTENTS ONLINE.

42   *Lewis's quarterly list*. London: H. K. Lewis. Quarterly.
Lists new scientific and medical books on sale. Many of the titles are available on loan from the lending library which the company operates.

Whitaker's book list. (See [59].)

Bibliographies (Chapter 6)

43   *American book publishing record*. New York: Bowker. Annual.
Covers all books published in the USA in the year. Catalogue entries (more than 38,000 in the 1987 edition) are in Dewey sequence. There are author and title indexes. The subject guide gives Dewey and Library of Congress numbers for each subject. Monthly and weekly updates are available and there are cumulations for the periods 1970–4, 1975–9, 1980–4.

44   *Books at Boston Spa*. Boston Spa: British Library. Microfiche. Issued bimonthly.
Lists in one author/title alphabetical sequence all English language and Western European language books, published in 1980 or later, that are held by the British Library Document Supply Centre. Has over 250,000 entries. The BLDSC catalogue, BNB [49], and the Science Reference Library catalogue [47] are available online on BLAISE-LINE.

45   *Books in English*. London: British Library, 1971–. Annual subscription with a new edition every two months. Microfiche.
Lists over 100,000 titles annually. Produced from records of the British Library and Library of Congress. Cumulations are available for 1971–80 and 1981–5. The titles of the books are listed by catalogue headings.

46   *Books in print*. New York: Bowker. Annual with midyear supplement.
The 1988–9 edition comprises seven volumes and includes details on almost

800,000 titles. Subject access to the information is provided by [58]. Available online.

47 *Books at the Science Reference Library.* London: British Library. Microfiche. Issued bimonthly.

48 *British books in print.* London: Whitaker. 4 vols. Annual.
Titles, authors and editors are given in a single alphabetical sequence.

49 *British national bibliography.* 1950–. London: British Library. Weekly.
New and forthcoming books are listed in subject order using the Dewey classification and catalogued according to AACR. There are also author and subject indexes. Cumulations are published four-monthly and annually. The online file is known as UK MARC.

50 *Catalogue of Lewis's medical, scientific and technical lending library.* London: H. K. Lewis, 1975. 2 vols.
Author and subject listings of hardback books written in English. Supplements have been issued covering: 1973–5, 1976–8, 1979–81, 1982–4 and 1985–7.

51 *Cumulative book index: a worldwide list of books in the English language.* 1898–. New York: H. W. Wilson. Monthly with annual cumulations.

52 *German books in print.* Munich: K. G. Saur. 5 vols. Annual.
Interfiles authors, titles and title keywords in a single listing. A separate *Subject guide* (4 vols, annual) lists the titles under subject headings.

53 **Gray, D. E.** *Veterinary books: a subject guide.* Alnwick: MAFF, 1983. 78pp. (MAFF Booklet 2437.)
Lists about 600 books and serial publications in classified order.

54 *International books in print.* Munich: K. G. Saur. 2 vols. Annual.
Lists English language titles published outside the USA and UK.

55 *Medical and health care books and serials in print.* New York: Bowker. 2 vols. Annual.

56 *Pure and applied science books 1876–1982.* New York: Bowker, 1982. 6 vols. 7784 pp.
Lists 220,000 titles under Library of Congress headings with author and title indexes. A companion work is *Health science books 1876–1982* (4 vols, 4601 pp.).

57 *Scientific and technical books and serials in prints.* New York: Bowker. 3 vols. Annual.

58 *Subject guide to books in print.* New York: Bowker. Annual.
The 1988–9 edition indexes almost 700,000 non-fiction titles from *Books in print* using Library of Congress subject headings. A bimonthly supplement, *Forthcoming books*, updates the work.

59 *Whitaker's book list.* 12 Dyott Street, London WC1A 1DF, England: Whitaker. Annual.
Single volume list of all books published in the UK during the year. In a single alphabetical arrangement of authors, titles, and keywords from the titles.

Review Journals and Series (Chapter 5)

60 *Advances in veterinary science and comparative medicine.* 1953–. San Diego: Academic Press. Annual.
Previously (1953–68) *Advances in veterinary science.* Each volume has about a dozen reviews on a variety of topics, although some consists of reviews on a single subject: **23** (1979) *Veterinary immunology,* **26** (1982) *The respiratory systems,* **28** (1984) *Research on nonhuman primates,* **31** (1987) *Experimental and comparative toxicology,* **32** (1988) *Immunodeficiency disorders and retroviruses* and **33** (1989) *Vaccine biotechnology.* The contents of volumes **1–23** are listed in volume **24** (1980); updates appear in subsequent volumes.

61 *Annual review of . . .* 4139 El Camino Way, PO Box 10139, Palo Alto, California 94306: Annual Reviews.
The titles from this series likely to be of interest to veterinary scientists are: *Biochemistry* (1932–), *Genetics* (1967–), *Immunology* (1983–), *Neuroscience* (1977–), *Nutrition* (1981–), *Microbiology* (1947–), *Pharmacology and toxicology* (1961–) and *Physiology* (1939–).

62 *Compendium on continuing education for the practicing veterinarian.* 1979–. Lawrenceville: Veterinary Learning Systems. Monthly.
Formerly entitled *Compendium on continuing education for the small animal practitioner.* Each issue has sections devoted to small animals, equines, and food animals. There are about four refereed review articles in each section and each has a set of review questions for the reader to check his knowledge. Also included are case reports.

63 **Foundation for Continuing Education of the New Zealand Veterinary Association.** *Publications.* Massey University, Palmerston North, New Zealand (Tel. 69–079): Centre for Veterinary Continuing Education.
Each volume comprises the papers presented at a course. Recent titles include:

    120 *Avian veterinary handbook.* 118pp.
    119 *Small animal gastroenterology and nutrition.* 313pp.
    118 *Slaughter of stock.* 137pp.

117 *Equine seminar 1988.* 241pp.
116 *Small animal urology.* 165pp.
115 *Goat seminar 1987.* 124pp.
114 *Equine reproduction.* 196pp.
113 *Small animal dermatology.* 286pp.
112 *Zoonoses in New Zealand.* 107pp.
111 *Small animal orthopaedics.* 196 + 61pp.
110 *Feline medicine.* 115pp.
109 *Clinical neurology of small animals.* 90pp.
108 *Clinical neurology of farm animals.* 47pp.
107 *Ectoparasites of sheep in New Zealand and their control.* 79pp.
106 *Goat husbandry and medicine.* 213pp.
104 *Clinical immunology.* 334pp.
102 *The veterinary handbook (of diseases affecting animals in New Zealand).* 269pp.
101 *Dairy cattle medicine.* 322pp.

64 *In practice.* 1979–. London: BVA. Bimonthly.
Issued as a supplement to *Veterinary record* and intended to update the practising
veterinary surgeon in clinical matters. Contains five or six articles which are
liberally illustrated in colour.

65 **Office International des Épizooties.** *Technical Series.* Paris: OIE.
The following reviews have been published:

No. 8. *Update on avian diseases.* 1988. 78pp.
No. 7. *Enzyme immunoassay techniques, ELISA, in animal and plant diseases.* 2nd ed.
    1987. 54pp.
No. 6. *Brucellosis in cattle, sheep and goats.* 1987. 282pp.
No. 5. *Cryptosporidiosis: a cosmopolitan disease in animals and in man.* 2nd ed. 1988.
    122pp.
No. 4. *Diseases transmissible by semen and embryo transfer techniques.* 1985. 117pp.
No. 3. *Animal health and economics.* 1983. 381pp.
No. 2. *Infectious laryngotracheitis.* 1982. 104pp.
No. 1. *Rift Valley fever.* 1981. 63pp.

66 **Post-Graduate Committee in Veterinary Science, University of Sydney.**
Proceedings. Sydney: the Committee. Occasional.
Each volume contains the proceedings of a conference, seminar or refresher course
for veterinarians. Although not intended as textbooks they usually provide a
reasonable survey of the field. Recent titles include:

1988 **110** *Sheep health and production.* 606pp.
1988 **108** *Small companion animal reproduction.* 534pp.
1988 **106** *Fish diseases.* 365pp.
1988 **104** *Australian wildlife.* 1052pp.

1987 **103**   *Veterinary clinical toxicology.* 630pp.
1987 **100**   *Teeth 'Open wide' (dentistry in dogs and cats).* 201pp.
1987   **97**   *'Through the naked eye' – Gross pathology of domestic animals.* 638pp.
1987   **96**   *Artificial breeding in sheep and goats.* 67pp.
1987   **95**   *Pig production.* 2 vols. 1203pp.
1987   **94**   *The stallion: artificial breeding and embryo transfer.* 359pp.
1986 **93A**   *Clinical pathology case reports.* 68pp.
1986   **93**   *Clinical pathology.* 306pp.
1986   **92**   *Poultry health.* 827pp.
1986   **87**   *Orthopaedic surgery: dogs and cats.* 457pp.
1986   **85**   *Soft tissue surgery: dogs and cats.* 522pp.
1986   **83**   *Equine surgery.* 389pp.
1985   **82**   *Equine exercise physiology seminar.* 86pp.
1985   **81**   *Symposium and workshop on ultrasound.* 94pp.
1985   **79**   *Symposium on computer and business management.* 530pp.
1985   **78**   *Dairy cattle production.* 630pp.
1985   **74**   *Equine gastroenterology.* 400pp.
1984   **73**   *Goats.* 600pp.
1984   **72**   *Deer refresher course.* 762pp.
1984   **71**   *Clinical pharmacology & therapeutics.* 522pp.
1984   **70**   *Embryo transfer.* 278pp.
1984   **69**   *Clinical oncology.* 373pp.
1984   **68**   *Beef cattle production.* 642pp.
1983   **67**   *Sheep: production and preventive medicine.* 567pp.
1983   **66**   *Disease prevention and control in poultry production.* 340pp.
1983   **65**   *Equine practice – diagnosis and therapy.* 848pp.
1983   **64**   *Greyhounds.* 755pp.
1983   **63**   *Nutrition.* 1028pp.
1983 **62A**   *Veterinary anaesthesia.* 169pp.
1983   **62**   *Anaesthesia and intensive care.* 526pp.
1982   **61**   *Nephrology, urology and diseases of the urinary tract.* 403pp.
1982   **60**   *Advances in veterinary virology.* 541pp.
1981   **55**   *Aviary and caged birds.* 664pp.

67   Post-Graduate Committee in Veterinary Science, University of Sydney. *Veterinary Review Series.* Sydney: the Committee.

Each review contains extensive reference lists and often has much tabulated data and fine illustrations. The titles are revised at regular intervals. Recent titles are:

28 1985 *Parasitic diseases of the horse.* 150pp. J. H. Arundel.
27 1985 *Veterinary clinical enzymology.* 28pp. P. J. Canfield, D. B. Church and
         C. H. Gallagher.
26 1985 *Veterinary anthelmintics.* 118pp. J. H. Arundel.
25 1985 *Diseases of aquarium fish.* 116pp. G. L. Reddacliffe.
24 1984 *Parasitic diseases of the cat in Australia.* 113pp. C. W. Prescott.
23 1984 *Skin diseases of the pig.* 55pp. R. D. A. Cameron.

22 1981 *Equine dermatoses.* 130pp. R. R. Pascoe.
21 1981 *Canine dermatoses.* 52pp. J. M. Keep.
20 1981 *Feline dermatoses.* 51pp. J. M. Keep.
19 1980 *Avian anaesthesia.* 14pp. A. Kirkby.
17 1977 *Canine parasitology.* 110pp. J. D. Kelly.

68 *Problems in veterinary medicine.* 1989–. Hagerstown: J. B. Lippincott.
Quarterly.
Devoted to aspects of small animal practice. The first issue has articles on
urogenital surgical conditions.

69 *Progress in Veterinary Microbiology and Immunology.* Edited by R. Pandey. 1985–.
Basel: Karger. Occasional.
Each volume contains about eight reviews.

1989 **5** *Nononcogenic avian viruses.*
1988 **4** *Moving frontiers in veterinary microbiology and immunology.*
1987 **3** *Biotechnology and comparative medicine.*
1986 **2** *Veterinary microbiology: molecular and clinical perspectives.*
1985 **1** *Infection and immunity in farm animals.*

70 *Veterinary annual.* 1959–. Edited by G. S. G. Grunsell, M-E. Raw and
R. W. G. Hill. Bristol: Scientechnica. Annual.
Each issue has about forty articles primarily by authors from the UK.

71 *Veterinary clinics of North America: equine practice.* 1985–. Philadelphia: W. B.
Saunders. Three a year.
With the next two titles succeeds *Veterinary clinics of North America* (1971–79).
Recent issues have been devoted to:

1989 **5** 3 Urogenital surgery
       2 Abdominal surgery
       1 The equine foot
1988 **4** 3 Urogenital surgery
       2 Reproduction
       1 Management of colic
1987 **3** 3 Clinical pathology
       2 Neurologic diseases
       1 Clinical pharmacology

72 *Veterinary clinics of North America: food animal practice.* 1985–. Philadelphia:
W. B. Saunders. Three a year.
From 1979–84 subtitled *large animal practice.* Also published in Spanish. Recent
issues have dealt with:

1989 **5** 3 Dairy practice management
       2 Clinical toxicology
       1 Llama medicine

1988	**4**	3	Stress and disease in cattle
		2	Metabolic diseases of ruminant livestock
		1	Investigation of disease outbreaks and impaired productivity
1987	*3*	3	Bovine reproduction
		2	Farm animal behavior
		1	Bovine neurologic diseases
1986	**2**	3	Anesthesia
		2	Parasites: epidemiology and control
		1	Necropsy techniques
1985	**1**	3	Calf diarrhea
		2	Bovine respiratory disease
		1	Bovine lameness and orthopedics

73   *Veterinary clinics of North America: small animal practice.* 1979–. Philadelphia: W. B. Saunders. Monthly.

Also published in Japanese by Gakusosha, Italian by Antonio Delfino Editore and Spanish by Editorial Inter-Medica. Recent issues have been devoted to:

1989	**19**	6	Critical care
		5	Clinical pathology part II
		4	Clinical pathology part I
		3	Clinical nutrition
		2	Fluid and electrolyte disorders
		1	Geriatrics and gerontology
1988	**18**	6	Clinical pharmacology
		5	Puritis
		4	Diseases of the ear canal
		3	Common neurologic problems
		2	Tropical fish medicine
		1	Hemostasis
1987	**17**	6	Parasite infections
		5	Exotic pet medicine
		4	Orthopedic salvage procedure
		3	Pediatrics
		2	Non-cardiac surgical diseases of the thorax
		1	Zoonotic diseases
1986	**16**	6	Viral diseases
		5	Dentistry
		4	Computers
		3	Reproduction and periparturient care
		2	Canine urolithiasis II
		1	Canine urolithiasis I

An index to volumes **14** and **15** appears in **15** (1985): (6).

74 *Veterinary medicine report*. St Louis: C. V. Mosby. Three a year.
Covers new developments in clinical practice with discussions of new products and techniques. Each issue has review articles on three or four themes each supplemented with discussion papers and case reports.

75 *Veterinary reviews and annotations*. 1955–61. **1–7** (2). Farnham Royal: CAB.
Since the cessation of this title reviews have been published in *Veterinary bulletin*.

Lists of Journals (Chapters 2 and 6)

76 *AGLINET union list of serials*. Rome: FAO, David Lubin Memorial Library, 1985. 145pp.
Has a list of addresses of AGLINET libraries and indicates their holdings.

77 **Boyd, C. T., Hull, D. C., MacNeil, K. J., Malamud, J.** and **Anderson, D. C.** 'Basic list of veterinary medical serials, 2nd edition, 1981, with revisions to April 1, 1986'. *The serials librarian* **11** (1986): 5–39.
As well as lists of indexing, abstracting and veterinary medical serials gives an adjunct list of core human medical and general science serials.

78 *British union catalogue of periodicals: a record of the periodicals of the world, from the seventeenth century to the present day, in British libraries*. London: Butterworths, 1955–8. 4 vols.
Updated by supplements until 1980 and subsequently by *Serials in the British Library* (London: British Library Bibliographic Services Division, 1981–. Quarterly with microfiche cumulations).

79 *CAB International serials checklist 1988 edition*. Wallingford: CAB International, 1988. 511pp.
Lists the serials, annual reports and conferences proceedings covered by CAB International in compiling their database. For each entry the title, country of publication, publisher and ISSN are listed. There is an index of ISSNs and a list of publishers which gives their addresses.

80 *Current serials received*. Boston Spa: British Library Document Supply Centre. Annual.
Only includes current titles but useful since it indicates availability of the journal from the BLDSC.

81 'List of serials abstracted'. *Veterinary bulletin* **58** (1988): i–v.
Changes to the list are noted in some of the January issues of *Veterinary bulletin*.

82 *New serial titles: a union list of serials commencing publication after December 31,*

1949. Washington DC: Library of Congress. 1953–. Monthly with annual cumulations.
Entries are arranged alphabetically by title and the holdings of major North American libraries are indicated. Continues the *Union list of serials in libraries of the United States and Canada* (edited by E. B. Titus. New York: H. W. Wilson, 1965, 5 vols).

83   *Serial sources for the BIOSIS database.* Philadelphia: BIOSIS. Annual.
Entries are listed in alphabetical order according to abbreviated title (derived using the ANSI rules). There is also a listing of publishers' addresses.

84   *The standard periodical directory.* New York: Oxbridge Communications. Annual.
The most comprehensive source of information on US and Canadian periodicals. The last edition covered more than 65,000 periodicals.

85   *Ulrich's international periodicals directory.* New York: Bowker. Annual with quarterly updates.
The best source of prices, publishers' addresses and frequency information on more than 110,000 regularly and irregularly issued serials. Available online. A directory of similar scope is *The serials directory* (3rd ed., Birmingham, Alabama: Ebsco Publishing, 1988, 3 vols).

86   *World list of scientific periodicals published in the years 1900–1960.* 4th ed. Edited by P. Brown and G. B. Stratton. London: Butterworths, 1963–5. 3 vols. 1824pp.
Entries are arranged in alphabetical order of the important words in the titles and the '*World list*' abbreviated title is given. The location of the periodicals in a number of UK libraries is indicated and the publishing history of each journal is given.

Major Journals (Chapter 6)

The contents of the journals can be assumed to be in the language of the country of publication. Most of the major journals issue annual author and subject indexes.

87   *Acta veterinaria (Beograd).* 1951–. Veterinarski fakultet, Bulevar JNA 18, 11000 Belgrade, Yugoslavia. Bimonthly.
Articles are in English.

88   *Acta veterinaria (Brno).* 1922–. Palackeho 1–3, 612 42 Brno, Czechoslovakia: University of Veterinary Science, Central Library. Quarterly.
Articles are in English.

89 *Acta veterinaria Hungarica* 1948–. H-1389 Budapest, PO Box 149, Hungary, KULTURA Foreign Trading Company. Quarterly.
The contents are in English. Formerly entitled *Academiae scientiarium Hungaricae: acta veterinaria.*

90 *Acta veterinaria Scandinavica.* 1960–. Copenhagen: Danish Veterinary Association. Quarterly.
With *Nordisk veterinærmedizin* published jointly with other Scandinavian societies. Publishes manuscripts from Nordic veterinarians and institutes. Has about fifteen papers in English per issue. Most volumes have supplements containing theses or conference proceedings.

91 *American journal of veterinary research.* 1940–. Schaumberg: AVMA. Monthly.
One of the most prestigious research journals. Each issue has about forty reports of original work.

92 *Animal production.* 1959–. 33 Montgomery Street, Edinburgh EH7 5JX, Scotland: Scottish Academic Press. Bimonthly.
Most issues have a few dozen papers on aspects of basic and applied sciences relevant to animal production. Journal of the British Society of Animal Production.

93 *Annales de médecine vétérinaire.* 1849–. 45 Rue des Vétérinaires, 1070 Brussels, Belgium: Imprimerie Bietlot. Eight a year.
Official journal of the Faculty of Veterinary Medicine of the University of Liège. Contents page and summaries are in English. Has a review article and about four clinical and research papers in each issue.

94 *Annales de recherches vétérinaires.* 1970–. 29 Rue Buffon, 75505 Paris, France: Éditions Scientifiques Elsevier. Quarterly.

95 *Archiv für experimentelle Veterinärmedizin.* 1950–. Postfach 506, 701 Leipzig, Democratic Republic of Germany: S. Hirzel Verlag. Bimonthly.
Contents page and summaries in English and Russian. Publishes about twenty articles in each issue across the whole span of veterinary medicine. Official journal of the Akademie de Landwirtschaftswissenschaften der Deutschen Demokratischen Republik.

96 *Australian veterinary journal.* 1925–. 272 Brunswick Road, Brunswick, Victoria 3056, Australia: Australian Veterinary Association. Monthly.
Often includes a review article and most issues have seven or eight original articles plus a similar number of short communications. Contains *AVA news* as an insert.

97   *Berliner und Münchener tierärztliche Wochenschrift*. 1888–. Berlin: Paul Parey. Fortnightly.
Summaries are in English and German.

98   *Biologizace a chemizace živočisné výroby – veterinaria*. 1964–. Smĕcky 30, Prague 1, Czechoslovakia: ARTIA. Bimonthly.
Articles in Czech or Slovak, contents page and abstracts in English.

99   *British veterinary journal*. 1875–. London: Baillière Tindall. Bimonthly.
Published on behalf of the British Veterinary Association. Most issues have seven or eight research papers plus a few short communications. Also has viewpoint articles and those in the Veterinary Professional Development Series review topics for practitioners. From 1875 to 1948 published as *Veterinary journal*.

100   *Bulletin de l'Academie Vétérinaire de France*. 1928–. Paris: the Academy. Bimonthly.

101   *Canadian journal of veterinary research*. 1937–. Ottawa: Canadian Veterinary Medical Association. Quarterly.
Until 1986 published as the *Canadian journal of comparative medicine*. Much Canadian research also appears in the *Canadian journal of animal science*.

102   *Canadian veterinary journal*. 1960–. Ottawa: Canadian Veterinary Medical Association. Bimonthly.
Includes CVMA news, research and review articles plus a miscellany of other features and regular columns of interest to the practitioner.

103   *Clinical insight*. 1986–. 36 Belgrave Mews North, London SW1X 8RS, England: Practice Publications. Monthly.
Issued free to practising veterinarians in the UK.

104   *Comparative immunology, microbiology and infectious diseases*. 1978–. Oxford: Pergamon. Quarterly.

105   *Cornell veterinarian*. 1911–. New York State College of Veterinary Medicine, Ithaca, New York 14853: The Cornell Veterinarian. Quarterly.
Has editorials reviewing topics of current interest, a useful list of new books received plus occasional book reviews.

106   *Dansk veterinærtidsskrift*. 1918–. Vanløse: Danish Veterinary Association. Fortnightly.
Normally has a few brief review or research articles in each issue but mostly comprises news items and stories of interest to practitioners.

107   *Deutsche tierärztliche Wochenschift.* 1893–. Hanover: M & H Schaper. Monthly.

Each issue has about fifteen original articles, normally in German, each with an English abstract. There is also a news section.

108   *Indian veterinary journal.* 1924–. 7 Chamiers Road, Madras 600 035, India: Indian Veterinary Association. Monthly.

About fifteen general research articles in each issue plus an equivalent number of clinical articles and short communications.

109   *Irish veterinary journal.* 1946–. Dublin: Irish Veterinary Association. Monthly.

Four or so articles in each issue.

110   *Japanese journal of veterinary research.* 1954–. Hokkaido University, Nishi-9-chome, Kita-18-jo, Sapporo-Shi 060, Japan: Faculty of Veterinary Medicine. Quarterly.

The contents are in English and other European languages. Includes lists of publications by faculty members and details of theses.

111   *Japanese journal of veterinary science.* 1939–. Faculty of Agriculture, University of Tokyo, 1-1-1 Yayoi, Bunkyo-ku, Tokyo 113, Japan: c/o Department of Veterinary Microbiology. Bimonthly.

All the articles are in English. Most issues have about forty papers across the whole span of veterinary medicine. Journal of the Japanese Society of Veterinary Science.

112   *Journal of the American Veterinary Medical Association.* 1869–. Schaumberg, Illinois: the Association. Fortnightly.

One of the foremost journals. As well as AVMA news each issue has about six research articles, six to eight clinical reports and several reports of retrospective studies. Regular features include review articles, abstracts of important recent literature, a 'What is your diagnosis?' column, book reviews, announcements and classified advertisements. From 1869 to 1915 published as *American veterinary review*.

113   *Journal of animal science.* 1942–. 309 West Clarke Street, Champaign, Illinois 61820: American Society of Animal Science. Eleven issues a year.

Issues contain about thirty articles on aspects of the science of animal production. Includes many papers on the physiology, biochemistry and nutrition of food animals. An annual supplement contains abstracts from the ASAS's annual meeting and from meetings of its regional sections. There is an author index to the supplement but no subject index although the abstracts from the annual meeting are printed in subject sections.

114 *Journal of comparative pathology.* 1888–. London: Academic Press. Eight a year.
Publisher a wide variety of research and descriptive papers on all aspects of disease and comparative pathology in vertebrates. From 1888–1964 published as *Journal of comparative pathology and therapeutics.*

115 *Journal of the Japan Veterinary Medical Association.* 1948–. Tokyo: the Association. Bimonthly.
All the articles are in English. There are about forty papers in each issue, most concerned with veterinary research. Many are studies with laboratory animals.

116 *Journal of the South African Veterinary Association.* 1927–. Pretoria: the Association. Quarterly.

117 *Journal of veterinary internal medicine.* 1987–. Hagerstown, Maryland: J. B. Lippincott. Quarterly.
Official journal of the American College of Veterinary Internal Medicine. Includes review articles and research papers plus retrospective surveys of cases..

118 *Journal of veterinary medicine.* 1953–. Berlin: Paul Parey. *Series A* and *B* ten issues a year, *Series C* quarterly.
Published as *Series A: Animal physiology, pathology and clinical veterinary medicine*, *Series B: Infectious diseases, immunology, food hygiene, veterinary public health* and *Series C: Anatomia, histologia, embryologia.* Previously known as *Zentralblatt für Veterinärmedizin: Reihe A, B* and *C.* Most of the contributions are in English with about ten articles in each issue. Supplements to the journal are published as *Advances in veterinary medicine (Fortschritte der Veterinärmedizin)* occasionally.

119 *Medycyna weterynaryjna.* 1945–. Al. Jerozolimskie 28, Warsaw, Poland: Panstwowe Wydawnictwo Rolinicze i Lesne. Monthly.
Most articles have English abstracts. There is a contents page in English.

120 *Monatshefte für Veterinärmedizin.* 1946–. Jena: VEB Gustav Fischer Verlag. Fortnightly.
Contents page and summaries in Russian and English. Eight or so articles per issue on aspects of veterinary medicine of farm animals.

121 *New Zealand veterinary journal.* 1952–. Wellington: New Zealand Veterinary Association. Quarterly.
Changed to quarterly publication from monthly in 1988. Now contains approximately ten major articles per issue plus a similar number of letters to the

editor (brief communications). Display advertising, professional news and editorials no longer appear but are published in *New Zealand vet script* which is a general news magazine.

122   *Nordisk veterinærmedicin.* 1949–. Frederiksberg: Danish Veterinary Association. Monthly.
Also known as *Scandinavian journal of veterinary medicine.* Most of the articles are in English.

123   *Onderstepoort journal of veterinary research.* 1933–. Private Bag X144, Pretoria 0001, Republic of South Africa: Department of Agriculture and Water Supply, Directorate of Agricultural Information. Quarterly.
During 1933–50 published as *Onderstepoort journal of veterinary science and animal husbandry.*

124   *Le point vétérinaire.* 1973–. Maisons Alfort: Le Point Vétérinaire. Monthly.
Contains seven or eight brief, well illustrated review articles for the practising veterinarian.

125   *Der praktische Tierärzt.* 1921–. Hanover: Schlütersche Verlagsanstalt. Monthly.
Has special issues on continuing education topics.

126   *Recueil de médecine vétérinaire.* 1824–. 7 Avenue du Général de Gaulle, 94704 Maison Alfort, France: APRMV. Monthly.
Journal of l'École National Vétérinaire d'Alfort. A blend of review articles, clinical and research papers, book reviews, official announcements and other news items. Includes lists of French theses. Two or three of the issues each year are special issues with articles on a topic of general interest.

127   *Research in veterinary science.* 1960–. London: BVA. Bimonthly.
Principal British journal for the publication of veterinary research especially experimental studies.

128   *Revue de médecine vétérinaire.* 1838–. 23 Chemin des Capelles, 31076 Toulouse, France: École Nationale Vétérinaire de Toulouse. Monthly.
Similar format to *Recueil de médecine vétérinaire.* Contains six to eight research and clinical papers, news on new books, official documents and information relevant to French veterinarians.

129   *Revue scientifique et technique de l'Office International des Épizooties.* 1982–. Paris: OIE. Quarterly.
Publishes reviews and original articles of interest to those concerned with the international control of animal disease.

130 *Schweizer Archiv für Tierheilkunde.* 1859–. Dietzingerstrasse 3, CH-8036 Zurich, Switzerland: Orell Füssli AG. Monthly.
Official organ of the Gesellschaft Schweizerischer Tierärzte. Five or six articles per issue.

131 *State veterinary journal.* 1945–. Alnwick, Northumberland: MAFF. Biannual.
The official journal of the State Veterinary Service. Each issue contains about eight mainly review type papers, often concerned with epidemiology, plus reports on the research and advisory activities of the Central Veterinary Laboratories and of the various Regional Laboratories and Centres.

132 *Tijdschrift voor diergeneeskunde.* 1863–. Utrecht: Royal Netherlands Veterinary Association. Fortnightly.
In Dutch with English abstracts. Includes some papers in English reproduced from *Veterinary quarterly.* Also has a comprehensive section of news for practitioners in the Netherlands.

133 *Tierärztliche Umschau.* 1948–. Neuhauser Strasse 21, Postfach 1222, D-7750 Konstanz, Federal Republic of Germany: Terra-Verlag Heizmann. Monthly.
About six research papers mostly on farm animal topics in each issue. Articles are in German with English abstracts. A Spanish edition *Panorama veterinario* is published by Editorial Eco (Calle de la Cruz 44, Barcelona 34, Spain).

134 *Vaccine.* 1983–. Guildford: Butterworth. Bimonthly.
Papers on immunoprophylaxis plus a topical news section including a section on new patents. Butterworth also publish *Molecular biotherapy* (1988–, quarterly), which like *Vaccine* includes items on the application of biologicals in veterinary practice.

135 *Veterinariya.* 1924–. Sadovaya-Spasskaya, 18, 107807. Moscow B–53, USSR: Ministerstvo Sel'skogo Khozyaistva. Monthly.
Only the contents page in English. Has about twenty-five articles in each issue.

136 *Veterinarski glasnik.* 1949–. Post. preg. 422, Bulevar JNA 18, 11001 Belgrade, Yugoslavia: Savez Veterinaria i Veterinarskih Tehnicara. Monthly.
Contents page is in English, abstracts are provided in Russian and English.

137 *Veterinary medicine.* 1905–. Lenexa, Kansas: Veterinary Medicine Publishing. Monthly.
Specializes in brief, well-illustrated continuing education articles. Published under various titles up to 1920 and then until 1964 published as *Veterinary medicine.* From 1964 to 1985 known as *Veterinary medicine – small animal clinician (VM-SAC).*

138 *Veterinary practice.* 1966–. Epsom: A. E. Morgan. Fortnightly.
Issued free to veterinary surgeons in practice and to veterinary libraries and

colleges in the UK. Contains news about the profession and brief technical articles.

139   *Veterinary quarterly*. 1979–. Dordrecht: Kluwer. Quarterly.
Published for the Royal Netherlands Veterinary Association. All the contents are in English.

140   *Veterinary record*. 1888–. London: British Veterinary Association. Weekly.
Essential reading for veterinary surgeons in the UK and one of the foremost journals. Most issues have several research papers and a number of short communications. The journal deals with the practical aspects of veterinary medicine and the editorials, news section, correspondence and topical features give a complete record of the UK veterinary scene.

141   *Veterinary research communications*. 1977–. Dordrecht: Kluwer. Bimonthly.
Formerly *Veterinary science communications*.

142   *Veterinary times*. 1972–. Ryde House, Ripley, Surrey, England: Henderson
    Group One. Monthly.
A similar newspaper style journal to *Veterinary practice*. Until 1984 called *Veterinary drug*.

143   *Vlaams diergeneeskundig tijdschrift*. 1932–. Casinoplein 24, B-9000 Ghent,
    Belgium: Faculteit Diergeneeskunde. Bimonthly.

144   *Wiener tierärztliche Monatsschrift*. 1914–. Wienerstrasse 21–23, 3580 Horn,
    Austria: Ferdinand Berger & Söhne. Monthly.
Contents page and abstracts in English. Has about six articles in each issue. Journal of the Österreichische Gesellschaft der Tierärzte.

145   *Zimbabwe veterinary journal*. 1970–. PO Box A 195, Avondale, Harare,
    Zimbabwe: Zimbabwe Veterinary Association. Quarterly.
Until 1980 known as the *Rhodesian veterinary journal*.

Medical Journals of Special Interest

146   *British medical journal*. 1857–. Tavistock Square, London WC1H 9JR,
    England: British Medical Association. Weekly.
A forum for the discussion of medical matters in their social context as well as for the publication of clinical research. More research-orientated articles are published in the *Lancet*.

147   *New England journal of medicine*. 1812–. 1440 Main Street, Waltham,
    Massachusetts 02254: Massachusetts Medical Society. Weekly.

Information on Theses (Chapter 6)

International

148 *Dissertation abstracts international. Section C: European abstracts.* 1976-. 300 North Zeeb Road, Ann Arbor, Michigan 48106: University Microfilms International. Quarterly.
Available with [152-155] online as DISSERTATION ABSTRACTS ONLINE.

United Kingdom

149 *British reports, translations and theses.* 1981-. Boston Spa: British Library Document Supply Centre. Monthly.
Successor to the *BLLD announcement bulletin* (1971-80) and indexes over 5,000 items per year. Materials from the Republic of Ireland and selected non-HMSO official publications are included as well as theses and other documents from British universities, government insitutions, industry and learned societies. Online in the SIGLE database on BLAISE-LINE.

150 *Index to theses with abstracts.* 1950/51-. London: Aslib. Quarterly.
To become available online. Previously entitled *Index to theses accepted for higher degrees by universities of Great Britain and Ireland,* for which the companion *Abstracts of theses* provided abstracts on microfiche.

151 *Retrospective index to theses of Great Britain and Ireland, 1716-1950.* Edited by R. R. Bilboul with F. L. Kent. Santa Barbara: ABC-Clio, 1975-7. 5 vols.
Precedes the *Index to theses with abstracts* [150].

United States

152 *American doctoral dissertations.* 1934-. Ann Arbor: University Microfilms International. Annual.
Gives a full list of all doctoral dissertations accepted by US and Canadian universities.

153 *Comprehensive dissertations index.* 1973-. Ann Arbor: University Microfilms International. Annual.
Covers all American doctoral dissertations from 1861 to date.

154 *Dissertation abstracts international. Section B: Sciences and engineering.* 1969-. Ann Arbor: University Microfilms International. Monthly.
Only includes theses of US and Canadian insitutions which allow copying of their theses and copies of these items are available from UMI. The publication began as *Microfilm abstracts* (1938).

155 *Masters abstracts.* 1962-. Ann Arbor: Universities Microfilms International. Quarterly.

Dictionaries and Thesauri

156 *Animal disease thesaurus*. Fourteenth revision. Room 740, Federal Building, Hyattsville, Maryland 20782: Veterinary Services, APHIS, USDA, 1988. 233pp.
An expansion of the *Veterinary multilingual thesaurus* with about 4,000 terms presented in both alphabetical and hierarchical listings.

157 *Black's veterinary dictionary*. 16th ed. Edited by G. P. West. 35 Bedford Row, London WC1R 4JH, England: A & C Black, 1988. 703pp.
An illustrated dictionary providing a great deal of background information useful to all those who may be involved with animals. The entries are more than simple definitions and the dictionary serves as a useful reference work for non-veterinarians. The same publishers issue similar dictionaries on medicine and agriculture.

158 Blood, D. C. and **Studdert, V. P.** *Baillière's comprehensive veterinary dictionary*. London: Baillière Tindall, 1988. 1124pp.
Admirably comprehensive, containing over 52,000 entries covering every facet of veterinary science. Appendices give much numerical, anatomical and clinical data.

159 *CAB thesaurus 1988 edition*. Wallingford: CAB, 1988. 2 vols. 1127pp.
Contains 56,000 terms, about 85 percent of which are preferred terms. Represents the controlled terminology now used for indexing the AGRICOLA and CAB ASTRACTS databases and includes about 85 percent of the terms in AGROVOC [167].

160 *Concise veterinary dictionary*. General Editor: R. S. Hine. Consultant editors: C. M. Brown, D. A. Hogg and D. F. Kelly. Oxford: OUP, 1988. 890pp.

161 *Controlled vocabulary*. Wallingford: Commonwealth Bureau of Animal Health. Revised periodically.

162 Jablonski, S. *Dictionary of medical acronyms and abbreviations*. St Louis: C. V. Mosby, 1987. 205pp.
A similar guide is S. B. Sloane's *Medical abbreviations and eponyms* (Philadelphia: W. B. Saunders, 1987, 410pp.).

163 Logan, C. M. and **Rice, M. K.** *Logan's Medical and scientific abbreviations*. Philadelphia: J. B. Lippincott, 1987. 673pp.

164 Mason, I. L. *A world dictionary of livestock breeds, types and varieties*. 2nd ed. Farnham Royal: CAB, 1969. 268pp. (Commonwealth Bureau of Animal Breeding and Genetics Technical Communication, no. 8.)

Entries list the ancestry of each breed and the place and date of origin. A third edition is in preparation. American livestock is described in *Modern breeds of livestock* (4th ed., H. M. Briggs and D. M. Briggs, New York: Macmillan, 1980, 802pp.).

165   *SNOVET: systematized nomenclature of medicine – microglossary for veterinary medicine.* Schaumberg, Illinois: AVMA, 1984. 200pp. plus new additions lists.
A list of preferred words and phrases each with a unique numeric code. Provides a controlled vocabulary for indexing medical records. A new edition is due shortly.

166   *Veterinary subject headings for use in Index veterinarius and the Veterinary bulletin.* Compiled by R. Mack. Farnham Royal: CAB, 1972. 44pp.
Has an alphabetical listing of terms and a useful section in which the terms are listed in classified order.

Multilingual and Non-English Dictionaries and Thesauri

167   *AGROVOC: a multilingual thesaurus of agricultural terminology.* D. Leatherdale with G. Eric Tidbury and R. Mack. Rome: Apimondia, 1986. 530pp.
Lists terms used in indexing AGRIS. Also available in monolingual versions in French, German, Italian and Spanish and there are two trilingual (English, French, Spanish) and (English, German, Italian) indexes to the main work.

168   Carrasco, C. *Diccionario de medicina, farmacia, veterinaria y química.* Madrid: Garsi, 1977. 1027pp.

169   Castelló, J. A. *Diccionario avicola-ganadero inglés–español.* Barcelona: Real Escuela Oficial y de Superior Avicultura, 1986. 135pp.

170   Commission of the European Communities. *Veterinary multilingual thesaurus.* Munich: K. G. Saur, 1979, 5 vols.
The five volumes comprise *1. German, 2. English, 3. French, 4. Italian* versions and *5. Quadrilingual index* to all the descriptors (preferred terms).

171   *Dictionary of agriculture in six languages: German, English, French, Spanish, Italian, Russian.* 5th ed. Compiled by G. Haensch and G. Haberkamp de Antón. Amsterdam: Elsevier, 1986. 1264pp.

172   *Elsevier's dictionary of pharmaceutical science and techniques in six languages: English, French, Italian, Spanish, German, Latin. Volume 1: Pharmaceutical technology. Volume 2: Materia medica.* Compiled by A. Sliosberg. Amsterdam: Elsevier, 1968 and 1980. 686 + 552pp.

173   *Elsevier's encyclopaedic dictionary of medicine in five languages: English, French, German, Italian and Spanish.* Compiled by A. F. Dorian. Amsterdam: Elsevier, 1987–. 4 vols.

The four parts will deal with: A. *General medicine*, B. *Anatomy*, C. *Biology, genetics and biochemistry* and D. *Therapeutic substances*. The terms are both translated and defined (in English). So far parts A and B have appeared.

174   *Elsevier's lexicon of parasites and diseases in livestock.* Compiled and arranged by M. Merino-Rodriguez. Amsterdam: Elsevier, 1964. 125pp. (Elsevier Lexica no. 3.)
Provides 663 terms in Latin, English, French, Spanish, Italian and German. There are two sections; a systematic list, grouping the terms under the English version by taxonomic group, and six alphabetical listings of all the terms in each of the languages.

175   **European Association for Animal Production.** *Dictionary of animal production terminology, in English, French, Spanish, German and Latin.* Amsterdam: Elsevier, 1985. 683pp. (EAAP Publication, no. 30.)
The most up-to-date multilingual dictionary on animal science. Compiled by the EAAP in collaboration with FAO. Contains approximately 9,000 entries.

176   **International Dairy Federation.** *Dictionary of dairy terminology in English, French, German and Spanish.* Amsterdam: Elsevier, 1983. 328pp.

177   **Kozlovsky, V. G.** and **Rakipov, N. G.** (eds) *English–Russian dictionary of agriculture.* Oxford: Pergamon, 1985. 875pp.

178   **Mack, R.** *Dictionary for veterinary science and biosciences: German/English and English/German.* Berlin: Paul Parey, 1988. 321pp.
Includes trilingual appendices which define Latin anatomical and medical terms and animal and plant names.

179   **Mack, R.** *Russian–English veterinary dictionary.* Farnham Royal: CAB, 1972. 104pp.
Six thousand terms are listed, including abbreviations, acronyms, drug and chemical names. Veterinary helminthology is covered in *Russian–English dictionary of helminthology and plant nematology* (G. I. Pozniak, Farnham Royal: CAB, 1979, 108pp.).

180   **Navarro Pruneda, G.** *Diccionario tecnológico de ciencias veterinarias y zootécnica: inglés–español.* Havana: Editorial Científico-Técnica, 1982. 167pp.

181   **Organisation for Economic Co-operation and Development.** *Multilingual dictionary of fish and fish products.* 2nd ed. Farnham: Fishing News, 1978. 430pp.

182   **Shishkov, V. P.** *Veterinarnyi entsiklopedicheskii slovar'.* Moscow: Izd-vo 'Sov. entsiklopediia', 1981. 639pp.
Russian language veterinary dictionary.

183   Trabing, M. E. *Diccionario panamericano de ganadería. Inglés–español, español–inglés medicina veterinaria.* Montevideo: Editorial Hemisferio Sur, 1978. 286pp.

184   Villemin, M. *Dictionnaire des termes vétérinaires et zootechniques.* 3rd ed. Paris: Vigot, 1984. 472pp.

185   Wiesner, E. and **Ribbeck, R.** (eds) *Worterbuch der Veterinärmedizin. A–K, L–Z.* 2nd ed. Stuttgart: Gustav Fischer, 1983. 1362pp.
Defines over 47000 terms.

Directories: General and Biographical (Chapter 3)

International

186   *The ABPI guide to acronyms and abbreviations in animal health and agriculture.* Compiled by J. M. Kirkness. 12 Whitehall, London SW1A 2DY, England: The Association of the British Pharmaceutical Industry, 1985. 43pp.
Addresses are given for organizations and associations included in the guide. Inanimate acronyms are also defined.

187   *Agricultural research centres: a world directory of organizations and programmes.* 9th ed. London: Longman, 1988. 2 vols. 1065pp.
A directory of around 7,500 industrial, academic and government laboratories in more than 130 countries. There are indexes to titles of establishments and to subjects. A companion work, *Medical research centres* (8th ed., 1988, 2 vols, 1150pp.) covers the medical specialities.

188   *Agricultural & veterinary sciences international who's who.* 3rd ed. London: Longman, 1987. 2 vols. 1195pp.
Gives profiles of about 7,500 senior scientists. There is a country and subject index listing the personnel included. The previous edition was entitled *Who's who in world agriculture* and had about 12,000 entries.

189   *European research centres: a world directory to organizations and programmes.* 7th ed. London: Longman, 1988. 2 vols. 2110pp.
The USSR is excluded but the work provides information on 20,000 laboratories in EEC, EFTA and COMECON countries. A companion work is *Pacific research centres* (2nd ed., 1988, 526pp.).

190   *List of research workers 1981 in the agricultural sciences in the Commonwealth.* Farnham Royal: CAB, 1981. 658pp.
Gives the names and contact points for research workers in government and state-aided institutions (including universities). Their research interests are indicated in a few words. A new guide: *Directory of research workers in agriculture and related*

fields in Commonwealth countries is in preparation and will be published by CAB International shortly.

191   *Tropical agriculture information sources. Volume 1. European Community.* Wageningen: Technical Centre for Agricultural and Rural Cooperation, 1987. 181pp.
Gives data on institutes in nine of the EEC countries and indicates their subject interests and library resources. A companion volume *Information sources on tropical agriculture. Volume II. ACP countries* (1988, unpaginated) describes 337 agriculture information services in African, Caribbean and Pacific countries.

192   *Who's who in science in Europe.* 5th ed. Harlow: Longman, 1987. 3 vols. 2880pp.
Has personal and professional information and details of the publications of over 22,000 scientists.

193   *World directory of veterinary schools 1971.* 3rd ed. Geneva: WHO, 1973. 260pp.
Provides descriptions of undergraduate education in sixty-eight countries with brief notes on the postgraduate training which is available. A *World directory of schools for animal health assistants 1971* (Geneva: WHO, 1974, 195pp.) gives information on the training of non-professional staff in fifty-two countries.

Australia

194   *Yearbook.* Artarmon: Australian Veterinary Association. Annual.
Includes a list of member veterinarians. Some of the state licensing bodies also issue lists, e.g. *The veterinary list for Victoria* (272 Brunswick Road, Brunswick: Veterinary Board of Victoria) and the *Veterinary surgeons roll as at . . .* (Department of Agriculture, McKell Building, Rawson Place, Sydney, New South Wales 2000: Board of Veterinary Surgeons of New South Wales). Both these lists give basic address details with information on degrees held and date of registration.

Canada

195   *Directory of Canadian veterinarians 1984–85.* Ottawa: Canadian Veterinary Medical Association, 1984. 155pp.
Issued as a supplement to the *Canadian veterinary journal* for September 1984. Has alphabetical listings by province. There are details of veterinary schools and of provincial licensing bodies and veterinary associations.

France

196   *Annuaire vétérinaire roy.* 50 Avenue de Clichy, F–75018 Paris, France: Édition et Publicité R. Walter. Annual.
Lists veterinarians, classified under region and specialization, institutes and research centres.

197   *Vade-mecum du vétérinaire.* Compiled by M. Fontaine. 15th ed. Paris: Vigot, 1987. 1664pp.
Mostly concerned with drugs and dosages but also quotes normal values and gives details of legislation.

Federal Republic of Germany

198   *Adressbuch der deutschen Tierärzteschaft.* Hanover: Schlütersche Verlagsanstalt. Triennial.
Official and professional organizations are listed. The names, addresses and specialities of all veterinarians are given according to geographic area. Published on behalf of the Deutsche Tierärzteschaft.

199   *Forschungsstatten der Landbauwissenschaften, Ernährungswissenschaften, Forst-wissenschaften, Holzwirtschaftswissenschaften, des Naturschutzes, der Landschaftspflege, der Veterinärmedizin in der Bundesrepublik Deutschland 1984.* Postfach 201415, Villichgasse 17, 5300 Bonn 2, FRG: Zentralstelle für Agrardokumentation und -information (ZADI), 1984. 611pp.
Lists research centres. ZADI also publish a list of current research projects: *Forschungsvorhaben im Bereich der Landbau-, Ernährungs-, Forst- und Holzwirt-schaftswissenschaften sowie der Veterinärmedizin. Teil 2: Tierische Produktion/Veterinär-medizin.*

200   *Mitglieder der Deutschen Veterinärmedizinischen Gesellschaft eV.* Geissen: Deutsche Veterinärmedizinische Gesellschaft, 1986. 189pp.
An address list of members.

201   *Tierärzteadressbuch.* Wiesbaden: Deutsche Tierärzteschaft. Occasional.

Ireland

202   *Veterinary register of Ireland.* Dublin: Veterinary Council. Annual.

The Netherlands

203   *Diergeneeskundig jaarboek.* Utrecht: Royal Netherlands Veterinary Association. Annual.

New Zealand

204   *Veterinary surgeons in New Zealand.* 1957–. Wellington: Government Printing Office. Annual.

Poland

205   *Polish agricultural research completed in 1986. 8. Veterinary medicine.* Warsaw: Osrodek Informacji Naukowej Polskiej Akademii Nauk, 1986. 231pp.
These are indexes to both the scientists and research institutes involved.

United Kingdom

206 *Registers and directory*. London: RCVS, 1987. 425pp.
Lists all registered veterinary surgeons and also has geographical indexes and details of staff holding government and academic appointments. Published biennially with an *Amendments booklet* in intervening years.

207 *The Report of the Chief Veterinary Officer: animal health*. London: HMSO. Annual.
Reviews the activities of the State Veterinary Service. The disease situation is reviewed and the work of the Central Veterinary Laboratory and Veterinary Investigation Service is described. There is a summary of changes to legislation and a list of selected publications by the Service's staff.

United States of America

208 *American men and women of science: physical and biological sciences*. 17th ed. New York: Bowker, 1989. 8 vols. Published triennially.
Includes biographical and contact information on nearly 140,000 American and Canadian scientists. Available online.

209 *Directory of American research and technology*. New York: Bowker. Annual.
Profiles corporate and academic R&D facilities. Includes details of key personnel. The *Research centers directory* (Detroit: Gale Research Company) is a similar guide which gives contact details and indicates the research activities of institutions.

210 *Directory of animal disease diagnostic laboratories*. Washington, DC: US Government Printing Office, 1982. 233pp.

211 *Directory: caring for animals*. Schaumberg, Illinois: American Veterinary Medical Association. Annual.
The 1988 edition lists over 44,380 members of the AVMA and 2,646 non-member veterinarians practising in the United States. In total 48,646 individuals are listed. There is an extensive reference section which includes a directory of information sources. The AVMA also compile an annual *Media guide to veterinary sources and information* for journalists.

212 *Media resource book: a guide to animal health information*. Alexandria, Virginia: Animal Health Institute, 1988. 44pp.
Gives contact points in AHI member firms, federal and state agencies, state departments of agriculture, universities, and in groups relating to the veterinary profession.

213 *Veterinarian directory*. 5639 S. 86th Circle, Omaha, Nebraska 68127: American Business Directories. Annual.
Provides a geographical listing of about 25,000 veterinarians.

Trade and Drug Directories

International

214 *'Animal health international' directory.* 2nd ed. London: IMSWORLD Publications, 1986. 682pp.
Gives names and addresses for animal healthcare companies and lists trade names in use. There is a separate listing of biological products and a listing of products by company.

215 *Biological substances: international standards and reference reagents.* Geneva: WHO, 1987. 94pp.
Has lists of standards for antibiotics, antibodies, antigens, blood products and related substances, endocrinological and related substances and miscellaneous biological products.

216 Council of Europe. *European pharmacopoeia.* 2nd ed. London/Sainte-Ruffine: Pharmaceutical Press/Maisonneuve, 1980–. Four 'cycles' each of several parts.
The standards given have been accepted by the eight Council of Europe members and by the Nordic countries for their own pharmacopoeias. The first volume covers general matters, the second consists of monographs published in series and issued twice a year. The three volumes and two supplements of the first edition (1969–77) remain in force until new texts replace them. *Pharmeuropa* (1988–, BP 431 R 6, 67006 Strasbourg, France: Council of Europe) is a newsletter publishing material relevant to the work of the *European pharmacopoeia.*

217 *Handbook of pharmaceutical excipients.* London: Pharmaceutical Press, 1986. 375pp.
A joint publication of the American Pharmaceutical Association and The Pharmaceutical Society of Great Britain. Gives monographs on 145 of the most commonly used excipients. An invaluable reference for formulation chemists, and others requiring data on 'inactive ingredients' in drug formulations.

218 *Intenational animal health directory.* 2nd ed. Richmond: V&O Publications, 1988. 312 + 34pp. index.
Organized by country and gives address information for animal health companies. Also lists government organizations, including regulatory bodies, and relevant associations. The data are available online in PHARMACONTACTS which also contains data from similar directories covering the pharmaceutical, agrochemical, and medical device and diagnostic industries.

219 *The international pharmacopoeia.* 3rd ed. Geneva: WHO, 1979, 1981, 1988. 3 vols. 223 + 342 + 407pp.

Volume 1 describes forty-two general methods of analysis. Volumes 2 and 3 contain quality specifications for 283 pharmaceutical substances, including all those in the WHO model list of essential drugs.

220 *Martindale: the extra pharmacopoeia.* 28th ed. London: The Pharmaceutical Press, 1982. 2024pp.
Prepared by the editorial staff of the Royal Pharmaceutical Society. A thorough and concise summary of the properties, actions and uses of medical drugs used throughout the world. Also covers ancillary substances. Available online. The twenty-ninth edition is in the press.

221 *The Merck index. An encyclopedia of chemicals, drugs and biologicals.* 10th ed. Rahway, New Jersey: Merck, 1983. 2194pp.
Has brief but detailed entries for over 10,000 chemicals. A good source of data on patents, method of synthesis, uses, structure, toxicity and nomenclature. Available online.

222 *The pesticide manual. A world compendium.* 8th ed. Edited by C. R. Worthing. 20 Bridport Road, Thornton Health, Surrey CR4 7QG, England: British Crop Protection Council, 1987. 1081pp.
Gives information on nomenclature, development, properties, uses, toxicology, formulations, and analysis of chemical and microbiological agents used in pest control. The databank is available online.

223 **Rossof, I.S.** *Handbook of veterinary drugs: a compendium for research and clinical use.* New York: Springer-Verlag, 1974. 730pp.
Provides information on about 1800 drugs. Lists synonyms and the uses of the drug. Recommended dosages are given with warnings about possible adverse effects.

224 **Sittig, M.** *Veterinary drug manufacturing encyclopedia.* Park Ridge, Illinois: Noyes, 1981. 507pp.
Gives manufacturing processes for 512 veterinary drugs. A more recent volume by the same author and publisher (*Pharmaceutical manufacturing encyclopedia*, 2nd ed. 1988, 2 vols, 1752pp.) gives information on about 1,300 medical drugs including many with veterinary uses.

225 **Slack, R.** and **Nineham, A. W.** *Medical and veterinary chemicals.* Oxford: Pergamon, 1968. 2 vols. 4 + 208pp.
The first volume contains a history of the development of various classes of drugs. The second is a tabulated listing of the drugs in classified order with details of chemical structure, year of introduction and early literature references.

Argentina

226 *Vademecum específicos veterinarios argentinos.* Virrey Loreto 2544-4°B, Capital Federal: Avila-Galloni. Annual.

Australia

227 *IVS annual 1988/89.* 100 Alexander Street, Crows Nest, New South Wales 2065: IMS Publishing. Annual.
Has full data sheet information on available products.

228 *Veterinary prescribers index.* PO Box 278, Balgowlah 2093, New South Wales: PVP Publications. Annual.

Belgium

229 *Compendium des spécialités pharmaceutiques vétérinaires.* 4th ed. Square Marie-Louise 49, 1040 Brussels: Association Générale de l'Industrie du Médicament, 1985. 443pp.

Brazil

230 *Compêndio veterinário.* Caixa Postal 4989, São Paulo: Organização Andrei Editora.

Canada

231 *Canadian veterinary pharmaceuticals and biologicals 1984/85.* Edited by D. J. Campbell. Media, Pennsylvania: Harwall Publishing, 1984.
Compilation of drug information on the drugs available in Canada.

232 *Veterinary pharmaco-therapeutic compendium.* 2nd ed. Edited by J. C. Panisset. 2999 Choquette, St-Hyacinthe, Quebec: CDMV, 1986. Sections paginated separately.
Describes over 2,000 drugs available though CDMV Inc.

Colombia

233 *Vademecum veterinario.* 4th ed. Apartado Aereo 54000, Bogotá: APROVET, 1985. 335pp.

Denmark

234 *Den danske Dyrlægeforening: Lommebog.* Venløse: Danish Veterinary Association. Annual.

Finland

235 *Pharmaca fennica veterinaria.* Iso-Roobertinkatu 4-6A, PL 320, 00121 Helsinki: Lääketietokeskus. Annual.

France

236 *Dictionnaire des médicaments vétérinaires.* 4th ed. Compiled by E. Meissonnier, P. Devisme and P. Join-Lambert. Maisons-Alfort: Point Vétérinaire, 1987. 1040pp. 4 appendices.

Gives datasheets on 2,412 products supplied by seventy-three animal health companies with appropriate indexes. There are several useful appendices including one on legislation.

German Democratic Republic

237 *Veterinary drugs from the German Democratic Republic.* Wilhelm-Pieck-Strasse 35, 8122 Radebeul: VEB Pharmaceutisches Kombinat GERMED Dresden. Undated. 281pp.

Federal Republic of Germany

238 *Lexicon der Tierärzneimittel.* Postfach 51 04 50, Berlin 51: DELTA Verlag. Annual.

Lists the available proprietary preparations and gives basic data sheet information. Two companion publications, *Delta Liste* and *Delta Index*, give price details and an index by approved names.

India

239 *Vetindex.* 1986–. 90 Nehru Place, New Delhi 110 019: A. E. Morgan Publications (India) Private Limited. Annual.

M. P. Verma's *Veterinary drugs and biologicals* (Anand: Kusum) is another guide produced annually.

Italy

240 *Guida di veterinaria e zootecnia.* 6th ed. Edited by L. Marini. Milan: Organizzazione Editoriale Medico Farmaceutica, 1987. 490pp.

The Netherlands

241 *Repertorium diergeneesmiddelen.* Postbus 576, 2003 RN Haarlem: De Toorts. Annual.

New Zealand

242 *Index of veterinary specialities annual.* PO Box 3397, Auckland 1000: IMS (NZ). Annual with updates in March and July.

Norway

243 *Felleskatalog.* Sørligaten 8, 0577 Oslo 5: Felleskatalogens redaksjon. Biannual.

Portugal

244   *Guia de productos veterinários.* Apartado 5392, 1708 Lisbon: José Arrais. Annual.

South Africa

245   *Index of veterinary specialities.* PO Box 2059, Pretoria 0001: IVS. Quarterly.

Spain

246   *Guia de productos zoosanitarios VETERINDUSTRIA.* Almagro 44, 3.°dcha, Madrid 28010: Veterindustria. Annual.

Sweden

247   *Fass vet.* Box 1319, 111 83 Stockholm: Lakemedelsinformation AB. Annual.

Union of Soviet Socialist Republics

248   **Dostoevskii, P. P.** (ed.) *Spravochnik veterinarnykh preparotov.* Kiev: 'Urozhai', 1986. 352pp.
Describes 376 veterinary drugs and 130 biological products available in the USSR.

United Kingdom

249   *Animal health news and index.* 10 Gymnasium Street, Ipswich IP1 3NX: John C. Alborough. Bimonthly.
Similar to *Index of veterinary specialities* but concentrates on products for farm animals and horses. Includes a news section and covers some non-medicinal products, for example, probiotics.

250   *Annual register of merchants' premises 1988.* London: Pharmaceutical Press, 1988. 226pp. plus monthly amendments.
Register of agricultural merchants, saddlers and similar premises. For pharmaceutical wholesalers and others who sell medicines to registered prmises.

251   *Anthelmintics for cattle, sheep, pigs, horses and poultry.* Alnwick: MAFF. Revised periodically. (MAFF Booklet 2412.)

252   *British pharmacopoeia (veterinary) 1985.* London: HMSO, 1985. 213pp. plus appendices. *British pharmacopoeia (veterinary) 1985. Addendum 1988.* London: HMSO, 1988. 219–317pp. plus appendices.
The Pharmacopoeia gives standards for the quality of substances, preparations and immunological products, together with information on action, use, dose, solubility, analysis, storage and labelling. The *British veterinary codex* (London: Pharmaceutical Press, 1965, 843pp.) and its *Supplement* (1970, 317pp.) are also useful for details of older compounds. Companion works, the *British pharmacopoeia*

1988 (London: HMSO, 2 vols, 1142pp. plus appendices) and the *British pharmacopoeia 1988 addendum 1989* (pp. 1143–1206 plus appendices) cover substances used in human medicine and pharmacy. The British approved names used in the pharmacopoeias are listed in *British approved names 1986* (London: HMSO, 1986, 136pp.). Supplements are issued biannually by the Department of Health.

253 *Compendium of data sheets for veterinary products.* 12 Whitehall, London SW1A 2DY: Datapharm Publications. Annual.
Compiled by the National Office of Animal Health. Contains data sheets supplied by NOAH members for each of their products. These have been prepared to comply with the requirements of the Medicines Act 1968. Also includes the NOAH Code of practice for the promotion of animal medicines. The same publishers also issue the *ABPI data sheet compendium* which describes medical products.

254 *Directory of UK animal health companies.* Richmond: V&O Publications, 1988. 145pp.
Profiles forty-two companies and gives brief data on forty-nine others.

255 **Ewing, W.** and **Haresign, W.** *Probiotics UK: the guide to probiotics in the United Kingdom 1989.* Marlow: Chalcombe Publications, 1989. 124pp.
Data sheet information on all the available products. A related work from the same publishers, *Probiotics: theory and applications* (edited by B. A. Stark and J. M. Wilkinson, 1989, 45pp.), gives further information on the nature of probiotics.

256 *A guide to veterinary pesticides: a key for veterinary workers to pesticides nomenclature in the literature and commerce, with notes on usage.* 2nd ed. London: HMSO, 1984. 104pp. (MAFF Reference Book 245.)

257 *Handbook of medicinal feed additives.* Baslow, Derbyshire: HGM Publications. Annual.
Gives comprehensive data on the feed additives available in the UK and describes the conditions of usage within the EC.

258 *The Henston veterinary vade mecum (large animals). Part I 1986/87 Disease and conditions. Part II 1989 Therapeutic products (summary tables).* Friary Court. 13–21 High Street, Guildford GU1 3DX, England: Update-Siebert Publications. 2 vols. Part I, 2nd ed. 1986, 332pp. Part 2, 5th ed. 1988, 256pp.
The first part is divided by species and each section lists diseases and conditions alphabetically with notes on their aetiology, diagnosis, treatment and control. Part 2 has tables grouping veterinary products according to their therapeutic class and giving basic details on each product.

259   *The Henston veterinary vade mecum (small animals) 1988/89*. Guildford: Update-Siebert Publications, 1988. 416pp.
Describes the diseases, conditions and clinical signs encountered in dogs and cats and describes the available therapeutic agents. There are directories of pharmaceutical companies and wholesalers and a variety of other data useful to small animal practitioners, for example, directories of laboratory diagnostic services, information on breeds etc. Each issue has some brief contributed articles on small animal practice. Update-Siebert Publications also compile and distribute the VETFAX audio tapes. These are sponsored by animal health companies and distributed to veterinary surgeons in the UK.

260   *Index of veterinary specialities*. Epsom: A. E. Morgan. Bimonthly.
Gives basic data on the composition, price and recommended uses of the available ethical pharmaceuticals. New preparations are listed in a special section, existing products are listed according to their pharmacological activity. A similar directory, *MIMS: monthly index of medical specialities* (30 Lancaster Gate, London W2 3LP) gives similar information on medical drugs.

261   *The UK pet trade year book and buyers guide*. London: Pet Trade and Industry Association. Annual.
Lists members of the PTIA, the Professional Groomers Association, manufacturers and wholesalers. Gives general information of interest to the pet trade.

United States of America

262   *Code of Federal Regulations. Title 21*. Washington, DC: US Government Printing Office. Annual.
Includes all the regulations affecting the use and development of pharmaceuticals in the United States. Amendments are noted in the *Federal register*.

263   *The complete handbook of approved new animal drug applications in the United States*. 1980–. 2925 LBJ Freeway, Suite 251, Dallas, Texas 75234: Shottwell & Carr. Updated by quarterly loose-leaf supplement.
Lists all approved drugs. Data on a selection of drugs used in daily practice is given in the *Veterinary practitioner's guide to approved new animal drugs* (1986, 164pp.).

264   Cornell Research Foundation. *Veterinary drug formulary*. Baltimore: Williams & Wilkins, 1985. 168pp.
Lists the drugs available in the pharmacy of the New York State College of Veterinary Medicine Teaching Hospital. There are lists of drugs by trade name, therapeutic action and generic name. The entries in the latter list give dosage information.

265 *Crop protection chemicals reference.* 4th ed. New York: John Wiley, 1988.
   2122pp.
Some veterinary pesticides are included.

266 *FARAD – the food animal residue avoidance databank trade name file: a
   comprehensive compendium of food animal drugs.* 2nd ed. By S. F. Sundlof, J. E.
   Riviere and A. L. Craigmill. Building 664, University of Florida, Gainesville,
   Florida 32611: Institute of Food and Agricultural Sciences, 1988. 609pp.
Arranged by generic drug name. All products containing the drug are then
described. There are indexes to trade name, to trade names according to the class
of livestock in which the product is to be used, and to trade names according to the
company marketing the product. The most complete and up-to-date list of
products approved by the Center for Veterinary Medicine for use in food animals.

267 *Feed additive compendium.* 12400 Whitewater Drive, Suite 160, Minnetonka,
   Michigan 55343: Miller Publishing. Annual with monthly supplements.
Gives listings of medicated feed additives and information on their use with
guidelines on regulatory, compliance and quality control guidelines. The monthly
update covers news in the medicated feed industry.

268 **Lewis, B. P.** and **Wilken, L. O.** *Veterinary drug index.* Philadelphia: W. B.
   Saunders, 1982. 327pp.
Covers veterinary pharmaceuticals, premixes and biologicals. Each entry gives
manufacturer details, data on type of formulation and route of administration and
on indications for use and dosages.

269 *List of FDA approved animal drug products.* Edited by R. B. Talbot, A. H.
   Fernandez and L. V. Melendez. Blacksburg: Laboratory of Veterinary
   Medical Informatics, Virginia–Maryland Regional College of Veterinary
   Medicine, 1987. (Information Series 87–1.) Monthly supplements.
Gives basic data on each product and has indexes to trade names, manufacturers,
distributors and active ingredients. There are lists of products approved for use in
particular species. Includes products for cats, dogs and horses as well as food
animals.

270 **United States Department of Agriculture. Food Safety and Inspection
   Service. Science Program.** *Compound evaluation and analytical capability national
   residue program plan.* Room 602, Cotton Annes Building, Washington, DC
   20250: Residue Evaluation and Planning Division. Annual.
Quotes residue tolerance and action levels for the compounds included in the
programme. Indicates and gives references on the methods of analysis. A chart
lists the compounds included in the programme over a ten year period. A final
section describes the activities planned for the current year.

271   *Veterinary biological products: licensees and permittees.* Hyattsville, Maryland: USDA-APHIS. Annual.
Lists establishments holding US veterinary licences to produce biological products.

272   *Veterinary pharmaceuticals and biologicals 1989/90.* 6th ed. Lenexa, Kansas: Veterinary Medicine Publishing, 1988. 1131pp.
Published biennially. Gives full data on over 1,300 products from forty-five manufacturers under various headings. One of the appendices lists FDA-approved New Animal Drug Applications including many products not described in the rest of the text. A complete desk reference for veterinarians.

Venezuela

273   *Productos farmaceuticos veterinarios.* 4th ed. Cátedra de Farmacología, Facultad de Ciencias Veterinarias, Maracay: Dr Paul Silvestrig, 1987. 472pp.

Research Directories (Chapter 3)

274   *AGREP: permanent inventory of agricultural research projects in the European Communities.* Farnham Royal: CAB, 1982. 2 vols. (+ supplement, 1983. 384pp.).
The first volume has the main list of research projects. The second consists of indexes.

275   **Agricultural and Food Research Council.** *Index of agricultural and food research 1986–87.* London: the Council, 1987. 210pp.
Each of the 1,458 entries summarizes the work of an individual researcher. The researchers are listed under the institute and department in which they work. There are subject and name indexes. Brief details are also given of research grants made by the council to universities and other bodies.

276   **Agricultural and Food Research Council.** *Programme of agricultural and food research.* London: the Council. 11 vols. Annual.
Indicates the background to each project, the research objectives and the researchers involved.

277   *Current research in Britain: biological sciences.* Boston Spa: British Library. Annual.
Three companion volumes deal with *The humanities, Social sciences* and *Physical sciences.* The latter volume also notes research of veterinary interest being undertaken in some departments of biochemistry, medicine etc. Overall 65,000 projects are described. The data are available online in CRIB.

278   *Directory of research grants.* Phoenix: Oryx Press. Annual.
More than 3,000 funding programmes are described.

279   *Foundation grants index.* 79 Fifth Avenue, New York 10003: Foundation Center. Annual.
Lists over 43,000 grants awarded in the United States in excess of $5,000 with details of the awarding institution and the project. *Foundation grants index bimonthly* provides current information. The *Foundation directory* is a biennial listing of the most important funding bodies.

280   *Grants register.* Edited by R. Turner. London: Macmillan. Biannual.
Complete guide to the international availability of grants for research, professional and advanced training and travel and vacation awards.

281   *ICAR: inventory of Canadian agricultural research.* Ottawa: Canadian Agricultural Research Council. Annual.
Available online from CISTI.

282   *Répertoires des opérations de recherches dans les établissements membres.* 7 Avenue du Général de Gaulle, F–94704 Maisons Alfort, France: Association des Établissements d'Enseignement Vétérinaire Totalement ou Partiellement de Langue Française, 1986. 79pp.
Lists research projects underway in veterinary schools in Canada, France, Belgium, Senegal and Morocco.

283   *The Wellcome Trust. Sixteenth Report 1984–86.* London: the Trust, 1987. 306pp.

Statistics (Chapter 7)

284   *Animal disease occurrence.* 1980–. Wallingford: CAB International. Two a year.
Provides abstracts of about 1,000 publications each year which contain disease incidence information. Data tables gives access to the relevant statistical data tabulated according to the animal affected, location of the outbreak and the pathogen or parasite involved.

285   *Animal health yearbook.* 1957–. Rome: FAO. Annual.
A joint publication by the FAO, OIE and WHO giving information on disease incidence and veterinary manpower.

286   *Animal production: quarterly statistics.* Luxembourg: Office for Official Publications of the European Communities. Quarterly.
Gives monthly statistics on animal populations, numbers slaughtered and trade in live animals for countries in the EEC. Also gives statistics on poultry and milk production. Production figures for the United States are given in *US Department of Agriculture: livestock and poultry outlook and situation* (Washington, DC: US GPO,

quarterly) and in the annual *Agricultural statistics* (Washington, DC: US GPO). UK animal production statistics are given in MAFF's *Agricultural statistics: United Kingdom* (London: HMSO, annual).

287   *Animal salmonellosis 1987*. Weybridge: Central Veterinary Laboratory, 1988. 76pp.
Figures and tables give data on the isolation of *Salmonella* from animals over a ten year period and on the resistance pattern encountered. The report is updated annually.

288   *Beef yearbook*. Bletchley: Meat and Livestock Commission. Annual.
Gives a comprehensive range of facts and figures on beef cattle in the United Kingdom including information on the incidence of infectious diseases. The *Sheep yearbook* and *Pig yearbook* contain similar data for those animals.

289   *Bulletin de l'Office International des Épizooties*. 1927–. Paris: OIE. Monthly.
Lists information received each month from national veterinary services on outbreaks of new animal disease especially those on the OIE's List A. Also gives information about the activities of the OIE and has a summary of List A outbreaks for the previous twelve months. Brief notes on outbreaks of disease and on current matters of interest is also published in *Disease information* (1988–). This is a weekly newsletter on reports of outbreaks of emergency animal diseases.

290   *EEC dairy facts and figures*. Thames Ditton, Surrey: Milk Marketing Board. Annual.

291   *FAO production yearbook*. 1958–. Rome: FAO. Annual.
Presents information on world agriculture and food including data on livestock populations and livestock products.

292   *FAO trade yearbook*. 1958–. Rome: FAO. Annual.
Gives data on international trade in livestock, meat products and other agricultural commodities.

293   *Farm management pocketbook*. 19th ed. By John Nix with Paul Hill. Ashford, Kent TN25 5AH, England: Wye College, Department of Agricultural Economics, 1988. 208pp.
Has quantitative data likely to be of value to those managing farm enterprises including gross margin data and information on labour costs. Relates to the UK scene only. A similar guide is *The agricultural budgeting and costing book* (The Old Vicarage, Church Lane, Twyford, Melton Mowbray, Leicestershire LE14 2HW, England: Agro Business Consultants, two issues a year).

294   *United Kingdom dairy facts and figures*. Thames Ditton, Surrey: Federation of United Kingdom Milk Marketing Boards. Annual.

With [290] provides a comprehensive range of statistics on dairy farming and milk production and utilization.

295   *Veterinary investigation diagnosis analysis II 1987 and 1980–87.* Weybridge: Central Veterinary Laboratory, 1988. 44pp.

Gives disease statistics on almost 200,000 submissions of material to the Veterinary Investigation Centres. Historical data are also given. The report is updated annually. Prepared by the Epidemiology Unit at Weybridge. A summary of the disease situation in the United Kingdom with regard to the major diseases is published annually by MAFF (*Return of proceedings under the Animal Health Act for the year* . . . London: HMSO).

296   *World animal health. No. 1: new animal disease outbreaks – statistics. No. 2: animal health status and disease control methods – Part one: reports, Part two: tables.* 1985–. Paris: OIE. Annual.

Comprehensive data on the health status of livestock in OIE member countries.

Organizations and Publications Concerned with Marketing Information

297   AGRA EUROPE, 25 Frant Road, Tunbridge Wells, Kent TN2 5JT, England. Tel. (0892) 33813. Telex: 95114 AGRATW G. Fax: (0892) 24593
Development of the animal feed industry in Europe 1985–1994. 1985. 61pp.

Also produce a wide variety of newsletters giving news and statistical information on aspects of European agriculture: *AGRA Europe* (weekly), *Green Europe* (monthly), *Milk products* (ten a year), *East Europe agriculture* (monthly), *CAP monitor* (updated loose-leaf guide), *Agrafile* (has separate titles on *Dairy products* and *Livestock and meat,* monthly) and *CAP weekly* (weekly with monthly summary). Some of these data are available online.

298   American Veterinary Medical Association [2013]
Have recently published *The US market for food animal veterinary medical services* (prepared by J. K. Wise of Wisemark Associates, 1987, 200pp.) covering the beef, dairy, swine and sheep markets. This has market estimates and details on surveys of livestock producers' attitudes. *The veterinary services market for companion animals* (prepared by Charles, Charles Research Group, 1988, 79pp.) deals with cats and dogs, equines, birds and exotic pets. The major findings from this report appeared in five articles published in *Journal of the American Veterinary Medical Association* in 1988.

299   Business Communications Company, 25 Van Zant Street, Suite 13, Norwalk, Connecticut 06855, USA. Tel. (203) 853 4266. Telex: 6502934929 (via WUI). Fax: (203) 853 0348.
Animal healthcare products for the 1990s. 1989.

The pet industry: the outlook for food, accessories, health products and services. 1989.
Pesticides used on agricultural animals. 1986.
Applied biology and biotechnology for livestock. 1984.

300   CARG – Research Services, Station House, Harrow Road, Wembley, Middlesex HA9 6DE, England. Tel. 01–903 1399. Telex: 923755 IPORES G. Fax: 01–900 1399

Produce FARM-TRAK, which covers the on-farm use of medicinal and nutritional products by dairy, beef, sheep and pig farmers in the United Kingdom.

301   County NatWest Securities Limited incorporating Wood Mackenzie, Kintore House, 74–77 Queen Street, Edinburgh EH2 4NS, Scotland. Tel. 031–225 8525. Telex: 72555. Fax: 031–243 4434

16th Floor, 535 Madison Avenue, New York 10022, USA. Tel. (212) 644 4200. Telex: 669117

The *Animal health and nutrition service* includes a quarterly newsletter, an executive summary of the market and four reference works giving: an overview of the industry (*Economic overview* – April/May), reviews on each major therapeutic area (*Product groups – February*), reviews on the major companies (*Company profiles* – August) and profiles of the top markets (*Country markets* – November). The organization also produce an *Agrochemical service* which deals with the world agrochemical industry in the same way.

302   Database International, PO Box 62, Maidstone, Kent ME14 2LB, England. Tel. (0622) 65743. Telex: 96433

Produce surveys on the market for feeds for domestic animals.

303   Doane Marketing Research, 555 No. New Ballas Road, PO Box 41902, St Louis, Missouri 63141, USA. Tel. (314) 993 4949.

Compile *Animal health market study*, a quarterly survey of the market in the United States.

304   Frost & Sullivan Inc., 106 Fulton Street, New York 10038–2786, USA Tel. (212) 233 1080. Telex: 235986. Fax: (212) 619 0831

Frost & Sullivan Ltd, Sullivan House, 4 Grosvenor Gardens, London SW1W 0DH, England. Tel. 01–730 3438. Telex: 261671. Fax: 01–730 3343

Recent market research reports have included:

Veterinary products market in the US. 1989. 200pp.
The feed additive market in Europe. 1988. 342pp.
Pet foods and pet products market in Europe. 1988. 411pp.
The pre-mixed feed products market in Europe. 1987. 338pp.
The impact of biotechnology on animal feeds and health products. 1986. 255pp.
Feed additives: impact of biotechnology. 1985. 255pp.

305   Hewin International Inc., van Leyenberghlaan 159, PO Box 7813, 1008 AA Amsterdam, The Netherlands. Tel. (020) 42 23 22. Telex: 15651. Fax: (020) 42 44 78

Have produced eight reports surveying existing markets under the general heading *Opportunities for development in agricultural animal health markets*. The most recent (6th, 7th and 8th) are *The use of chemicals in the European and North American fish farming industry*, *Biotechnology in animal health and nutrition* and *Additives and supplements for animal feeds*. Five other titles are in preparation.

306   HGM Publications, Abney House, Baslow, Derbyshire DE4 1RZ, England. Tel. (024688) 2329/2470

Feed industry review: a structural and financial analysis of the United Kingdom animal feedingstuffs industry. 1988.

307   ICC Information Group, 28–42 Banner Street, London EC1Y 8QE, England. Tel. 01–253 9736. Telex: 23678. Fax: 01–250 3084

Animal and pet food manufacturers and distributors. 10th ed. 1988.

308   Information Research Limited, 262 Regent Street, London W1R 5DA, England. Tel. 01–434 4536. Telex: 24224 (ref 3251)

Specific opportunities for suppliers of veterinary drugs in future world markets. 2nd ed. 1988. 151pp. This provides an overview of the world animal drug industry.

309   Intercontinental Medical Statistics, IMS House, 107 Marsh Road, Pinner, Middlesex HA5 5HQ, England. Tel. 01–868 4444. Telex: 922722

IMS America, Plymouth Meeting Executive Campus, 660 West Germantown Pike, PO Box 905, Plymouth Meeting, Pennsylvania 19462, USA. Tel. (215) 284 5000. Telex: 6851007

Compile EASYVET, an online database which has time series for sales of animal health products in the USA. It corresponds to the printed *US pharmaceutical market: animal and poultry*. IMS produces similar compilations of sales data for the UK (*British veterinary index*), The Netherlands and Italy. They also compile surveys of sales of veterinary products through pharmacies in France and Spain. Users in the United Kingdom have access to all this data online via FLEXIVET. IMS is to introduce audits covering Belgium and New Zealand shortly.

310   Jordan and Sons (Surveys), Jordan House, 47 Brunswick Place, London N1 6EE, England. Tel. 01–253 3030.

British animal and pet food companies. 1984.

311   Key Note Publications, 28–42 Banner Street, London EC1Y 8QE, England. Tel. 01–253 3006. Fax: 01–250 3084

Key Note reports: market information on industry sectors have been produced on:

Animal feedstuffs. 6th ed. 1988.
Battery farming. 3rd ed. 1987.
Pesticides and crop protection chemicals. 6th ed. 1988.
Pet foods. 7th ed. 1988.
Veterinary products. 3rd ed. 1987.

312   Landell Mills, 4 Miles Buildings, Bath, Avon BA1 2QS, England. Tel. (0225) 444646. Telex: 445675 LANMAR G. Fax: (0225) 447937

Prepare a variety of syndicated studies on selected sectors of the animal health market.

313   Marketing Strategies for Industry (UK), 32 Mill Green Road, Mitcham, Surrey CR4 4HY, England. Tel. 01-640 6621. Telex: 27950

Pet foods. 1989. 29pp. + 21 tables.
Animal feeds. 1988. 30pp. + 32 tables.

314   MILPRO, 1 & 2 Berners Street, London W1P 3AG, England. Tel. 01-637 1444. Telex: 25206. Fax: 01-631 4819

Compile the *National veterinary index* of sales of ethical veterinary pharmaceuticals products to veterinary surgeons in the UK.

315   Produce Studies, Northcroft House, West Street, Newbury, Berkshire RG13 1HD, England. Tel. (0635) 46112. Telex: 849228 PROMAR G. Fax: (0635) 43945

Prepare *Omnifarm,* a farm omnibus survey carried out at least twice a year among a representative sample of farms in the United Kingdom.

316   PJB Publications (Animal Pharm Bookshop), 18-20 Hill Rise, Richmond, Surrey TW10 6UA, England. Tel. 01-948 3262. Telex: 8951042. Fax: 01-948 5598

Each report is generally 100-150 pages and contains overview sections and quantitative data on the topic. The following reports have been issued recently:

1989   *The Japanese market for animal health products*
The sheep market for animal health products
Veterinary drug residues
Who owns whom in the world animal health industry
1988   *Acquisitions and mergers in the animal health industry*
Animal health company performance analysis
Animal health facts and figures. 3rd ed.
The Canadian market for animal health products
CAP – the livestock sector
Control of reproduction
Endoparasites: the veterinary market
The equine market for animal health products

        Feed additives – the market
        Feed additives – mode of action and applications
        The pig market for animal health products
        The poultry market for animal health products
        Veterinary antibiotics – new product profiles
        Veterinary biotechnology
        Veterinary product distribution in the European Community
        The world animal health industry: the way ahead
1987   *Bovine mastitis*
        Clorsulon: a product profile
        The economics of animal disease
        The hormone file
        Veterinary product registration in the EEC
        Veterinary product regulations in the Americas
        Veterinary vaccines
1986   *Developments in animal drug delivery*
        The French animal health products market
        Veterinary diagnostics – a perspective

317 Technology Management Group, 25 Science Park, New Haven, Connecticut 06511, USA. Tel. (203) 786 5445. Fax: (203) 786 5449

Emerging aquaculture markets: a worldwide study on feeds and veterinary products. 1988.
Veterinary drug delivery: a worldwide study on the impact of new drug delivery technologies. 1988.
The impact of biotechnology on animal care: an assessment of worldwide opportunities in diagnostics, vaccines, drugs, growth enhancers and other products. 1986.

318 Vivash Jones Consultants, Down Ampney House, Down Ampney, Cirencester, Gloucestershire GL7 5QW, England. Tel. (0793) 750521. Telex: 445753 AMPNEY G. Fax: (0793) 751648. London offices: 36 Belgrave Mews North, Belgrave Square, London SW1X 8RS. Tel. 01–235 9071

World animal health productivity and nutrition products market study update (annual) is the most general report. Vivash Jones also prepare studies on sectors of the market, e.g. aquaculture, antibacterials and antibiotics, parasiticides, reproduction control and veterinary biologicals, and studies on the market for products for particular species, on the animal health market in particular countries and profiles of all the major animal health companies. A seminar and project consultation service is available.

Journals

319 *Agricultural supply industry.* 1971–. Chislehurst: Veratbrite. Weekly.

320 *Agricultural and veterinary chemicals.* 1960–. 53 High Street, Totnes, Devon TQ9 5NP, England: Chandler Publications. Bimonthly.

321   *Animal health international.* 1980–7. London: IMSWORLD Publications. Quarterly with monthly newsletter.
Although no longer published back data can be searched online on IMSBASE.

322   *Animal pharm.* 1982–. Richmond. PJB Publications. Fortnightly.
An annual issue reviewing developments over the past year is published in January. Online in PHIND.

323   *Canadian vet supplies.* 1984–. 1 Philipsburg Street, C. P. 1320 Bedford, Quebec J0J 1A0, Canada: Selc Publishing. Bimonthly.

324   *What's new in farming.* 1977–. London. Morgan-Grampian. Monthly.

Conferences (Chapter 4)

Announcements of forthcoming events

325   *Baillière's veterinary diary.* Edited by T. Collins. London: Baillière Tindall. Annual.
A one page per day diary which also has an information section listing useful addresses, normal physiological values, notifiable diseases etc. Forthcoming events in the UK are noted in the diary section.

326   *Bulletin of the World Veterinary Association.* 1984–. Madrid: WVA. Three times a year.
Includes news from national member associations and an extensive *Calendar of meetings and congresses.*

327   'Calendar'. In: *Feedstuffs.* Minnetonka: Miller Publishing. Weekly.
Includes most American and international meetings in animal nutrition and animal production.

328   'Coming meetings'. In: *American journal of veterinary research.* Schaumberg, Illinois: AVMA. Monthly.
In addition to this list a *Veterinary meeting planning calendar* is produced annually by the AVMA and is available from Irene Jansons. This lists state and national association meeting dates.

329   'Coming meetings' and 'Foreign meetings'. In: *Journal of the American Veterinary Medical Association.* Schaumberg, Illinois: AVMA. Fortnightly.

330   'Diary'. In: *Veterinary record.* London: BVA. Weekly.
The *Veterinary record* also publish a more extensive 'Calendar of events' at regular intervals. These data are collected and held by the RCVS/BVA Continuing

Professional Development Committee based at the RCVS (Secretary: Mrs J. Plumb. Tel. 01-235 4971).

331   *Farm Diary*. Royal Works, Royal Parade, Chislehurst, Kent BR7 6NR, England: Veratbrite. Monthly.
Each issue includes between 150 and 200 agricultural events mostly taking place in Britain.

332   *National calendar of events*. Stoneleigh, Kenilworth: Royal Agricultural Society of England. Annual.
Comprehensive guide to all the agricultural shows, sales and open days, horse and dog shows and trials, general shows and conferences taking place in Britain. There is also a list of international events.

Guide to published proceedings

333   *Index of conference proceedings received*. 1964–. Boston Spa: British Library Document Supply Centre. Monthly.
Covers over 18,000 conferences each year. There are annual cumulations from 1974 and cumulative indexes covering 1964–81 (on microfiche). Available online as CONFERENCE PROCEEDINGS INDEX.

Standards (Chapter 7)

334   *Annual book of ASTM standards*. Philadelphia: Society for Testing and Materials. Annual. Many vols.
Details of standards in [336] and this catalogue are available online in the STANDARDS & SPECIFICATIONS database.

335   *BSI standards catalogue*. Linford Wood, Milton Keynes, Bucks MK14 6LE, England: British Standards Institution. Annual.
Standards are listed in numerical order and there is a subject index. Available online in BSI STANDARDLINE.

336   *Catalog of American national standards*. New York: American National Standards Institute. Annual.

337   *ISO catalogue*. Geneva: International Organization for Standardization. Annual.

Audiovisual Materials (Chapter 7)

International

338   FAO Film Library and FAO Photo Library. Information Division, Department of General Affairs and Information (address in Part III).

The libraries have published several lists of audiovisual materials: *FAO film loan catalogue*, *FAO photo library catalogue*, *FAO photo library colour diapositives* and *FAO photo library picture selection sheets*.

339   *World catalogue of veterinary films/video tapes and films/video tapes of veterinary interest.* 3rd ed. Madrid: World Veterinary Association, 1983. 114pp.
Gives synopses of 397 items with details of their provenance and availability.

340   *XXIII World Veterinary Congress videolibrary.* Montreal: World Veterinary Association, 1987. 14pp.
A catalogue distributed at the congress listing the items available for viewing and giving full details of their source.

Australia

341   Post-Graduate Committee in Veterinary Science. University of Sydney [2258].
A wide range of audio cassette tapes are available for many of the topics dealt with in the meetings organized by the Committee.

France

342   Association pour la Formation Continue des Vétérinaires Libéraux, 10 Place Léon Blum, 75011 Paris. Tel. (01) 43 79 11 52

343   École National Vétérinaire d'Alfort – Service Audiovisuel, 7 Avenue du Général de Gaulle, 94704 Maisons Alfort. Tel. (01) 43 96 71 00

344   École National Vétérinaire de Lyon – Service Audiovisuel, Marcy l'Étoile, BP 31, 69752 Charbonnières. Tel. (078) 87 00 84

345   Vidéo Magazine Vétérinaire (Éditions du Point Vétérinaire), 25 Rue Bourgelat, BP 233, 94700 Maisons-Alfort. Tel. (01) 43 53 20 01

Federal Republic of Germany

346   Videovet, Radlbäckstrasse 42, 8032 Gräfelfing. Tel. (089) 85 35 32

Italy

347   Unione Tipografico-Editrice Torinese – UTET, Corso Rafaelo 28, 10125 Turin. Tel. (011) 165291

United Kingdom

348   Allan White Memorial Video Library, Majorie Taylor, 101 Higher Lane, Rainford, St Helens, Lancashire WA11 8BQ, England. Tel. (0744) 883409
Tapes are available for purchase and hire. They are fully described in the library's *Catalogue*.

349   British Film Institute. *Catalogue.* 1963–. 21 Stephen Street, London W1P
   1PL: the Institute. Quarterly with annual cumulation.
Available in most large reference libraries. There is some overlap with the
BUVFC's *Catalogue* but has a broader coverage, i.e. records all films and videos
available for non-theatrical loan or sale in the UK, not just materials for higher
education purposes.

350   British Universities Film and Video Council. *Catalogue.* 55 Greek Street,
   London W1V 5LR: the Council. Annual.
Lists titles in subject order. Available in the HELPIS database on BLAISE-LINE.
This, and the National Library of Medicine's catalogue [357], are of use in
identifying titles produced for medical practitioners and students.

351   *Practice.* 50 Molyneux Street, London W1H 5HW, England: Practice
   (Tel. 01–724 0376). Five times a year.
Distributed free to veterinary surgeons in practice in the UK. Has a blend of items
on surgical and medical topics and on practice management.

352   Unit for Veterinary Continuing Education, The Royal Veterinary College, Royal College Street, London NW1 0TU, England. Tel. 01–387 2898
   (ext. 380/351)
Produce a wide range of videotapes, and audiotapes/transparency sets usually
with accompanying workbooks. These are described in three catalogues for large
animal practitioners, small animal practitioners and veterinary nurses. The
catalogues list other sources of audiovisual material in Britain. The Unit has
received funding from the European Commission to act as an international centre
for veterinary distance learning in Europe.

United States of America

353   American Animal Hospital Association [2033]
Produce a variety of videotapes on small animal medicine and surgery.

354   American Veterinary Medical Association [2013]
The AVMA runs a free-loan library of films. Details of available titles are given in
the *AVMA directory* [211]. The AVMA has also compiled a *Veterinary and audiovisual
catalogue* (1986) which lists the items available from veterinary schools and colleges
in the United States.

355   Audio Veterinary Medicine (Insta-tape), 810 South Myrtle Avenue, PO
   Box 1729, Monrovia, California 91016. Tel. (818) 303 2531
Produces audiotapes of contributions made at many American conferences,
meetings and symposia, including those of the AVMA, AAHA, Eastern States
Veterinary Association and Western Veterinary Conference. Also offer
subscriptions to species-oriented services entitled: *Small animal, Equine medicine*

(both monthly) and *Avian/exotic cage bird medicine, Dairy medicine* (both bimonthly).

356   International Veterinary Pathology Slide Bank, Department of Veterinary Pathology, College of Veterinary Medicine, The University of Georgia, Athens, Georgia 30602. Tel. (404) 542 5837
Co-ordinates a library of 35 mm transparencies and produces a videodisc providing a catalogue of the holdings. Involves over fifty collaborating institutions.

357   *National Library of Medicine audiovisuals catalog.* 1978–. Bethesda: NLM. Quarterly with annual cumulations.
Available online on AVLINE.

358   *Practice veterinary video.* 1988–. 2936 Brunswick Pike, PO Box 5818, Lawrenceville, New Jersey 08638: Video Learning Systems. Quarterly.
Each video lasts an hour and has about six segments featuring practical demonstrations. Some items are shared with the *Practice* videos produced in the UK.

359   Vetcare Video, 5121 West Ehrlich Road, Suite 104A, Tampa, Florida 33624. Tel. (800) 431 8838, (813) 963 6898

REFERENCE WORKS

360   *Handbook of veterinary procedures and emergency treatment.* Edited by R. W. Kirk and S. I. Bistner. 4th ed. Philadelphia: W. B. Saunders, 1985. 1000pp.
A compilation of numerical data, key facts, instructions and advice. Mainly intended for the small animal practitioner. Sections deal with emergency care, interpreting signs of disease, medical records and examination technique, clinical procedures, and the interpretation of laboratory tests. A useful companion to the Merck manual.

361   *International encyclopedia of veterinary medicine.* Editor in chief Sir T. Dalling. Edinburgh: W. Green & Son, 1966. 5 vols. 3168pp.
Useful compendium which consists of brief articles on each of the topics included. The final volume contains a detailed index in English and indexes in French, Spanish and German to the main topics.

362   *The Merck veterinary manual.* 6th ed. Edited by C. M. Fraser. Rahway, New Jersey: Merck, 1986. 1677pp.
The subtitle of *A handbook of diagnosis, therapy, and disease prevention and control for the veterinarian* indicates the broad scope of the work. A vast amount of descriptive information is presented and many tables provide much quantitative data. An invaluable desk reference. Available in the UK from Baillière Tindall/W. B. Saunders.

363   *Veterinary encyclopedia: diagnosis and treatment.* Edited by K. Wamberg. English edition edited by E. A. Macpherson. Copenhagen: Medical Book Company, 1968. 4 vols. Looseleaf: 2542pp. (+ supplement, 1972, 200pp.).
The length of the articles varies considerably, although many consist of three to four pages, some are considerably longer. German and French editions have also been published.

MULTIVOLUME WORKS AND SERIES

364   **Commission of the European Communities.** *Reports Series.* Luxembourg: Office for Official Publications of the European Communities.
Reports are numbered in the EUR series. The numbers, titles and details of the editors of a selection of recent reports is given below.

11353	*EEC directives and animal testing.* 1988. 66pp.
11285	*Disease in farm livestock: economics and policy.* K. S. Howe and J. P. McInerney. 1987. 190pp.
10984	*Contagious agalactia and other mycoplasmal diseases of small ruminants.* G. E. Jones. 1987. 118pp.
10983	*Rabbit production systems, including welfare.* T. Auxilia. 1987. 285pp.
10820	*Environmental aspects of respiratory disease in intensive pig and poultry houses, including the implications for human health.* J. M. Bruce and M. Sommer. 1987. 191pp.
10777	*Welfare aspects of housing systems for veal calves and fattening bulls.* M. C. Schlichting and D. Smidt. 1987. 174pp.
10776	*Welfare aspects of pig rearing.* D. Marx, A. Grauvogl and D. Smidt. 1987. 172pp.
10653	*Definition of the summer infertility problem in the pig.* E. Seren and M. Mattioli. 1987. 162pp.
10238	*Pestivirus infections of ruminants.* J. W. Harkness. 1987. 280pp.
10237	*Bluetongue in the Mediterranean region.* W. P. Taylor. 1987. 119pp.
10056	*Chlamydial diseases of ruminants.* I. D. Aitken. 1986. 162pp.
10054	*New developments and future perspectives in research on rumen function.* A. Niemann-Sorensen. 1986. 286pp.
10048	*Investigation on the possible effect of electrical stimulation on pH and survival of foot-and-mouth disease virus in meat and offals from experimentally infected animals.* 1986. 44pp.
9744	*Factors affecting the survival of newborn lambs.* G. Alexander, J. D. Barker and J. Slee. 1985. 198pp.
9742	*Assessing pain in farm animals.* I. J. H. Duncan and V. Molony. 1986. 92pp.
9741	*Studies on beef production from females.* H-J. Langholz. 1987. 263pp.
9739	*Campylobacter.* K. P. Lander. 1985. 145pp.
9737	*Immunity to herpesvirus infections of domestic animals.* P-P. Pastoret, E. Thiry and J. Saliki. 1985. 332pp.

9197   *Priority aspects of salmonellosis research.* H. E. Larsen. 1984. 342pp.

9180   *Commission of the European Communities, Directorate-General Agriculture. Farm animal welfare programme. Evaluation report 1979–83.* P. V. Tarrant. 1984. 89pp.

9000   *Paratuberculosis, diagnostic methods, their practical application and experience with vaccination.* J. B. Jorgensen and O. Aalund. 1984. 159pp.

8898   *Cell mediated immunity.* P. J. Quinn. 1984. 367pp.

8675   *Adjuvants, interferon and non-specific immunity.* F. M. Cancellotti and D. Galassi. 1984. 227pp.

8643   *Atrophic rhinitis in pigs.* K. B. Pedersen and N. C. Nielsen. 1983. 205pp.

8471   *Fifth international symposium on bovine leukosis.* O. C. Straub. 1984. 657pp.

8076   *Slow viruses in sheep, goats and cattle.* J. M. Sharp and R. Hoff-Jorgensen. 1985. 361pp.

365   *Current Topics in Veterinary Medicine and Animal Science.* 1978–. Dordrecht: Martinus Nijhoff.

The titles are the proceedings from seminars in the various CEC Programmes of Co-ordination of Research and are also given numbers in the EUR Reports Series. Volume numbers are not usually used to identify the works. Titles and authors/editors of the volumes issued thus far are as follows.

48 1988 *The management and health of farmed deer.* H. W. Reid. 205pp.

47 1988 *Increasing small ruminant productivity in semi-arid areas.* E. F. Thomson and F. S. Thomson. 296pp.

46 1988 *Modelling of livestock production systems.* S. Korver and J. A. M. van Arendonk. 215pp.

45 1987 *Summer mastitis.* G. Thomas, H. J. Over, U. Vecht and P. Nansen. 224pp.

44 1987 *Energy metabolism in farm animals: effects of housing, stress and disease.* M. W. A. Verstegen and A. M. Henken. 500pp.

43 1987 *Helminth zoonoses.* S. Geerts, V. Kumar and J. Brandt. 240pp.

42 1987 *Biology of stress in farm animals: an integrative approach.* P. R. Wiepkema and P. W. M. van Adrichem. 198pp.

41 1987 *Physiological and pharmacological aspects of the reticulo-rumen.* L. A. A. Ooms, A. D. Degryse and A. S. J. P. A. M. van Miert. 318pp.

40 1987 *Cattle housing systems, lameness and behaviour.* H. K. Wierenga and D. J. Peterse. 187pp.

39 1987 *Follicular growth and ovulation rate in farm animals.* J. F. Roche and D. O'Callaghan. 265pp.

38 1987 *Evaluation and control of meat quality in pigs.* P. V. Tarrant, G. Eikelenboom and G. Monin. 498pp.

37 1986 *Acute virus infections of poultry.* J. B. McFerran and M. S. McNulty. 242pp.

36 1986 *The present state of leptospirosis diagnosis and control.* W. A. Ellis and T. W. A. Little. 247pp.

35 1985 *Social space for domestic animals.* R. Zayan. 291pp.

34 1986 *Embryonic mortality in farm animals.* J. M. Sreenan and M. G. Diskin. 280pp.

33 1986 *Diagnosis of mycotoxicoses.* J. L. Richard and J. R. Thurston. 411pp.

32 1985 *Brucella melitensis.* J. M. Verger and M. Plommet. 270pp.

31 1985 Endocrine causes of seasonal and lactational anestrus in farm animals. F. Ellendorf and F. Elsaesser. 248pp.

30 1984 *The male in farm animal reproduction.* M. Courot. 377pp.

29 1984 *Recent advances in virus diagnosis.* M. S. McNulty and J. B. McFerran. 213pp.

28 1984 *Grassland beef production.* W. Holmes. 195pp.

27 1984 *Latent herpes virus infections in veterinary medicine.* G. Wittmann, R. M. Gaskell and H-J. Rziha. 522pp.

26 1984 *Manipulation of growth in farm animals.* J. F. Roche and D. O'Callaghan. 306pp.

25 1983 *Stunning of animals for slaughter.* G. Eikelenboom. 227pp.

24 1983 *Farm animal housing and welfare.* S. H. Baxter, M. R. Baxter and J. A. D. MacCormack. 343pp.

23 1983 *Indicators relevant to farm animal welfare.* D. Smidt. 251pp.

22 1982 *The ELISA: enzyme-linked immunosorbent assay in veterinary research and diagnosis.* R. C. Wardley and J. R. Crowther. 319pp.

21 1982 *Beef production from different dairy breeds and dairy beef crosses.* G. J. More O'Ferrall. 395pp.

20 1982 *Factors influencing fertility in the postpartum cow.* H. Karg and E. Schallenberger. 585pp.

19 1982 *Welfare and husbandry of calves.* J. P. Signoret. 246pp.

18 1982 *Transport of animals intended for breeding, production and slaughter.* R. Moss. 258pp.

17 1982 *Aujeszky's disease.* G. Wittman and S. A. Hall. 308pp.

16 1982 *Muscle hypertrophy of genetic origin and its use to improve beef production.* J. W. B. King and F. Ménissier. 658pp.

15 1982 *Fourth international symposium on bovine leukosis.* O. C. Straub. 614pp.

14 1981 *Advances in the control of theileriosis.* A. D. Irvin, M. P. Cunningham and A. S. Young. 427pp.

13 1981 *Laboratory diagnosis in neonatal calf and pig diarrhoea.* P. W. de Leeuw and P. A. Guinée. 200pp.

12 1981 *The mucosal immune system.* F. J. Bourne. 560pp.

11 1981 *The welfare of pigs.* W. Sybesma. 334pp.

10 1981 *The problem of dark-cutting in beef.* D. E. Hood and P. V. Tarrant. 504pp.

9 1981 *Epidemiology and control of nematodiasis in cattle.* P. Nansen, R. J. Jørgensen and E. J. L. Soulsby. 606pp.

8 1980 *The laying hen and its environment.* R. Moss. 333pp.

7 1980 *Control of reproductive functions in domestic animals.* W. Jöchle and D. R. Lamond. 248pp.

6 1981 *Diseases of cattle in the tropics: economic and zoonotic relevance.* M. Ristic and I. McIntyre. 662pp.

5 1979 *The future of beef production in the European Community.* J. C. Bowman and P. Susmel. 653pp.

4 1979 *Calving problems and early viability of the calf.* B. Hoffmann, I. L. Mason and J. Schmidt. 593pp.

3 1978 *Respiratory diseases in cattle.* W. B. Martin. 562pp.

2 1978 *Patterns of growth and development in cattle.* H. de Boer and J. Martin. 767pp.

1 1978 *Control of reproduction in the cow.* J. M. Sreenan. 667pp.

366 *Decision making in veterinary medicine series.* Toronto: B. C. Decker, 1987–.
Each volume presents algorithms enabling decisions to be made about patient care. The algorithms are intended to aid diagnosis, suggest diagnostic investigation procedures and provide recommended therapies. Each is supplemented by explanatory text and selected references. Volumes available are:

Decision making in small animal radiology. C. S. Farrow (ed.) 1987. 212pp.
Decision making in small animal orthopaedic surgery. G. Sumner-Smith (ed.) 1988. 216pp.
Decision making in small animal soft tissue surgery. A. G. Binnington and J. R. Cockshutt (eds). 1988. 232pp.
Decision making in large animal alimentary tract surgery. D. Horney (ed.) 1988. 220pp.
Decision making in small animal surgery. A. G. Binnington and J. Cockshutt (eds). 1987. 220pp.

367 **Department of Primary Industries and Energy. Bureau of Rural Science.** *Animal health in Australia.* Canberra: Australian Government Publishing Service.
Although intended for those working in Australia the series is of general interest. Each volume reviews current knowledge in a selected field. The titles available are:

9. *Exotic diseases.* W. A. Geering and A. J. Forman. 1987. 260pp.
8. *Helminth parasites of sheep and cattle.* V. G. Cole. 1986. 255pp.
7. *Viral, bacterial and fungal diseases of poultry.* W. I. B. Beveridge and L. Hart. 1985. 159pp.
6. *Bacterial and fungal diseases of pigs.* J. R. Buddle. 1985. 247pp.
5. *Protozoal and rickettsial diseases.* L. L. Callow. 1984. 264pp.
4. *Bacterial diseases of cattle, sheep and goats.* W. I. B. Beveridge. 1983. 196pp.
3. *Nutritional deficiencies and diseases of livestock.* E. A. Campbell. 1983. 277pp.
2. *Chemical and plant poisons.* A. A. Seawright. 1982. 290pp.
1. *Viral diseases of farm livestock.* W. I. Beveridge. 1981. 197pp.

368 *Developments in Animal and Veterinary Sciences.* 1986–. Amsterdam: Elsevier. A number of the volumes are proceedings from conferences and some have also been published as special issues in one of the Elsevier journals.

1986 **20** *Future production and productivity in livestock farming: science versus politics.* DSA (Bureau Européen d'Information pour le Développement de la Santé Animale). 254pp.

1987 **19** *Animal breeding and production.* E. Sasimowski. 782pp.

1985 **18** *Reproductive and developmental behaviour in sheep: an anthology from 'Applied animal ethology'.* A. F. Fraser. 439pp.

1984 **17** *Safety and quality in food.* DSA. 258pp.

1984 **16** *Advances in veterinary immunology 1983.* F. J. Bourne and N. T. Gorman. 259pp.

1984 **15** *Impact of diseases on livestock production in the tropics.* H. P. Riemann and M. J. Burridge. 632pp.

1984 **14** *Straw and other fibrous by-products as feed.* F. Sundstøl and E. Owen. 604pp.

1984 **13** *Prostaglandins in animal reproduction.* L-E. Edqvist and H. Kindahl. 304pp.

1983 **12** *Advances in veterinary immunology 1982.* F. Kristensen and D. F. Antczak. 312pp.

1983 **11** *Constitutional disorders and hereditary diseases in domestic animals.* D. Hamori. 727pp.

1983 **10B** *Genetics and animal breeding. Part B: stock improvement methods.* J. Maciejowski and J. Zieba. 206pp.

1982 **10A** *Genetics and animal breeding. Part A: biological and genetical foundations.* J. Maciejowski and J. Zieba. 284pp.

1982 **9** *Advances in veterinary immunology 1981.* F. Kristensen and D. F. Antczak. 282pp.

1982 **8** *Livestock production in Europe.* R. D. Politiek and J. J. Bakker. 335pp.

1981 **7** *Veterinary toxicology.* M. Bartik and A. Piskač. 346pp.

1980 **6** *Trends in veterinary pharmacology and toxicology.* A. S. J. P. A. M. van Miert, J. Frens and F. van der Kreek. 363pp.

1979 **5** *Physiology and control of parturition in domestic animals.* P. Ellendorff, M. Taverne and D. Smidt. 348pp.

1979 **4** *Social structure in farm animals.* G. J. Syme and L. A. Syme. 200pp.

1979 **3** *Bacterial infection and immunity in domestic animals.* J. B. Woolcock. 254pp.

1978 **2** *Ethology of free-ranging domestic animals.* G. W. Arnold and M. L. Dudzinski. 198pp.

1976 **1** *Guide dogs for the blind: their selection, development and training.* C. J. Pfaffenberger, J. P. Scott, J. L. Fuller, B. E. Ginsberg and S. W. Biefelt. 225pp.

369   *Developments in Biological Standardization.* 1965–. Basel: Karger. Three or four a year.

Contains the proceedings of symposia organized by the International Association of Biological Standardization. Important to those working in veterinary microbiology, with diagnostics, vaccines and other biologicals. Recent titles include:

1987	**68**	*Cells, products, safety*
	66	*Advances in animal cell technology: cell engineering, evaluation and exploitation*
1986	**65**	*Use and standardization of combined vaccines*
	64	*Reduction of animal usage in the development and control of biological products*
	63	*Use and standardization of chemically defined antigens*
	62	*Diagnostics and vaccines for parasitic diseases*
1984	**56**	*Brucellosis*

Papers in the same subject area are published in the *Journal of biological standardization* (London: Academic Press).

370   *Easter Schools in Agricultural Science (Univerisity of Nottingham).* 1955–. London: Butterworths. Annual.

Each volume usually consists of both review papers on aspects of the topic supplemented by articles reporting on current research. The works in the series are identified by their titles and editors rather than by the volume number. Recent volumes concerned with animal production are:

46	*Nutrition and lactation in the dairy cow.* P. C. Garnsworthy. 1988. 429pp.
43	*Control and manipulation of animal growth.* P. J. Buttery, D. B. Lindsay and N. B. Haynes. 1986. 347pp.
42	*Computer applications in agricultural environments.* J. A. Clark, K. Gregson and R. A. Saffell. 1987. 304pp.
38	*Immunological aspects of reproduction in mammals.* D. B. Crichton. 1984. 540pp.
37	*Fats in animal nutrition.* J. Wiseman. 1984. 521pp.
35	*Sheep production.* W. Haresign. 1983. 576pp.
34	*Control of pig reproduction.* D. J. A. Cole and G. R. Foxcroft. 1982. 664pp.
31	*Environmental aspects of housing for animal production.* J. A. Clark. 1981. 511pp.
29	*Protein deposition in animals.* P. J. Buttery and D. B. Lindsay. 1980. 305pp.
26	*Control of ovulation.* D. B. Crichton, G. R. Foxcroft, N. B. Haynes and G. E. Lamming. 1978. 492pp.
25	*Antibiotics and antibiosis in agriculture.* M. Woodbine. 1977. 386pp.
23	*Principles of cattle production.* H. Swan and W. H. Broster. 1976. 438pp.
21	*Meat.* D. J. A. Cole and R. A. Lawrie. 1975. 596pp.

371   *FAO Animal Production and Health Papers.* 1977–. Rome: FAO.
Most volumes give an overview of the topic stressing the method and impact of improving animal productivity. Several deal with animal genetic resources and indigenous breeds of livestock. Titles of particular interest are:

1987	**68**	*Crossbreeding* Bos indicus *and* Bos taurus *for milk production in the tropics*
1987	**67**	*Trypanotolerant cattle and livestock development in West and Central Africa.* 2 vols.
1987	**66**	*Animal genetic resources: strategies for improved use and conservation*
1986	**61**	*The Przewalski horse and restoration to its natural habitat in Mongolia*
1986	**60**	*Sheep and goats in Turkey*
1986	**59**	*Animal genetic resources data banks 3: descriptor list for poultry, 2: descriptor lists for cattle, buffalo, pigs, sheep and goats, 1: computer systems for regional data banks.* 3 vols.
1986	**58**	*Small ruminant production in developing countries*
1985	**57**	*The Awassi sheep with special reference to the improved dairy type*
1985	**56**	*Sheep and goats in Pakistan*
1987	**54/5**	*Small ruminants in the Near East.* 2 vols.
1985	**53**	*Slaughterhouse cleaning and sanitation*
1985	**49**	*Manual for the slaughter of small ruminants in developing countries*
1985	**46**	*Livestock breeds of China*
1984	**44.2**	*Animal genetic resources: cryogenic storage of germplasm and molecular engineering*
1984	**44.1**	*Animal genetic resources: conservation by management, data banks and training*
1984	**42**	*Animal energy in agriculture in Africa and Asia*
1983	**40**	*Intensive sheep production in the Near East*
1982	**38**	*Diagnosis and vaccination for the control of brucellosis in the Near East*
1982	**34**	*Breeding plans for ruminant livestock in the tropics*
1982	**33**	*Haemorrhagic septicaemia*
1982	**31**	*Hormones in animal production*
1982	**30**	*Sheep and goat breeds of India*
1982	**29**	*Echinococcus/hydatidosis surveillance, prevention and control*
1982	**27**	*Deer farming: guidelines on practical aspects*
1982	**26**	*Camels and camel milk*
1982	**25**	*Reproductive efficiency in cattle*
1981	**23**	*Disease control in semen and embryos*
1979	**13**	*Buffalo reproduction and artificial insemination*
1978	**9**	*Slaughterhouse and slaughter slab design and construction*
1976	**2**	*Eradication of hog cholera and African swine fever*

372   *FAO Animal Production and Health Series.* 1960–. Rome: FAO.
The FAO *Animal health yearbook* is now published in this series. Other titles of interest are:

1986   **23**   *Manual on the diagnosis of rinderpest.* G. R. Scott, W. P. Taylor and
P. B. Rossiter. 187pp.

1986   **21**   *The rabbit: husbandry, health and production.* F. Lebas, P. Coudert,
R. Rouvier and H. de Rochambeau. 235pp.

1970   **14**   *Observations on the goat.* M. H. French. 204pp.

1981   **12**   *Tropical feeds: on feed information summaries and nutritive values.* B.
Göhl. 529pp.

1978   **10**   *Newcastle disease vaccines: their production and use.* W. H. Allan, J. E.
Lancaster and B. Toth. 163pp.

1977   **4**   *The water buffalo.* W. Ross Cockrill. 283pp.

373   *WHO Monograph Series.* 1951–. Geneva: WHO.

55   *Laboratory techniques in brucellosis.* 2nd ed. G. G. Alton, L. M. Jones and
D. E. Pietz. 1975. 163pp.

23   *Laboratory techniques in rabies.* 3rd ed. Edited by M. M. Kaplan and H.
Koprowski. 1973. 367pp.

374   *WHO Technical Reports Series.* Geneva: WHO. Occasional.

774   *Salmonellosis control: the role of animal and product hygiene: report of a WHO
Expert Committee.* 1988. 83pp.

771   *WHO Expert Committee on Biological Standardization: thirty-eighth report.*
1988. 221pp.

763   *Evaluation of certain veterinary drug residues in food: thirty-second report of the
Joint FAO/WHO Expert Committee on Food Additives.* 1988. 40pp.
Monographs summarizing residue data on the compounds discussed at
the meeting (chloramphenicol and five growth promoters) are presented
in *Residues of some veterinary drugs in animals and foods* (Rome: FAO, 1988,
49pp., FAO Food and Nutrition Paper no. 41). Toxicological
monographs on some of the compounds are published in *Toxicological
evaluation of certain veterinary drugs in foods* (Geneva: WHO, 1989, 165pp.,
WHO Food Additives Series no. 23).

759   *Evaluation of certain food additives and contaminants: thirty-first report of the
Joint FAO/WHO Expert Committee on Food Additives.* 1987. 53pp.

748   *WHO Expert Committee on Specifications for Pharmaceutical
Preparations: thirtieth report.* 1987. 50pp.

740   *Joint FAO/WHO Expert Committee on Brucellosis: sixth report.* 1986. 132pp.

739   *Epidemiology and control of African trypanosomiasis: report of a WHO Expert
Committee.* 1986. 127pp.

709   *WHO Expert Committee on Rabies: seventh report.* 1984. 104pp.

701   *The leishmaniases: report of a WHO Expert Committee.* 1984. 140pp.

682   *Bacterial and viral zoonoses: report of a WHO Expert Committee. 1982. 146pp.*

637   *Parasitic zoonoses: report of a WHO Expert Committee.* 1979. 107pp.

573   *The veterinary contribution to public health practice: report of a Joint FAO/WHO
Expert Committee on Veterinary Public Health.* 1975. 80pp.

375 *World animal science.* Editors-in-chief A. Neimann-Sørensen and D. E. Tribe. 1981–. Amsterdam: Elsevier. 34 vols planned.

The series will provide a comprehensive overview of the literature on animal production science. The titles and editors of the volumes published so far are as follows:

Subseries A: Basic information

A1 1983   *Domestication, conservation and use of animal resources.* L. J. Peel and D. E. Tribe

A2 1984   *The development of animal production systems.* B. Nestel

A3 1983   *Dynamic biochemistry of animal production.* P. M. Riis

A4 1985   *General and quantitative genetics.* A. B. Chapman

A5 1985   *Ethology of farm animals.* A. F. Fraser

Subseries B: Disciplinary approach

B1 1981   *Grazing animals.* F. H. W. Morley

B2 1985   *Parasites, pests and predators.* S. M. Gaafar, W. E. Howard and R. E. Marsh

B3 1988   *Meat science, milk science and technology.* H. R. Cross and A. J. Overby

B4 1988   *Feed science.* E. R. Ørskov

B5 1987   *Bioclimatology and the adaptation of livestock.* H. D. Johnson.

B5 1987   *Animal production and environmental health.* D. Strauch

Subseries C: Production-system approach

C1 1982   *Sheep and goat production.* I. E. Coop

C2 1986   *Laboratory animals: laboratory animal models for domestic animal production.* E. J. Ruitenberg and P. W. J. Peters

C3 1987   *Dairy cattle production.* H. O. Gravert.

GENERAL VETERINARY BOOKS

376 **Aspinall, K. W.** *First steps in veterinary science.* London: Baillière Tindall, 1976. 213pp.
Introduction to veterinary science and practice for non-professional readers.

377 **Baker, J. K.** and **Greer, W. J.** *Animal health: a layman's guide to disease control.* Danville: Interstate Printers and Publishers, 1980. 402pp.

378 **Ellis, P. R.** *The management of animal health and productivity.* Oxford: Blackwell. Forthcoming.

379 **Hungerford, T. G.** *Diseases of livestock.* 8th ed. Sydney: McGraw-Hill, 1975. 1318pp.

380   Kelly, W. R. *Veterinary clinical diagnosis.* 3rd ed. London: Baillière Tindall, 1984. 440pp.
Describes history taking and the general examination of patients. Has sections on different body systems and on diagnostic tests.

381   Kirkbride, C. A. *Control of livestock diseases.* Springfield: C. C. Thomas, 1986. 152pp.
An outline of the effects of animal diseases, the predisposing factors and on methods for their prevention, control and eradication.

382   Parker, W. H. *Health and disease in farm animals: an introduction to farm animal medicine.* 3rd ed. Oxford: Pergamon, 1980. 307pp.
General introduction to animal health and medicine for farmers and agricultural students. Also describes basic animal anatomy and physiology.

383   Phillipson, A. T., Hall, L. W. and **Pritchard, W. R.** (eds) *Scientific foundations of veterinary medicine.* London: Heinemann, 1980. 438pp.
Has forty-nine chapters on aspects of veterinary physiology, metabolism and pathology. Attempts to outline the scientific basis underlying current clinical practice.

384   Sainsbury, D. *Animal health: health, disease and welfare of farm livestock.* London: Granada, 1983. 232pp.
For students and farmers. Describes how to maintain animals in good health in order to achieve maximum productivity.

385   Sainsbury, D. and **Sainsbury, P.** *Livestock health and housing.* 3rd ed. London: Baillière Tindall, 1988. 319pp.
Covers the factors (other than nutrition and genetics) that influence the production, health and welfare of housed animals. Disease prevention and animal welfare are emphasized throughout the text.

MATERIALS FOR ANCILLARY PERSONNEL

There is only a small body of literature available which is specifically intended for auxiliary personnel. Veterinary nurses and technicians will find useful information in many of the more detailed texts.

Dictionary

386   Handy-Marchello, B. *The veterinary technician's guide to medical terminology.* Reston, Virginia: Reston Publishing, 1984. 286pp.
A list of terms likely to be encountered with straightforward definitions. Abbreviations are included. US spelling is used.

Book Series

387 *Mosby's Fundamentals of Animal Health Technology.* 1983. Series editor R. G. Warren. St Louis: C. V. Mosby.
A series of basic texts for nurses and animal health technicians. Titles have appeared on:
  Principles of pharmacology. R. Giovanoni. 243pp.
  Small animal anesthesia. R. G. Warren. 367pp.
  Small animal radiography. L. J. Kleine. 178pp.
  Small animal surgical nursing. D. L. Tracey (ed.). 347pp.

Books

388 Alamargot, J. *Equipment for veterinary laboratories and clinics.* Maisons Alfort: IEMVT, 1986. 295pp. (Études et Synthèses de l'IEMVT, no. 17.)
Illustrated reference work for veterinary storekeepers and technicians.

389 Burton, N. R. (ed.) *A guide for receptionists in veterinary practice.* 2nd ed. Cheltenham: BSAVA, 1984. 84pp.

390 Heath, J. S. (ed.) in collaboration with the BSAVA RANA Committee. *Aids to nursing small animals and birds.* 2nd ed. London: Baillière Tindall, 1978. 198pp.
Designed as a pocket reference book for animal nurses.

391 Intravartolo, C. S. and **Richardson, R. C.** *The veterinary technician in small animal practice: patient management and client instructions.* Minneapolis: Burgess Publishing, 1983. 435pp.
Gives notes on each of the conditions which could be encountered in small animal practice, indicates the probable treatment and outlines the technician's role. History taking is discussed and the instructions to be given to the pet owner are indicated. Likely to be of use to both nurses and veterinary receptionists.

392 *Jones's Animal nursing.* 4th ed. Edited by D. R. Lane. Oxford: Pergamon, 1985. 706pp.
An essential text for those engaged in providing care for small animals. Covers both the principles and practice of the medical care of pet animals. Published on behalf of the BSAVA and is the standard textbook for those studying for qualifications in animal nursing. A new edition is in preparation.

393 McCurnin, D. M. (ed.) *Clinical texbook for veterinary technicians.* Philadelphia: W. B. Saunders, 1985. 511pp.
Intended as a reference text and textbook. Deals with large, small and exotic animals, medical and surgical nursing, restraint, anaesthesia, euthanasia and diagnostic techniques, record keeping and practice management.

394   *Manual for animal health auxiliary personnel.* Rome: FAO, 1983. 347pp.
Basic working manual for staff in developing countries.

395   Pratt, P. W. (ed.) *Laboratory procedures for animal health technicians.* Santa
Barbara: American Veterinary Publications, 1985. 486pp.
A manual for laboratory staff covering the use of laboratory equipment and
describing the range of tests, procedures and techniques which may be employed.

396   Pratt, P. W. (ed.) *Medical nursing for animal health technicians.* Santa Barbara:
American Veterinary Publications, 1985. 461pp.

397   Price, C. J. (ed.) *Practical veterinary nursing.* 2nd ed. Cheltenham: BSAVA,
1985. 200pp.
Covers the practical procedures laid down in the training scheme for nurses. Has
chapters on the nursing of birds, reptiles and wild mammals.

398   Solberg, V. *Laboratory manual for animal technicians.* Ames: Iowa State UP,
1985. 173pp.
Practical training manual with instructions on how to perform laboratory
procedures on animals. Includes lists of drugs, equipment and suppliers.

Journals

399   *The veterinary nursing journal.* 1986. c/o Editor, Mrs J. Gaymer, Model Farm,
Mentmore, Leighton Buzzard, Bedfordshire LU7 0QN, England: British
Veterinary Nursing Association. Bimonthly.
Includes brief articles, items of professional interest, reports of recent meetings
and details of forthcoming events.

400   *Veterinary technician.* 1970–. Lawrenceville: Veterinary Learning Systems.
Ten a year.
May be used with a formal continuing education programme.

Other Journal

New methods: the journal of animal health technology

Audiovisual Materials

401   *A catalogue of audio visual programmes for veterinary nurses, June 1987.* Edited by
J. Poland. London: Unit for Veterinary Continuing Education, 1987. 31pp.
Lists fifty-five items under four general headings, materials for the preliminary
nursing examination, for the final examination, for qualified veterinary nurses,
and for general background information. A new edition is in preparation.

10 Large Animals

GENERAL

Books

402 **Ashdown, R. R.** and **Done, S.** *Colour atlas of veterinary anatomy. Volume 1: The ruminants.* London: Baillière Tindall/Wolfe Medical Publications, 1984. Chapters paginated separately.
Deals with cattle, sheep and goats. Each photograph of a dissection is accompanied by a line drawing identifying the structures seen. Volume 2 deals with the horse. Volume 3, dealing with the dog, is in preparation.

403 **Blood, D. C.** and **Radostits, O. M.** with contributions by J. H. Arundel and C. C. Gay. *Veterinary medicine: a textbook of the diseases of cattle, sheep, pigs, goats and horses.* 7th ed. London: Baillière Tindall, 1989. 1502pp.
The standard reference work on large animal medicine. Each section in the book is supplemented by extensive reference lists to both review articles and original papers. The first section lists diseases according to body system; the second has sections on individual disease agents.

404 **Bogan, J. A., Lees, P.** and **Yoxall, A. T.** (eds) *Pharmacological basis of large animal medicine.* Oxford: Blackwell, 1983. 565pp.
Guide to the scientific principles underlying the rational use of drugs as therapeutic and managemental agents in large animal medicine.

405   Cox, J. E. *Surgery of the reproductive tract in large animals.* 3rd. ed. Liverpool: LUP, 1987. 194pp.
Concise illustrated handbook which arose from notes prepared for veterinary students.

406   *Current veterinary therapy: food animal practice – 2.* Edited by J. L. Howard. Philadelphia: W. B. Saunders, 1986. 1008pp.
Encyclopaedic reference work for the large animal practitioner. A vast amount of reference data is included in a text which reviews the prevention, therapy and management of disease in large animals.

407   Espinasse, J., Savey, M., Thorley, C. M., Toussaint Raven, E. and **Weaver, A. D.** *Atlas en couleur des affections du pied des bovins et des ovins – terminologie internationale.* Maisons Alfort: Éditions du Point Vétérinaire, 1984. 43pp.
A booklet, with text in English, Spanish and French, illustrating the classification of disorders of the ruminant digit which was proposed at the Fourth International Colloquium on Disorders of the Ruminant Digit held in 1982.

408   Jennings, P. B. (ed.) *The practice of large animal surgery.* Philadelphia: W. B. Saunders, 1984. 2 vols. 1233pp.
A comprehensive textbook covering all the procedures used in horses, cattle, sheep, goats and swine. Has a general section on basic principles and then surgical procedures are dealt with by body system.

409   Kersjes, A. W., Nemeth, F. and **Rutgers, L. J. E.** *A colour atlas of large animal surgery.* London: Wolfe Medical Publications, 1985. 143pp.
Illustrates 100 procedures mostly in cattle and horses. There is a brief accompanying text describing the conditions and the surgical techniques used. The book is intended to complement standard textbooks of surgery.

410   Oehme, F. W. (ed.) *Textbook of large animal surgery.* 2nd ed. Baltimore: Williams & Wilkins, 1988. 714pp.
Standard American reference work on general techniques and procedures in horses, cattle, sheep and goats.

411   Scott, D. W. *Large animal dermatology.* Philadelphia: W. B. Saunders, 1988. 487pp.
Thorough work which is organized into chapters on the agents and processes causing the diseases and disorders. Each chapter has a comprehensive bibliography. There are many illustrations including forty-eight in colour.

412   Turner, A. S. and **McIlwraith, C. W.** *Techniques in large animal surgery.* 2nd ed. Philadelphia: Lea & Febiger, 1988. 381pp.

Describes procedures on horses, cattle, swine, goats and the llama. Preliminary chapters discuss general aspects of large animal surgery.

413   Walker, D. F. and **Vaughan, J. T.** *Bovine and equine urogenital surgery.* Philadelphia: Lea & Febiger, 1980. 277pp.
Describes and illustrates more than sixty techniques.

Conferences

414   *Fifth international symposium on disorders of the ruminant digit, August 24–25, 1986, Veterinary College, University College, Dublin, Ireland.* Edited by A. D. Weaver. College of Veterinary Medicine, Columbia, Missouri 65211: Prof. A. D. Weaver, 1986. 106pp.

415   *Proceedings. Sixth international conference on production disease in farm animals, September 1986, Belfast, Northern Ireland.* Veterinary Research Laboratory, Stoney Road, Stormont, Belfast BT4 3SD, Northern Ireland: Dr D. A. Rice, 1986. 340pp.
Over sixty contributions concerned with disease and the improvement of productivity in cattle, sheep and pigs. The next conference is to be held in 1989 at Cornell University.

Journal

416   *Large animal veterinarian: covering health & nutrition.* 1945–. Mount Morris: Watt Publishing. Bimonthly.
Has eight or so brief review-type articles in each issue and news of new products. Previously known as *Animal health & nutrition: for large animal veterinarians* and *Animal health & nutrition for food animal veterinarians*.

CATTLE

There is a large amount of literature on the husbandry of both beef and dairy cattle. The optimization of production systems and the manipulation of reproduction are important aspects. Mastitis in dairy cows is the most significant disease.

Abstracting Service

417   *Dairy science abstracts.* 1939–. Wallingford: CAB International. Monthly.
Covers the whole of the science and technology of milk production and use. Has sections on cattle husbandry, milk and public health, mastitis and on the physiology and biochemistry of lactation.

Bibliography

418 *Mastitis literature survey*. 1972–. Wallingford: CAB International. Annual. Compiled from items originally published in *Veterinary bulletin* and *Dairy science abstracts*. The 1986 volume has 600 abstracts with an author index. Ongoing research projects are listed in the *Mastitis research index* published by the IDF [2207].

Books

419 Allen, D. and **Kilkenny, B.** *Planned beef production*. 2nd ed. London: Granada, 1984. 229pp.
Review of modern beef production techniques under British conditions.

420 Amstutz, H. E. (ed.) *Bovine medicine and surgery*. 2nd ed. Santa Barbara: American Veterinary Publications, 1980. 2 vols. 1269pp.
The only detailed work covering both the medicine and surgery of cattle and the standard American reference for bovine practitioners. About one-sixth of the text is devoted to surgical procedures.

421 Andrews, A. H. *Calf management and disease notes*. 25 Mardley Hill, Welwyn, Hertfordshire AL6 0TT: the Author, 1983. 284pp.
Gives brief but detailed notes on all aspects of calf management and disease. There are summary tables of differential diagnoses and of drug dosages.

422 Andrews, A. H. *Growing cattle management and disease notes. Part 1: management. Part 2: disease*. Welwyn: the Author, 1985–6. 2 vols. 167 + 372pp.
The first volume describes the management systems used for cattle from three months old to their entry to the dairy or suckler herd or their slaughter for beef. There are brief notes on the veterinary problems encountered. The second volume describes all the diseases occurring in British growing cattle. Appendices deal with the diseases grouped by common signs and there is a list of commonly used therapeutic agents quoting route of administration and dosage.

423 Armour, J. and **Ogbourne, C. P.** *Bovine ostertagiasis: a review and annotated bibliography*. Farnham Royal: CAB, 1982. 93pp. (Commonwealth Institute of Parasitology Miscellaneous Publication, no. 7.)
The review is supplemented by a bibliography of 379 papers all of which have abstracts.

424 *Badgers and bovine tuberculosis – a review of policy*. London: HMSO, 1986. 73pp.
The report of the Dunnet Committee. Indicates research needs, outlines action to reduce the risk of disease transmission and reconsiders badger removal operations

as a method for control. Further reviews are: *Bovine tuberculosis in badgers: twelfth report* (Surbiton: MAFF, 1988, 23pp.) and *The badger control policy: an economic assessment* (London: MAFF, 1987, 41pp. By A. P. Power and B. G. A. Watts. Government Economic Service Working Paper, no. 96).

425   Bargai, U., Pharr, J. W. and **Morgan, J. P.** *Bovine radiology.* Ames: Iowa State UP, 1989. 198pp. (Venture Series in Veterinary Medicine.)

426   Bath, D. L. *Dairy cattle: principles, practices, problems, profits.* 3rd ed. Philadelphia: Lea & Febiger, 1985. 473pp.

427   Belschner, H. G. and **Edwards, M. J.** *Cattle diseases.* 5th ed. London: Angus & Robertson, 1984. 378pp.
Introductory work for students and farmers.

428   Blowey, R. W. *A veterinary book for dairy farmers.* Ipswich: Farming Press, 1985. 397pp.
Stresses preventive medicine.

429   *British cattle.* Tring: National Cattle Breeders' Association, 1980. 132pp.
Descriptions and photographs of the breeds with details of breed societies.

430   Broster, W. H., Phipps, R. H. and **Johnson, C. L.** *Principles and practice of feeding dairy cows.* Reading: National Institute for Research in Dairying, 1986. 322pp. (NIRD Technical Publications, no. 8.)

431   Butterworth, M. H. *Beef cattle nutrition and tropical pastures.* London: Longman, 1985. 500pp.
Describes the nature of tropical grasslands and the nutritional characteristics of tropical forages. Nutritional deficiencies are discussed in depth.

432   *Calf rearing.* 6th ed. London: HMSO, 1984. 48pp. (MAFF Reference Book 10.)
Covers feeding, environment and housing, husbandry and disease control and has recommendations on the treatment of the in-calf cow.

433   Castle, M. E. and **Watkins, P.** *Modern milk production: its principles for students and farmers.* 2nd ed. London: Faber, 1984. 310pp.

434   *The cattle industry and welfare in Great Britain.* Alnwick: MAFF, 1984. 56pp. (MAFF Booklet 2482.)
Describes husbandry practices in Britain and reviews current knowledge on environmental control and cattle behaviour in relation to welfare.

435   Cooper, M. McG. and **Willis, M. B.** *Profitable beef production.* 4th ed. Ipswich: Farming Press, 1984. 200pp.

436   *Dairy herd fertility.* London: HMSO, 1984. 80pp. (MAFF Reference Book 259.)
A guide to reproductive physiology and the use of hormones in controlled breeding. Also describes various fertility recording systems.

437   Diggins, R. V., Bundy, C. E. and **Christensen, V. W.** *Beef production.* 4th ed. Englewood Cliffs: Prentice-Hall, 1984. 256pp.

438   Diggins, R. V., Bundy, C. E. and **Christensen, V. W.** *Dairy production.* 5th ed. Englewood Cliffs: Prentice-Hall, 1984. 326pp.

439   England, R. B. *A guide to age determination of cattle: incisor tooth eruption, development and attrition.* Santa Barbara: Veterinary Practice Publishing, 1984. 10pp.

440   Ensminger, M. E. *Beef cattle science.* 6th ed. Danville: Interstate Printers and Publishers, 1987. 1030pp.

441   Ensminger, M. E. *Dairy cattle science.* 2nd ed. Danville: Interstate Printers and Publishers, 1980. 625pp.

442   Esslemont, R. J., Bailie, J. H. and **Cooper, M. J.** *Fertility management in dairy cattle.* London: Collins, 1985. 143pp.
Complete review of fertility management including preventive veterinary medicine schemes, record keeping and the physiology of reproduction.

443   Etgen, W. M. (ed.) *Dairy cattle: feeding and management.* 7th ed. New York: John Wiley, 1987. 598pp.

444   Faull, W. B., Hughes, J. W., Clarkson, M. J. and **Walton, G. S.** *Mastitis notes for the dairy practitioner.* 4th ed. Liverpool: LUP, 1987. 82pp.
Deals with clinical mastitis and outlines the basics of mastitis control.

445   Felius, M. *Genus* Bos: *cattle breeds of the world.* Rahway, New Jersey: MSD AGVET, 1985. 234pp.
Provides an illustration and brief details on each breed. Cattle breeds are also described in J. Friend and D. Bishop's *Cattle of the world* (Poole: Blandford Press, 1978, 198pp.).

446   Fuller, R. *Suckled calf production.* Hurley: Chalcombe Publications, 1988. 85pp.
Guide to the management of suckler cows and their calves.

447   Greenough, P. R., MacCallum, F. J. and **Weaver, A. D.** *Lameness in cattle.* 2nd ed. Edited by A. D. Weaver. Bristol: Wright/Scientechnica, 1981. 471pp.
Comprehensive profusely illustrated work on bovine locomotor disorders. Has a bibliography of 917 items.

448   Hardy, R. and **Meadowcroft, S.** *Indoor beef production.* Ipswich: Farming Press, 1986. 159pp.

449   Hill, D. *Cattle and buffalo meat production in the tropics.* London: Longman. Forthcoming.

450   Hinks, W. *Breeding dairy cattle.* Ipswich: Farming Press, 1983. 106pp.

451   Jensen, R. and **Mackey, D. R.** *Diseases of feedlot cattle.* 3rd ed. Philadelphia: Lea & Febiger, 1979. 300pp.
The majority of cattle in the United States are finished for fattening in feedlots. This book concentrates on diseases of the digestive and respiratory system.

452   Jørgensen, R. J. and **Ogbourne, C. P.** *Bovine dictyocauliasis: a review and annotated bibliography.* Farnham Royal: CAB, 1985. 104pp. (Commonwealth Institute of Parasitology Miscellaneous Publication, no. 8.)
A review of current knowledge on *Dictyocaulus viviparus* parasitic bronchitis in cattle. There is bibliography of 383 abstracts of papers published since 1968.

453   Juergenson, E. M. *Approved practices in beef cattle production.* 5th ed. Danville: Interstate Printers and Publishers, 1980. 467pp.

454   Juergenson, E. M. and **Mortenson, W. P.** *Approved practices in dairying.* 4th ed. Danville: Interstate Printers and Publishers, 1977. 353pp.

455   Kahrs, R. F. *Viral diseases of cattle.* Ames: Iowa State UP, 1981. 299pp.

456   Kiley-Worthington, M. and **De La Plain, S.** *The behaviour of beef suckler cattle* (Bos taurus). Basel: Birkhauser, 1983. 196pp. (Tierhaltung/Animal Management, vol. 14.)

457   Ladds, P. W. *A colour atlas of lymph node pathology in cattle.* Ames: Iowa State UP, 1986. 80pp.
Has 246 photographs of nodal changes caused by diseases and likely to be encountered in the post-mortem laboratory and slaughterhouse.

458   Lean, I. *Nutrition of dairy cattle.* Sydney: Post-Graduate Committee in Veterinary Science, 1987. 485pp.
Survey of the theory and practice of the nutrition of dairy cattle written for both

the livestock producer and veterinary surgeon. The diseases and disorders associated with nutritional problems are covered.

459   Leaver, J. D. *Milk production: science and practice.* London: Longman, 1983. 173pp. (Longman Handbooks in Agriculture.)

460   Miller, W. J. *Dairy cattle feeding and nutrition.* New York: Academic Press, 1979. 411pp. (Animal Feeding and Nutrition.)

461   Neumann, A. L. and **Lusby, K. S.** *Beef cattle.* 8th ed. New York: John Wiley, 1986. 326pp.
Guide to the science and practice of beef cattle husbandry with particular reference to conditions in the United States.

462   Noakes, D. E. *Fertility and obstetrics in cattle.* Oxford: Blackwell, 1986. 139pp. (Library of Veterinary Practice.)
Review in note form for the student and practitioner.

463   Owen, J. B. *Cattle feeding.* Ipswich: Farming Press, 1983. 170pp.

464   Pasquini, C. (ed.) *Atlas of bovine anatomy.* Eureka: Sudz Publishing, 1982. 335pp.
Consists of line drawings labelled with terms from the *Nomina anatomica veterinaria*.

465   Pavaux, C. *A color atlas of bovine visceral anatomy.* London: Wolfe Medical Publications, 1983. 168pp.
Uses 220 photographs of dissections to demostrate the visceral anatomy of the cow.

466   Payne, J. M. *Metabolic and nutritional diseases of cattle.* Oxford: Blackwell, 1989. 149pp. (Library of Veterinary Practice.)

467   Payne, W. J. A. *Cattle production in the tropics. Volume 1: General introduction and breeds and breeding.* London: Longman, 1970. 336pp. (Tropical Agriculture Series.)
Describes cattle husbandry systems in the tropics with discussions of breeding methods and fertility. Includes detailed descriptions of the breeds.

468   Perry, T. W. *Beef cattle feeding and nutrition.* New York: Academic Press, 1980. 383pp. (Animal Feeding and Nutrition.)

469   Peters, A. R. and **Ball, P. J. H.** *Reproduction in cattle.* London: Butterworths, 1987. 191pp.

The most recent text providing an introduction to the subject of bovine reproduction for both agriculturalists and veterinarians.

470   Preston, T. R. and **Willis, M. B.** *Intensive beef production*. 2nd ed. Oxford: Pergamon, 1974. 567pp.

471   Rosenberger, G. (ed.) *Clinical examination of cattle*. Translated by R. Mack. Berlin: Paul Parey, 1979. 453pp.
Guide to the techniques and procedures used in the diagnosis of diseases and disorders in cattle. There many illustrations and colour plates. A companion volume, *Krankheiten des Rindes* (1970, 1,390pp.) on cattle diseases proper, is available only in German.

472   Rouse, J. E. *World cattle*. Norman: University of Oklahoma Press, 1970–3. 3 vols. 1046 (vols 1 & 2) + 650pp.
The status of the cattle industry in each country is reviewed with information on the cattle breeds and cattle diseases.

473   Roy, J. H. B. *The calf*. 4th ed. London: Butterworths, 1980. 442pp. (Studies in the Agricultural and Food Sciences.)
Comprehensive discussion of the management and rearing of calves which discusses nutrition in detail and has sections on calf mortality and diseases.

474   Russell, K. and **Slater, S.** *The principles of dairy farming*. 10th ed. Ipswich: Farming Press, 1985. 316pp.

475   Schalm, O. W., Carroll, E. J. and **Jain, N. C.** *Bovine mastitis*. Philadelphia: Lea & Febiger, 1971. 360pp.

476   Schmidt, P. J. and **Yeates, N. T. M.** *Beef cattle production*. 2nd ed. Sydney: Butterworths, 1985. 338pp.

477   Sloss, V. and **Dufty, J. H.** *Handbook of bovine obstetrics*. Baltimore: Williams & Wilkins, 1980. 208pp.
Covers obstetrical anatomy, physiology and pathology and describes specific obstetric procedures.

478   Stansfield, M. *The new herdsman's book*. Ipswich: Farming Press, 1983. 179pp.
Basic manual of stockmanship.

479   Straiton, E. *Calving the cow and care of the calf: The TV Vet book series for stock farmers No. 2*. 3rd ed. Ipswich: Farming Press, 1988. 164pp.

480   Straiton, E. *Cattle ailments – recognition and treatment: The TV Vet book series for stock farmers No. 1*. 5th ed. Ipswich: Farming Press, 1987. 167pp.

481   Thickett, W., Mitchell, D. and **Hallows, B.** *Calf rearing*. Ipswich: Farming Press, 1986. 139pp.

482   Thomas, V. M. *Beef cattle production: an integrated approach*. Philadelphia: Lea & Febiger, 1986. 270pp.
Overview of current US practice. Concentration on bovine reproduction.

483   Thompson, G. B. and **O'Mary, C. C.** (eds.) *The feedlot*. 3rd ed. Philadelphia: Lea & Febiger, 1983. 306pp.
Reviews the husbandry and feeding methods used in feedlots in the intensive production of beef cattle in North America. Has a chapter on diseases and parasites.

484   Toussaint Raven, E. *Cattle footcare and claw trimming*. Ipswich: Farming Press, 1985. 126pp.
A practical manual on claw trimming and a general discussion of foot ailments.

485   Weaver, A. D. *Bovine surgery and lameness*. Oxford: Blackwell, 1986. 237pp. (Library of Veterinary Practice.)
Information is presented in note form on surgical procedures and on lameness.

486   Webster, A. J. F. *Understanding the dairy cow*. Oxford: Blackwell, 1987. 357pp.
A basic text on the reproductive biology, physiology, behaviour and health of the dairy cow. Written for the stockman and student in order to develop good practice in dairy cow husbandry.

487   Webster, J. *Calf husbandry, health and welfare*. London: Granada, 1984. 202pp.
Introductory work explaining the scientific basis of calf rearing. Common diseases and their recognition are discussed. Alternatives to traditional veal calf production systems are described.

488   Wenkoff, M. S. *The evaluation of bulls for breeding soundness*. Ottawa: Canadian Veterinary Medical Association, 1987. 48pp.

489   Whittemore, C. T. *Lactation of the dairy cow*. London: Longman, 1980. 94pp. (Longman Handbooks in Agriculture.)

490   Wilkinson, J. M. *Beef production from silage and other conserved forages*. London: Longman, 1985. 140pp.

491   Wilson, P. N. and **Brigstocke, T. D. A.** *Improved feeding of cattle and sheep.* London: Granada, 1981. 238pp.

Conferences

492   *Bovine respiratory disease: a symposium.* Edited by R. W. Loan. College Station: Texas A & M University Press, 1984. 520pp.
Contains review papers on the causative agents and on aspects of the immunology of respiratory disease.

493   *The British Mastitis Conference: jointly organised by the Milk Marketing Board, AFRC Institute for Animal Health and Ciba-Geigy Agrochemicals.* Animal Health Department, Whittlesford, Cambridge CB2 4QT, England: Ciba-Geigy Agrochemicals, 1988. 64pp.
The conference held on 20 October 1988 was the first in what are intended to be annual events.

Journals

494   *Agri-practice.* 1980–. Santa Barbara: Veterinary Practice Publishing. Bimonthly.
The majority of the eight or so papers in each issue concern cattle, some deal with pigs. Most are on aspects of reproduction or nutrition, frequently they are on pharmacological or clinical evaluations of new products. Volumes **1–3** were entitled *Bovine practice.*

495   *Dairy farmer.* 1929–. Ipswich: Farming Press. Monthly.

496   *Hoard's dairyman.* 1885–. 28 Milwaukee Avenue West, Fort Atkinson, Wisconsin 53538: Hoard's Dairyman. Fortnightly.

497   *Journal of dairy research.* 1929–. Cambridge: CUP. Quarterly.
Has some articles on the physiology and biochemistry of lactation and on mastitis but is mostly concerned with the science of the utilization of milk.

498   *Journal of dairy science.* 1917–. 309 West Clark Street, Champaign, Illinois 61820: American Dairy Science Association. Monthly.
Each issue has many papers on the physiology and biochemistry of milk production. Supplements contain abstracts from the ADSA's annual and branch meetings.

Other Journals

Australian dairy farmer
Drovers journal
Journal of the Society of Dairy Technology
Milk producer
New Zealand journal of dairy science and technology
Science African journal of dairy science

BUFFALOES

Buffaloes are multipurpose animals providing both meat and milk, and are the classic draught animals of Asia.

Bibliography

499 *Bibliography on swamp buffalo 1976–85.* Bangkok: International Buffalo Information Center, 1987. 274pp.
Has abstracts of 564 items and updates Ross Cockrill's text. There are author and subject indexes.

Directory

500 *Directory of names in buffalo studies and research.* Bangkok: International Buffalo Information Center, 1984. 76pp.
Arranged by country. Gives the names and addresses of 626 individuals working on buffaloes in forty-one countries and the entries indicate their field of work. There is a name index and an index to fields of interest.

Books

501 **Basu, S. B.** *Genetic improvement of buffaloes.* New Delhi: Kalyani Publishers, 1985. 187pp.

502 **Cockrill, W. Ross** (ed.) *The husbandry and health of the domestic buffalo.* Rome: FAO, 1974. 993pp.
An encyclopaedic work on the biology and utilization of the water buffalo, *Bubalus bubalis*. The distribution and potential of the buffalo in various geographic regions is reviewed. There is a bibliography of over 4,000 references and many colour and black and white illustrations. An abridged but updated version has been published in the FAO's Animal Production and Health Series (no. 4, 1977).

503   Cockrill, W. Ross *The buffaloes of China*. Rome: FAO, 1976. 96pp.

504   Mloszewski, M. J. *Behavior and ecology of the African buffalo*. Cambridge: CUP, 1983. 256pp.

Conferences

505   *Proceedings of the buffalo seminar, 29 April–2 May 1985, Bangkok, Thailand*. Edited by C. Chantalakhana. Bangkok: International Buffalo Information Center, 1986. 355pp.

506   *The use of nuclear techniques to improve domestic buffalo production in Asia: proceedings of the final research co-ordination meeting organised by the Joint FAO/IAEA Division of Isotope and Radiation Applications of Atomic Energy for Food and Agriculture Development and held in Manila, Philippines, 30 January–3 February 1984*. Vienna: International Atomic Energy Agency, 1984. 218pp. (Panel Proceedings Series.)
Contains reports of research projects carried out using nuclear techniques and gives recommendations for further studies.

Journals

507   *Buffalo bulletin*. 1982–. Bangkok: International Buffalo Information Center. Quarterly.
Contains news, information and short articles.

508   *Buffalo journal*. 1986–. Faculty of Veterinary Science, Chulalongkorn University, Bangkok 10500, Thailand: Research Centre for Bioscience in Animal Production. Biannual.

509   *International Buffalo Association newsletter*. 1988–. 3811 SW 95th Avenue, Miami, Florida 33165: World Buffalo Association. Monthly.

DEER

The farming of deer has become popular over the last few decades. Venison is a lean meat which has proved attractive to consumers.

Bibliographies

510   Arora, B. M. *Disease of cervids: a bibliography*. 2nd ed. Izatnagar 243 122, India: Indian Veterinary Research Institute, 1986. 145pp.

511   Morton, J. K. and **Dieterich, R. A.** *Bibliography of reindeer/caribou investigators*. Fairbanks: Institute of Arctic Biology, University of Alaska, 1983. 55pp.

Books and Reviews

512   Alexander, T. L. (ed.) *Management and diseases of deer: a handbook for the veterinary surgeon*. London: Veterinary Deer Society, 1986. 254pp.
A comprehensive account, written in a concise form, of all aspects of deer in health and disease.

513   Blaxter, Sir K. L., Kay, R. N. B., Sharman, G. A. M., Cunningham, J. M. M., Eadie, J. and **Hamilton, W. J.** *Farming the red deer*. London: HMSO, 1988. 169pp.
Reports of joint investigations, over the period 1973–82, by the Rowett Research Institute and the Hill Farming Research Organisation into the farming of deer.

514   Chaplin, R. E. *Deer*. Poole: Blandford Press, 1977. 218pp.
Well illustrated discussion on the biology of deer. Covers all the world's deer.

515   Dasmann, W. *Deer range: improvement and management*. Jefferson, North Carolina: McFarland & Company, 1981. 168pp.
Reviews the management of deer habitats with reference to North American conditions. There is an extensive bibliography.

516   Davidson, W. R., Hayes, F. A., Nettles, V. F. and **Kellogg, F. E.** *Diseases and parasites of white-tailed deer*. Tallahassee, Florida: Tall Timbers Research Station, 1981. 458pp. (Miscellaneous Publication, no. 7.)
The twenty-nine chapters cover all the important diseases and parasites and review related aspects of health such as trauma, necropsy procedures, physiologic values and disease investigation, prevention and control.

517   de Nahlik, A. J. *Wild deer: culling, conservation and management*. 2nd ed. Southampton: Ashford Press Publishing, 1987. 264pp.

518   Fletcher, J. 'Veterinary aspects of deer management. 1: Management. 2: Disease.' *In practice* **9** (1987): (1) 4–7 and **9** (1987): (3) 94–7.

519   Rudge, A. J. B. (ed.) *The capture and handling of deer*. Peterborough: Nature Conservancy Council, 1984. 273pp.
Contains a review of the capture and handling of deer, guidelines on their safe and humane handling and detailed data sheets on seven species which are found wild in Britain.

520   Vipond, J. E. *Red deer farming in Scotland*. Cleeve Gardens, Oakbank Road, Perth PH1 1HF, Scotland: Scottish Agricultural Colleges, 1987. 47pp.
Gives general advice on the farm management of red deer.

521   Yerek, D. (ed.) *The farming of deer: world trends and modern techniques*. Wellington 1, New Zealand: Agricultural Promotion Associates, 1982. 176pp.
There are reviews of deer farming in various geographic regions and chapters on a number of aspects of deer farming as practised in New Zealand. A chapter is devoted to diseases.

522   Yerex, D. and **Spiers, I.** *Modern deer farm management*. Box 176, Carterton, New Zealand: Ampersand Publishing Associates, 1987. 168pp.

Conferences

523   *Biology of deer production: proceedings of the international conference held at Dunedin, New Zealand, 13–18 February 1983*. Edited by P. F. Fennessy and K. R. Drew. Wellington, New Zealand, 1985. 482pp. (Bulletin, Royal Society of New Zealand, no. 22.)

524   *Biology and management of the Cervidae*. Edited by C. M. Wemmer. Washington, DC: Smithsonian Institute Press, 1987. 577pp. (Research Symposia of the National Zoological Park.)

525   *Proceedings of a deer course for veterinarians, Dunedin, July 1987*. Auckland: Deer Branch of the New Zealand Veterinary Association, 1988. 194pp. (Deer Branch Course, no. 4.)
The courses are held annually.

526   *Proceedings of the fourth international reindeer/caribou symposium, Whitehorse, Yukon, Canada, 22–25 August 1985*. Edited by A. Gunn, F. L. Miller and S. Sjenneberg. Box 378, N-9401 Harstad, Norway: Nordic Council for Reindeer Research. *Rangifer* Special issue no. 1 (1986): 374pp.

Journals

527   *Deer* 1966– c/o Editor, Highland Water, The Drove, West End, Southampton SO3 3EF, England: British Deer Society. Three per year.
The society has also sponsored the publication of a *Field guide to British deer*. (3rd ed. by F. J. Taylor Page, Oxford: Blackwell, 1982, 95pp.). Most issues of *Deer* and *Deer farming* have two or three articles on health aspects.

528   *Deer farming*. 1981–. c/o Editor, Pantwgan Deer Farm, Llanarthney, Camarthen, Dyfed SA32 8NZ, Wales: British Deer Farmers' Association. Quarterly.

Other Journal

Deer talk

SHEEP

Sheep are farmed world-wide under many different production systems. Wool and meat have been the traditional products but the use of sheep for milk production is growing. Much of the research work on sheep is carried out in Australia and New Zealand.

Directory

529 *Directory of current research on sheep and goats.* Edited by J. W. B. King. Wallingford: CAB International, 1988. 271pp.
Lists current research projects together with details of publications arising from them. The basic organization is by the institute at which the work is being performed. There are author and subject indexes.

Books

530 **Barlow, R. M.** and **Patterson, D. S. P.** (eds) 'Border disease of sheep: a virus-induced teratogenic disorder'. *Fortschritte der Veterinärmedizin* **36** (1982): 90pp.

531 **Belschner, H. G.** *Sheep management and diseases.* 10th ed. London: Angus & Robertson, 1976. 838pp.

532 **Blunt, M. H.** (ed.) *The blood of sheep: composition and function.* Berlin: Springer-Verlag, 1975. 224pp.
Contains reviews on a variety of aspects of the cellular and biochemical constituents of sheep's blood.

533 **Botkin, M. P., Field, R. A.** and **Johnson, C. L.** *Sheep and wool: science, production and management.* Englewood Cliffs: Prentice-Hall, 1988. 451pp.

534 *British sheep.* 7th ed. Tring: National Sheep Association, 1987. 242pp.
An illustrated guide to British breeds. Includes a list of contact points for the Breed Societies. There is a glossary of sheep terms.

535 **Bryson, T.** *Sheep housing handbook.* Ipswich: Farming Press, 1984. 153pp.

536 **Carles, A. B.** *Sheep production in the tropics.* Oxford: OUP, 1983. 213pp. (Oxford Tropical Handbooks.)

537   **Clarkson, M. J.** and **Faull, W. B.** *Notes for the sheep clinician.* 3rd ed. Liverpool: LUP, 1987. 175pp.
Provides a clear summary of disease problems in sheep and relates this information to economics and production. The work evolved from notes written for veterinary students.

538   **Cooper, M. McG.** and **Thomas, R. J.** *Profitable sheep farming.* 5th ed. Ipswich: Farming Press, 1982. 192pp.
Has a chapter on ailments of sheep.

539   **Croston, D.** and **Pollott, G. E.** *Planned sheep production.* London: Collins, 1985. 211pp.
Uses the British sheep industry as a model for a discussion of methods of improving production schemes. Chapters discuss hill, upland and lowland sheep production systems.

540   **Davies, A. S., Garden, K. L., Young, M. J.** and **Reid, C. S. W.** *An atlas of X-ray tomographical anatomy of the sheep.* Wellington, New Zealand: Department of Scientific and Industrial Research, 1987. 118pp.

541   **Day, G.** and **Jessup, J.** (eds) *The history of the Australian merino.* Richmond, Australia: Heinemann, 1984. 180pp.

542   **Dolling, C. H. S.** *Breeding merinos.* Adelaide: Rigby, 1970. 266pp.

543   **Downing, E.** *Keeping sheep.* 2nd ed. London: Pelham Books, 1987. 144pp. (Garden Farming Series.)
A guide to small scale sheep farming. Other titles by the same author deal with goats, pigs and rabbits.

544   **Dubey, J. P.** and **Towle, A.** *Toxoplasmosis in sheep: a review and annotated bibliography.* Farnham Royal: CAB International, 1986. 152pp. (Commonwealth Institute of Parasitology Miscellaneous Publication, no. 10.)
A critical review of research on *Toxoplasma gondii* with an annotated bibliography of over 300 abstracts published since 1950.

545   **Eales, F. A.** and **Small, J.** with drawings by **D. M. Pollack.** *Practical lambing: a guide to veterinary care at lambing.* London: Longman, 1986. 132pp.
Intended for the shepherd and indicates throughout when veterinary assistance is required.

546   **Ensminger, M. E.** and **Parker, R. O.** *Sheep and goat science.* 5th ed. Danville: Interstate Printers and Publishers, 1986. 643pp.
A comprehensive work of particular relevance to those engaged in sheep and goat husbandry in the USA.

547   Fell, H. R. *Intensive sheep management.* 2nd ed. Ipswich: Farming Press, 1985. 260pp.
Up to date discussion of the methods used in intensifying sheep production in the UK.

548   Fraser, A. and **Stamp, J. T.** revised by **J. M. M. Cunningham** and **J. T. Stamp.** *Sheep husbandry and diseases.* 6th ed. London: Collins, 1987. 344pp.
An overview of sheep production in which eight of the twenty chapters provide straightforward discussions of sheep diseases.

549   Gatenby, R. M. *Sheep production in the tropics and sub-tropics.* London: Longman, 1986. 351pp. (Tropical Agriculture Series.)
Relates research results and knowledge obtained with breeds in temperate climates to the problems of improving sheep production in tropical areas. There is a directory of breeds of sheep in the tropics and an extensive bibliography,

550   Goodwin, D. H. *Sheep management and production: a practical guide for farmers and students.* 2nd ed. London: Hutchinson, 1979. 224pp.
Straightforward introduction to sheep production practices.

551   Hart, E. *Sheep: a guide to management.* Marlborough: Crowood Press, 1985. 121pp.
Introduction to the basics of sheep husbandry.

552   Hecker, J. F. *The sheep as an experimental animal.* London: Academic Press, 1983. 216pp.
A brief introduction to the topic but containing much factual data and a large bibliography. Chapters deal with anatomy, physiology and genetics, behaviour, breeds and supply of sheep, management, sampling and recording, and diseases and parasites.

553   Henderson, D. *A veterinary book for sheep farmers.* Ipswich: Farming Press. Forthcoming.

554   Johnston, R. G. *Introduction to sheep farming.* London: Collins, 1983. 266pp.

555   Juergenson, E. M. *Approved practices in sheep production.* 4th ed. Danville: Interstate Printers and Publishers, 1981. 455pp.
A practical guide to tried and tested methods currently in use in the husbandry of sheep in the United States.

556   Kimberling, C. V. (ed.) *Jensen and Swift's diseases of sheep.* 3rd ed. Philadelphia: Lea & Febiger, 1988. 394pp.

The most up-to-date veterinary text. Separate sections deal with the diseases of breeding sheep and nursing lambs, feedlot lambs and adult sheep. Each disease is reviewed with references to the literature.

557   Martin, W. B. (ed.) *Diseases of sheep.* Oxford: Blackwell, 1983. 282pp.
A comprehensive survey for the veterinary surgeon. Similar to Jensen and Swift's monograph but directed at veterinarians serving the sheep industry in Britain and Europe.

558   Mason, I. L. *Sheep breeds of the Mediterranean.* Farnham Royal: FAO/CAB, 1967. 215pp.
Includes 157 photographs of breeds.

559   May, N. D. S. *The anatomy of the sheep: a dissection manual.* 3rd ed. St Lucia, Australia: University of Queensland Press, 1970. 369pp.

560   Mills, O. *Practical sheep dairying: the care and milking of the dairy ewe.* Wellingborough: Thorsons, 1982. 224pp.

561   Owen, J. B. *Sheep production.* London: Baillière Tindall, 1976. 436pp.
A summary of knowledge on sheep production and the factors affecting efficiency in sheep production systems.

562   Owen, J. B. *Performance recording in sheep.* Farnham Royal: CAB, 1971. 132pp. (Commonwealth Bureau of Animal Breeding and Genetics Technical Communication, no. 20.)
Reviews the methods of performance recording used throughout the world and discusses the use of the information so obtained in sheep improvement.

563   Parry, H. B. *Scrapie disease in sheep: historical, clinical, epidemiological, pathological and practical aspects of the natural disease.* Edited by D. R. Oppenheimer. London: Academic Press, 1983. 192pp.

564   Ponting, K. *Sheep of the world.* Poole: Blandford Press, 1980. 155pp.
Gives a brief account of the early history of sheep and describes the breeds. There are fifty-two colour illustrations.

565   Ryder, M. L. *Sheep and man.* London: Duckworth, 1983. 846pp.
Comprehensive survey of the association of man with sheep from ancient to modern times.

566 *Sheep handling and dipping.* London: HMSO, 1984. 34pp. (MAFF Booklet 2332.)

567   *The shepherd's guide: a guide to the diseases of sheep and the care and training of sheepdogs.* 38 Elliot Street, Glasgow G3 8JT, Scotland: Robert Young & Co., 1985. 156pp.
The most recent edition of a standard work. A practical guide for the shepherd and sheep farmer. Intended as an adjunct to veterinary advice.

568   **Spedding, C. R. W.** *Sheep production and grazing management.* 2nd ed. London: Baillière Tindall, 1970. 435pp.

569   **Speedy, A. W.** *Sheep production: science into practice.* London: Longman, 1980. 195pp. (Longman Handbooks in Agriculture.)
A good introduction to the scientific principles of sheep production.

570   **Thedford, T. R.** *Sheep health handbook: a field guide for producers with limited veterinary services.* Morrilton: Winrock International, 1983. 132pp.

571   **Turner, H. N.** and **Young, S. S. Y.** *Quantitative genetics in sheep breeding.* South Melbourne, Victoria, Australia: Macmillan, 1969. 332pp.
A technical monograph with much detail on the mathematics of genetic variation.

572   *The TV Vet sheep book: recognition and treatment of common sheep ailments.* 5th ed. Ipswich: Farming Press, 1986. 192pp.

Conferences

573   *Efficient sheep production from grass. Proceedings of a symposium organised jointly with the National Sheep Association held at Harrogate, North Yorkshire 4–5 November 1986.* Edited by G. E. Pollott. c/o Institute for Grassland and Animal Production, Hurley, Maidenhead SL6 5LR, England: British Grassland Society, 1987. 212pp. (BGS Occasional Symposium, no. 21.)

574   *Footrot in ruminants. Proceedings of a workshop, Melbourne 1985.* Edited by D. J. Stewart, J. E. Peterson, N. M. McKern and D. L. Emery. Glebe, New South Wales 2037, Australia: CSIRO Division of Animal Health, 1986. 283pp.
Modern survey of the disease and of current knowledge on its causative agent *Bacteroides nodosus.*

575   *Immunogenetic approaches to the control of endoparasites, with particular reference to parasites of sheep. Proceedings of a workshop held at Sydney University, October 22–23, 1983.* Edited by J. K. Dineen and P. M. Outteridge. 314 Albert Street, East Melbourne, Victoria 3002, Australia: CSIRO, 1984. 169pp.
The papers deal with helminth parasites.

576   **Land, R. B.** and **Robinson, D. W.** (eds) *Genetics of reproduction in sheep.* London: Butterworths, 1985. 427pp.

Contains thirty-nine papers, mostly dealing with genetic variation and the Booroola gene, from a workshop held in Edinburgh.

577   Lindsay, D. R. and **Pearce, D. T.** (eds) *Reproduction in sheep*. Canberra: Australian Academy of Science, 1984. 403pp. (Australian Wool Corporation Technical Publication.)
Has twenty-three reviews and over sixty research papers on aspects of reproduction. Outside Australia distributed by Cambridge University Press.

578   *The management and diseases of sheep. Papers presented at a British Council special course, Edinburgh, 5–17 March 1978*. London/Slough: British Council/CAB, 1979. 469pp.
Comprises thirty-eight review papers on aspects of sheep health and production.

579   Marai, I. F. M and **Owen, J. B.** (eds) *New techniques in sheep production*. London: Butterworths, 1987. 292pp.
A collection of reviews on methods of improving sheep production. Among the techniques covered are: increasing fecundity, genetic improvement, breed development, reproductive management and health control, and on the performance of the current systems used for the production of wool, meat and milk.

580   Tomes, G. J., Robertson, D. E. and **Lightfoot, R. J.** (eds) *Sheep breeding*. 2nd ed. Revised by W. Haresign. London: Butterworths, 1979. 580pp. (Studies in the Agricultural and Food Sciences.)
Has sixty-five papers, ten of which review the sheep industries in particular countries.

Journals

581   *The sheep farmer*. 1971–. The Sheep Centre, Malvern, Worcestershire WR13 6PH, England: National Sheep Association. Ten a year.

582   *Sheep dairy news*. 1984–. Wield Wood, Alresford, Hampshire SO24 9RU, England: Secretary—BSDA. Three a year.
Journal of the British Sheep Dairying Association. Most issues usually include a brief article on a veterinary topic.

583   *Wool technology and sheep breeding*. 1954–. Box 1, Kensington, New South Wales 2033, Australia: Wool Technology Press. Quarterly.
Compiled by the Department of Wool Science of the University of New South Wales.

Other Journals

National wool grower
Sheep breeder and sheepman magazine
Sheep Canada

GOATS

Goats have always been important domestic animals in developing countries and they are becoming increasingly popular in developed countries as sources of meat, milk and highly prized cashmere and mohair fibre.

Books

584   Chatelain, E. *Atlas d'anatomie de la chèvre* (Capra hircus). Route de St-Cyr, 78000 Versailles, France: INRA Publications, 1987. 203pp.

585   *Code of practice: the hygienic production of goats' milk.* Alnwick: MAFF, undated. 32pp.

586   Devendra, C. and **Burns, M.** (eds) *Goat production in the tropics.* 2nd ed. Farnham Royal: CAB, 1983. 183pp.
Discusses the breeds, their husbandry and comparative performance. Contains a bibliography of about 750 items.

587   Devendra, C. and **McLeroy, G. B.** *Goat and sheep production in the tropics.* London: Longman, 1982. 271pp. (Intermediate Tropical Agriculture Series.)
The two species are given equal space in this work which, with its numerous photographs and practical approach, is suited to students and extension workers.

588   Downing, E. *Keeping goats.* 2nd ed. London: Pelham Books, 1984. 128pp. (Garden Farming Series.)

589   Dunn, P. *The goatkeeper's veterinary book.* 2nd ed. Ipswich: Farming Press, 1987. 198pp.
A popular reference work on the ailments of goats for both the goat-keeper and veterinary surgeon dealing with goats.

590   Gall, C. (ed.) *Goat production.* London: Academic Press, 1981. 619pp.
Comprehensive discussion of all aspects of goats and their uses by man worldwide. Has a chapter on diseases.

591   **Garrett, P. D.** *Guide to ruminant anatomy based on the dissection of the goat.* Iowa: Iowa State UP, 1988. 102pp.
Illustrations of the anatomy of the ox are included where appropriate.

592   **Guss, S. B.** *Management and diseases of dairy goats.* Scottsdale: Dairy Goat Journal Publishing, 1977. 222pp.

593   **Halliday, J.** and **Halliday, J.** *Practical goat-keeping.* London: Ward Lock, 1982. 104pp.

594   **Hetherington, L.** *All about goats.* 2nd ed. Ipswich: Farming Press, 1987. 200pp.
Has a sixty-eight page veterinary section by 'The TV Vet'.

595   **Luttmann, G.** *Raising milk goats successfully.* Charlotte: Williamson Publishing, 1986. 172pp.
Williamson Publishing have issued a number of other guides to small-scale livestock husbandry: *Raising pigs successfully* (K. Kellogg and B. Kellogg), *Raising rabbits successfully* (B. Bennett), *Raising poultry successfully* (W. Graves), *The sheep raiser's manual* (W. K. Kruesi) and *Keeping bees* (J. Vivian).

596   **Mackenzie, D.** *Goat husbandry.* 4th ed. Revised and edited by J. Laing. London: Faber, 1980. 375pp.
An established text on goat-keeping which was one of the first scientific textbooks on this subject.

597   **Morris, J., Hepburn, J., Wilkinson, M.** and **Stark, B.** *Goats for fibre: guide to producing mohair, cashmere and cashgora in Great Britain.* Bodmin, Cornwall: National Angora Stud, 1987. 107pp.

598   **Mowlem, A.** *Goat farming.* Ipswich: Farming Press, 1988. 198pp.
Comprehensive guide to commercial goat farming.

599   **Neal, J.** *Goatkeeping for profit.* Newton Abbot: David & Charles, 1988. 168pp.

600   **Owen, N. L.** *The illustrated standard of the dairy goat.* Rev. ed. Scottsdale: Dairy Goat Journal Publishing, 1973. 66pp.

601   **Sinn, R.** *Raising goats for milk and meat.* Little Rock: Heifer Project International, 1985. 110pp.
Originally written for a training course in West Africa and so deals with tropical goat husbandry.

602   Thear, K. *Goats and goat-keeping*, London: Merehurst Press, 1988. 176pp.

603   Thear, K. *Commercial goat farming*. Widdington, Saffron Walden, Essex CB11 3SP, England: Broad Leys Publishing, 1985. 42pp.

604   Thedford, T. R. *Goat health handbook: a field guide for producers with limited veterinary services*. Morrilton: Winrock International, 1983. 123pp.
Has a similar format to Thedford's other work on sheep. There are diagnostic guides to diseases and symptoms in the form of tables. Most of the book consists of descriptions of individual diseases.

605   Turner, M. *Goat care: a complete handbook*. Jefferson, North Carolina: McFarland, 1984. 186pp.

606   Weems, D. B. *Raising goats: the backyard dairy alternative*. Blue Ridge Summit, Pennsylvania: Tab Books, 1983. 202pp.
Complete practical guide to goat-keeping.

607   Wilkinson, J. M. and **Stark, B. A.** *Commercial goat production*. Oxford: Blackwell, 1987. 159pp.
Guide to the development of a goat herd as a business activity.

608   Yerex, D. *The farming of goats: fibre and meat production in New Zealand*. Carterton, New Zealand: Ampersand Publishing Associates, 1986. 200pp.
Discussion of the practicalities of goat husbandry with special reference to conditions in New Zealand. The author has edited a similar work on the farming of deer.

Conferences

609 *Goat production and research in the tropics: proceedings of a workshop held at the University of Queensland, Brisbane, Australia, 6–8 February 1984*. Edited by J. W. Copland. Canberra: Australian Centre for International Agricultural Research, 1985. 118pp. (ACIAR Proceedings Series, no. 7.)

610 *Les maladies de la chèvre: colloque international, Niort (France) 9–11 Octobre 1984*. Paris: Institut National de la Recherche Agronomique, 1984. 750pp. (Colloques de l'INRA, no. 28.)
The second colloquium is to be held in Niort in June 1989.

611 *Proceedings of the fourth international conference on goats. March 8 to 13, 1987, Brasília, Brazil*. Brasilia: Departamento de Difusão de Technologia, 1987. 2 vols. 805 + 744pp.
The third conference was held in Tucson, Arizona in 1982 and proceedings were published by the Dairy Goat Journal Publishing Company (1982, 620pp.).

612 *Sheep and goats in humid West Africa: proceedings of the workshop on small ruminant production systems in the humid zone of West Africa, held in Ibadan, Nigeria, 23–26 January 1984*. Edited by J. E. Sumberg and K. Cassaday. Addis Ababa: International Livestock Centre for Africa, 1985. 74pp.

613 *Small ruminant production systems in South and Southeast Asia: proceedings of a workshop held at Bogor, Indonesia, 6–10 October 1986*. Edited by C. Devendra. Ottawa: International Development Research Centre, 1987. 414pp. (IDRC Proceedings Series 256e.)

614 *Small ruminants in African agriculture = Les petits ruminants dans l'agriculture africaine: proceedings of a conference held at ILCA, Addis Ababa, Ethiopia, 30 September–4 October 1985*. Edited by R. T. Wilson and D. Bourzat. Addis Ababa: International Livestock Centre for Africa, 1985. 261pp.

615 **Smith, O. B.** and **Bosman, H. G.** (eds) *Goat production in the humid tropics*. Wageningen: PUDOC, 1988. 187pp.
Proceedings of a meeting held at the University of Ife, Nigeria in 1987.

Journals

616 *Goat Veterinary Society journal*. 1979–. c/o Dr S. Lloyd, Department of Clinical Veterinary Medicine, University of Cambridge, Madingley Road, Cambridge CB3 0ES, England: the Society. Biannual.
Contains the proceedings of the meetings plus other articles, news and information.

617 *Goat health and production*. 1987–. Palmerston North Animal Health Laboratory, PO Box 1654, Palmerston North: NZ Ministry of Agriculture and Fisheries. Quarterly.

618 *Small ruminant research*. 1988–. Amsterdam: Elsevier. Quarterly.
Journal of the International Goat Association. Publishes technical articles on goats, sheep and other small ruminants.

Other Journals

Australian goat world
Chèvre: revue des éleveurs de chèvres
Dairy goat journal
Goats today
Journées de la recherche ovine et caprine
United caprine news

PIGS

Swine are reared intensively. The major considerations are therefore adequate housing and environmental conditions, correct nutrition and close supervision of their reproductive status.

Abstracting Service

619   *Pig news and information.* 1980–. Wallingford: CAB International. Quarterly. Contains about 3,000 abstracts per year and each issue also contains news items, several review articles and a 'country report' describing an aspect of pig production in a single territory.

Directory

620   *Index of current research on pigs.* 1954–. Prepared by R. Braude. Wallingford: CAB International. Annual.
Lists research centres in over fifty countries. Each entry gives the titles of projects currently under way in each organization and there are lists of their publications during the previous year. There are author and subject indexes.

Books

621   Barron, N. S. *The pig farmer's veterinary book.* 10th ed. Ipswich: Farming Press, 1978. 180pp.

622   Baxter, S. *Intensive pig production: environmental management and design.* London: Granada, 1984. 588pp.

623   Belschner, H. G. and **Love, R. J.** *Pig diseases.* 3rd ed. London: Angus & Robertson, 1984. 152pp.
A revision of Belschner's book first published in 1967. Intended for pig farmers and students and describes briefly the nature, prevention and treatment of each of the important diseases. Has fifty-one figures and twelve colour plates.

624   Brent, G. *Housing the pig.* Ipswich: Farming Press, 1986. 248pp.

625   Brent, G. *The pigman's handbook.* 2nd ed. Ipswich: Farming Press, 1987. 244pp.
Guide to the management of pig units with a discussion of health problems.

626   Bundy, C. E., Diggins, R. V. and **Christensen, V. W.** *Swine production.* 5th ed. Englewood Cliffs: Prentice-Hall, 1984. 400pp.

627   Cunha, T. J. *Swine feeding and nutrition.* 2nd ed. New York: Academic Press, 1977. 352pp. (Animal Feeding and Nutrition.)

628   Drochner, W. *Aspects of digestion in the large intestine of the pig.* Berlin: Paul Parey, 1987. 84pp.

629   English, P. R., Fowler, V. R., Baxter, S., and **Smith, W. J.** *The growing and finishing pig: improving efficiency.* Ipswich: Farming Press, 1988. 555pp.

630   English, P. R., Smith, W. J. and **MacLean, A.** *The sow: improving her efficiency.* 2nd ed. Ipswich: Farming Press, 1982. 354pp.
Has a fifty-four page chapter on the diseases of the sow and piglets.

631   Ensminger, M. E. and **Parker, R. O.** *Swine science.* 5th ed. Danville: Interstate Printers & Publishers, 1984. 568pp.
An overview of the husbandry of pigs and of the swine industry with particular reference to US practice. The final chapter provides feed composition tables.

632   Eusebio, J. A. *Pig production in the tropics.* London: Longman, 1980. 115pp. (Intermediate Tropical Agriculture Series.)

633   Gilbert, S. G. *Pictorial anatomy of the fetal pig.* 2nd ed. Seattle: University of Washington Press, 1966. 77pp.

634   Goodwin, D. H. *Pig management and production: a practical guide for farmers and students.* London: Hutchinson, 1973. 203pp.

635   Hughes, P. E. and **Varley, M. A.** *Reproduction in the pig.* London: Butterworth, 1980. 241pp.

636   Johnson, G. *Profitable pig farming.* 5th ed. Ipswich: Farming Press, 1976. 208pp.

637   Kidder, D. E. and **Manners, M. J.** *Digestion in the pig.* Bristol: Scientechnica, 1978. 201pp.
Presents a large amount of factual data on the digestive physiology of the pig. Each chapter has an extensive list of references.

638   Krider, J. L., Conrad, J. H. and **Carroll, W. E.** *Swine production.* 5th ed. New York: McGraw-Hill, 1982. 679pp.

639   Leman, A. D., Straw, B., Glock, R. D., Mengeling, W. L., Penny, R. H. C. and **Scholl, E.** (eds) *Diseases of swine.* 6th ed. Ames: Iowa State UP, 1986. 930pp.

The standard reference work covering all aspects of swine medicine. Each of the seventy-seven chapters in the six sections has an extensive bibliography. Basic anatomy and physiology, differential diagnosis and veterinary techniques and practices are covered as well as pig diseases. Previous editions are still useful for the historical perspective they provide.

640   Mount, L. E. and **Ingram, D. L.** *The pig as a laboratory animal.* London: Academic Press, 1971. 175pp.
Intended as a brief practical guide for those working with pigs as laboratory animals.

641 *The nutrient requirements of pigs: technical review by an Agricultural Research Council Working Party.* Farnham Royal: CAB, 1981. 307pp.
Five chapters review in detail the energy, protein and amino acid, vitamin, mineral and water requirements. There is a glossary of terms used.

642   Odlaug, T. O. *Laboratory anatomy of the fetal pig.* 7th ed. Dubuque: W. C. Brown, 1984. 98pp.

643 *Pig health and production recording.* Revised ed. Alnwick: MAFF, 1983. 59pp. (MAFF Booklet 2075.)
A guide to the collection of on farm data. Includes definitions of terms used to describe reproductive events in pig herds.

644 *Pig production and welfare.* Alnwick: MAFF, 1984. 104pp. (MAFF Booklet 2483.)
Prepared by the Animal Welfare Group of ADAS to assist the Farm Animal Welfare Advisory Committee. Reviews current knowledge on pig behaviour and their environmental requirements and relates this to practice in the UK pig industry.

645   Pond, W. G. and **Houpt, K. A.** *The biology of the pig.* Ithaca: Cornell University Press, 1978. 371pp.

646   Pond, W. G. and **Maner, J. H.** *Swine production and nutrition.* Westport: AVI, 1984. 731pp.
More than half the book is devoted to feeds and feeding.

647   Sack, W. O. *Essentials of pig anatomy* and *Horowitz–Kramer atlas of musculoskeletal anatomy of the pig.* Ithaca: Veterinary Textbooks, 1982. 192pp.
The first part presents the essential features of the regional anatomy of the pig with supporting references and illustrations. The second part is an atlas of 113 anatomical plates depicting the musculoskeletal system.

648   **Sainsbury, D.** *Pig housing.* 5th ed. Ipswich: Farming Press, 1978. 222pp.

649   **Smith, W. J.** and **Taylor, D. J.** *A colour atlas of diseases of the pig.* London: Wolfe Medical Publications. Forthcoming.

650   **Stanton, H. C.** and **Mersmann, H. J.** (eds) *Swine in cardiovascular research.* Boca Raton: CRC Press, 1986. 2 vols. 400pp.

651   **Straiton, E.** *Pig ailments: recognition and treatment. TV vet book for pig farmers.* 6th ed. Ipswich: Farming Press, 1988. 160pp.

652   **Suarez, F. R.** and **Huang, H. K.** *Cross-sectional anatomy of the pig: an atlas for computerized tomography.* Iowa City: University of Iowa, 1982. 74pp.

653   **Swindle, M. M.** *Basic surgical exercises using swine.* New York: Praeger, 1983. 237pp.

654   **Taylor, D. J.** *Pig diseases.* 4th ed. 31 North Birbiston Road, Lennoxtown G65 7LZ, Scotland: the Author, 1986. 300pp.
A thorough review of the field appropriate for the veterinarian. Much practical and numerical data are included and these are references to recent literature. There are no illustrations and the text is typescript in an very ordered manner.

655   **Thornton, K.** *Outdoor pig production.* Ipswich: Farming Press, 1988. 206pp.

656   **Thornton, K.** *Practical pig production.* 3rd ed. Ipswich: Farming Press, 1981. 234pp.
Good overview of the economic and practical considerations in the rearing of pigs.

657   **Walker, W. F. Jr** *Anatomy and dissection of the fetal pig.* 4th ed. New York: W. H. Freeman, 1988. 116pp.

658   **Walton, J. R.** *A handbook of pig diseases.* 2nd ed. Liverpool: LUP, 1987. 166pp.
Provides information in note form on pig diseases occurring in the UK and has sections on general topics such as differential diagnosis, anaesthesia and surgical procedures.

659   **Whittemore, C. T.** *Elements of pig science.* Harlow: Longman, 1987. 181pp. (Longman Handbooks in Agriculture.)

660   **Whittemore, C. T.** and **Elsley, F. W. H.** *Practical pig nutrition.* 2nd ed. Ipswich: Farming Press, 1979. 190pp.

661   Wiseman, J. *History of the British pig.* London: Duckworth, 1986. 118pp.

662   Wrathall, A. E. *Reproductive disorders in pigs.* Corrected 2nd impression. Farnham Royal: CAB, 1975. 313pp. (Commonwealth Bureau of Animal Health, Review Series, no. 11.)
Reviews the literature and lists over 1,360 references.

Conferences

663   Cole, D. J. A and **Haresign, W.** (eds) *Recent developments in pig nutrition.* London: Butterworths, 1985. 321pp.
Reprints review papers originally presented at the Nutrition Conferences for Feed Manufacturers held at the University of Nottingham.

664 *Manipulating pig production. Proceedings of the inaugural conference of the Australasian Pig Science Association (APSA) held in Albury (NSW), on November 23 to 25, 1987.* c/o Dr D. P. Hennessy, VRI Attwood, Mickleton Road, Attwood, Victoria 3047, Australia: the Association, 1988. 242pp.
Has review papers on amino acid requirements, embryonic loss, energy and protein metabolism, welfare, transgenic pigs and immunological manipulation of reproduction. Also contains papers from symposia on seasonal infertility, estimating amino acid availability and control of pre- and post-weaning diarrhoea.

665 *Swine in biomedical research.* Edited by M. E. Tumbleson. New York: Plenum Press, 1986. 3 vols. 1988pp.
Proceedings of the conference held at the University of Missouri, Columbia, 17–24 June 1985.

Journals

666 *International pigletter.* 1981–. PO Box 21–505, St Paul, Minnesota 55121: Pig World. Monthly.
Four page newsletter on swine management.

667 *Pig farming.* 1953–. Ipswich: Farming Press. Monthly.

668 *Pig international.* 1971–. Mount Morris: Watt Publishing. Monthly.
There is a special American edition: *Pig American.*

669 *Pig unit newsletter.* 1982–. Stoneleigh, Kenilworth, Warwickshire CV8 2LZ, England: National Agricultural Centre. Quarterly.

670 *Pigs.* 1985–. Doetinchem: Misset International. Bimonthly.
Brief well-illustrated articles on pig production and has a news section.

671   *Pork '89*. 1981–. 7950 College Boulevard, PO Box 2939, Shawnee Mission, Kansas 66201: Vance Publishing. Monthly.
Publishes an annual guide to herd health and nutrition which lists products available in the United States. *Swine practitioner* is a quarterly supplement to *Pork*.

Other Journals

Australian pig bulletin
Australian pork journal
Canadian swine
Hog farm management
Hogs today
Industria porcina
Journées de la recherche porcine en France
National hog farmer

CAMELIDS

The world population has been increasing steadily, largely because of camelids' increased use as a source of meat and milk. Camelids are used as work animals but their traditional role in transportation has declined. The camelids native to South America are of particular importance to its rural economy.

Bibliographies

672   **Cockrill, W. Ross** (ed.) *The camel: an all-purpose animal Volume II. Bibliography*. PO Box 1703, S-751 47 Uppsala, Sweden: Scandinavian Institute of African Studies, 1985. 228pp.
A companion bibliography to [684]. Over 3,000 references are listed in author order there being no other index.

673   **Farid, M. F. A.** *Camelids bibliography*. PO Box 2440, Damascus, Syria: The Arab Centre for the Studies of Arid Zones and Dry Lands, 1981. 546pp. (ACSAD-AS-P15-1981.)
Contains 2,539 annotated references up to July 1981 and has indexes to subjects and species and a geographical index. Updates have appeared in the *Camel newsletter* published by the Centre. A second edition of the bibliography is in preparation.

Books and Reviews

674   'Diseases of camels'. *Revue scientifique et technique de l'OIE* **6** (1987): (2).
A special issue containing ten articles.

675   Escobar, R. C. translated by **J. Johnson**. *Animal breeding and production of American camelids*. Lima: Talleres Gráficos de Abril, 1984. 358pp.
Available from Roy Hennig, PO Box 1079, Mt Shasta, California 960067, USA.

676   Gauthier-Pilters, H. and **Dagg, A. I.** *The camel: its evolution, ecology, behaviour and relationship to man*. Revised ed. Chicago: University of Chicago Press, 1983. 240pp.

677   Higgins, A. J. (ed.) *The camel in health and disease*. London: Baillière Tindall, 1986. 168pp.
A modern concise guide to the husbandry, management and medical treatment of dromedary and Bactrian camels. Eight chapters are revisions of review papers first published in the *British veterinary journal* **140–2** (1984–6). The two additional chapters deal with anaesthetic management and intensive husbandry.

678   Mukasa-Mugerwa, E. *The camel (*Camelus dromedarius*): a bibliographical review*. Addis Ababa: International Livestock Centre for Africa, 1981. 147pp. (ILCA Monograph, no. 5.)
The reproductive performance and nutrition of the dromedary in Africa and Asia is reviewed. Disease, meat and milk production and utilization are discussed. There is an extensive bibliography.

679   Rathore, G. S. *Camels and their management*. New Delhi: Indian Council of Agricultural Research, 1986. 228pp.
Anatomy, physiology and psychology(!) are reviewed but the bulk of the work deals with the practical aspects of husbandry, disease control and surgery with special reference to Indian conditions.

680   Richard, D. *Le dromadaire et son élevage*. Maison Alfort: IEMVT, 1984. 161pp. (Études et Synthèses de l'IEMVT, no. 12.)
The author has compiled a bibliography on the camel (published as Études et Synthèses de l'IEMVT, no. 1). A new edition of this bibliography is in preparation by the staff of IEMVT. A bibliographic database is to be compiled in order to produce the bibliography.

681   Smuts, M. M. S. and **Bezuidenhout, A. J.** *Anatomy of the dromedary*. Oxford: Clarendon Press, 1987. 230pp.
Terminology from the *Nomina anatomica veterinaria* is used throughout this exceptionally well-illustrated reference work.

682   Wilson, R. T. *The camel*. London: Longman, 1984. 223pp.
An excellent, readable and comprehensive work on all aspects of the one-humped camel (*Camelus dromedarius*). Many figures and illustrations. A vast amount of numerical information is presented in over seventy tables. Over 2,000 references are listed in the bibliography.

683   Yagil, R. *The desert camel: comparative physiological adaptation.* Basel: Karger, 1985. 163pp. (Comparative Animal Nutrition, no. 5.)
A complete discussion of the physiology of the dromedary.

Conferences

684   Cockrill, W. Ross (ed.) *The camelid: an all-purpose animal. Volume I. Proceedings of the Khartoum workshop on camels December 1979.* Uppsala: Scandinavian Institute of African Studies, 1984. 544pp.
Thirty-two valuable papers reviewing camelid species, breeds and status, diseases, feeding, reproduction, physiology and meat and milk production. Contains a useful review of the Camelidae of South America (pp. 112–43) No index. Most of these papers were first published in the *International Foundation for Science*'s *Provisional Report no. 6: Camels (1979).*

685   *Llama medicine workshop for veterinarians, January 13–15, 1988.* College of Veterinary Medicine and Biomedical Sciences, Fort Collins, Colorado 80523: Department of Clinical Services, 1988. Unpaginated.

Journal

686   *Revista de camelidos sudamericanos.* 1986–. Apartado 4270, Lima, Peru: Centro de Información Científica de Camelidos Sudamericanos. Quarterly.
The Centre also produces *Technical bulletins* on specific topics and has compiled a *Bibliografia de camelidos sudamericanos* (1985).

HORSES

Horses are the recipients of some of the most sophisticated and expensive medical and surgical care given by veterinary surgeons. They are expensive companion animals and the monetary value of racehorses and animals on stud farms can be enormous.

Information Guide

687   Wells, E. B. *Horsemanship: a guide to information sources.* Detroit: Gale Research, 1979. 138pp. (Sports, Games and Pastimes Information Guide Series, vol. 4.)

Abstracting Service

688   Zentralblatt Pferd/Equine abstracts. 1984–. Warendorf: FN-Verlag. Quarterly.
The titles of the references included are in both German and English and about ten percent have abstracts in German.

Current awareness Lists

689   'Current equine papers'. In: *Journal of equine veterinary science.*
Lists papers on equine topics appearing in individual issues of journals. Page
numbers are not included but authors' addresses are given.

690   'Index of literature'. In: *Equine veterinary journal.*
Newly published articles are listed in classified order under a few dozen subject
headings. The language of the original article and summaries are indicated.

Review Series

Veterinary clinics of North America: equine practice [71]

Historical Bibliographies

691   **Grimshaw, A.** *The horse: a bibliography of British books 1851–1976.* London:
   Library Association, 1982. 474pp.
Over 3,000 entries, fully indexed and containing a commentary on the role of the
horse in British social history.

692   **Wells, E. B.** *Horsemanship: a bibliography of printed materials from the sixteenth
   century through 1974.* New York: Garland Publishing, 1985. 282pp. (Garland
   Reference Library of the Humanities, vol. 474.)

Dictionary

693   **Rossdale, P. D.** and **Wreford, S. M.** *The horse's health from A to Z: an equine
   veterinary dictionary.* Newton Abbot: David & Charles, 1974. 433pp.

Directory

694   *Index of equine research in the British Isles and Ireland. Volume 4 (1986).* Bath
   Lodge, Bath Road, Atworth, Melksham, Wiltshire SN12 8HS, England:
   British Equine Veterinary Association Trust, 1986. 72pp.
Gives the titles of projects, the address of the researchers involved and details of the
funding. Includes a directory of those organizations involved in equine research
and health. Contains details of similar indexes of equine research for Australia,
France and the USA.

Books

695   **Allen, W. E.** *Fertility and obstetrics in the horse.* Oxford: Blackwell, 1988.
   173pp. (Library of Veterinary Practice.)

Describes the diagnostic techniques employed and the therapeutic approaches available when dealing with the management of brood mares. Fertility problems in the stallion are also covered.

696   Ashdown, R. R. and **Done, S. H.** *Colour atlas of veterinary anatomy. Volume Two. The horse.* London: Baillière Tindall/Gower Medical Publishing, 1987. Chapters paginated separately.
Full-colour photographs of dissections are accompanied by line drawings which identify the structures. *Nomina anatomica veterinaria* nomenclature is used throughout.

697   Belschner, H. G. and **Rose, R. J.** *Horse diseases.* 3rd ed. London: Angus & Robertson, 1982. 252pp.

698   Blackmore, D. J. and **Brobst, D.** *Biochemical values in equine medicine.* Newmarket: Animal Health Trust, 1981. 108pp.
Pocket-book guide for the veterinarian and veterinary technician. Describes the tests and contains basic numerical data.

699   *Breeding management and foal development.* PO Box 9001, Tyler, Texas 75711: Equine Research, 1982. 700pp.

700   Bromiley, M. *Equine injury and therapy.* London: Blackwell, 1987. 159pp.
Describes the conditions encountered, appropriate first aid, and the methods of physiotherapy which can be employed.

701   Brown, C. M. *Problems in equine medicine.* Philadelphia: Lea & Febiger. Forthcoming.

702   Brown, J. H. and **Powell-Smith, V.** *Horse and stable management.* London: Granada, 1984. 240pp.
Introductory text for those who own or work with horses.

703   Butler, D. *The principles of horseshoeing II: an illustrated textbook of farrier science and craftsmanship.* Maryville, Missouri: the Author, 1985. 567pp.

704   Cassell, D. *The horse and the law.* Newton Abbot: David & Charles, 1987. 160pp.
For the horse owner. Covers all aspects of the law including a chapter on veterinary and other services.

705   Churchill, P. (ed.) *World atlas of horses and ponies.* Maidenhead: Sampson Low, 1980. 160pp.
Illustrates the types and varieties of animals found throughout the world.

706   Coffman, J. R. *Equine clinical chemistry and pathophysiology.* Bonner Springs: Veterinary Medicine Publishing, 1981. 275pp.

707   *Colours and markings of horses.* London: RCVS, 1984. 10pp.
Outlines a system for identifying individual animals using colours, body markings and other characteristics. Realistic illustrations of coat colours and body, limb and head markings are given in *The colours and markings of horses* (D. E. Packer and T. M. Ali, Ipswich: Farming Press, 1985, 70pp.). Colour is dealt with in detail in *Hair colour in the horse* (R. Guerts translated by A. Dent, London: J. A. Allen, 1977, 108pp.) and *Horse color* (D. P. Sponenberg and B. V. G. Beaver, College Station: Texas A & M University Press, 1983, 124pp.).

708   Cunha, T. J. *Horse feeding and nutrition.* Orlando: Academic Press, 1980. 292pp. (Animal Feeding and Nutrition.)

709   *Current therapy in equine medicine – 2.* Edited by N. E. Robinson. Philadelphia: W. B. Saunders, 1987. 761pp.
An essential reference work for equine practitioners describing the therapy and prevention of all the common medical disorders. The diseases and confirmatory diagnostic procedures are described. Appendices give normal clinical pathology data and the approximate doses of common drugs. The first edition is still of value for more detailed information on some of the topics.

710   Denny, H. R. *Treatment of equine fractures.* Bristol: Wright. Forthcoming.

711   Dietz, O. and **Wiesner, E.** (eds), translated by **T. C. Telger**, edited by **A. S. Turner**. *Diseases of the horse. A handbook for science and practice.* Basel: Karger, 1984. 3 vols. 1196pp.
Thirty-two authors provide a comprehensive manual. The first volume deals with the basics of the diagnosis and treatment of equine diseases. The second part (volumes 2 and 3) deals with specific disorders. The original edition was published in German in 1982.

712   Dik, K. J. and **Gunsser, I.** *Atlas of diagnostic radiology of the horse.* London: Wolfe Medical Publications. 1988–. 3 vols. Forthcoming.
Part 1 (204pp.) deals with diseases of the front limb, Part 2 will cover diseases of the hind limb and Part 3 the skull and vertebral column.

713   Edwards, E. H. *A standard guide to horse and pony breeds.* New York: McGraw-Hill, 1980. 352pp.

714   Fackelman, G. E. and **Nunamaker, D. M.** *Manual of internal fixation in the horse.* New York: Springer-Verlag, 1982. 106pp.

715   Frape, D. L. *Equine nutrition and feeding.* Harlow: Longman, 1986. 373pp.
Detailed account of a subject of interest to all dealing with horses. Covers all
nutritionally related problems.

716   Ginther, O. J. *Ultrasonic imaging and reproductive events in the mare.* 4343
Garfoot Road, Cross Plains, Wisconsin 53528: Equiservices, 1986. 378pp.
The principles and methodology of ultrasonic scanning are described but most of
the book is concerned with interpreting the results obtained. A supplement to the
author's *Reproductive biology of the mare: basic and applied aspects* (Ann Arbor:
McNaughton & Gunn, 1979, 413pp.).

717   Gordon, B. J. and **Allen, D. Jr** *Field guide to colic management in the horse: the
practitioner's reference.* Lenexa: Veterinary Medicine Publishing, 1988. 292pp.
Review of the mechanisms of gastrointestinal function in both health and disease.
Has sections on diagnostic procedures and interpretations, and medical and
surgical therapy.

718   Hayes, M. H. *Veterinary notes for horse owners: an illustrated manual of horse
medicine and surgery.* 17th ed. Revised by P. D. Rossdale. London: Stanley Paul,
1987. 740pp.
Straightforward text on equine medicine and surgery of value to new practitioners
and horse owners.

719   Hickman, J. (ed.) *Horse management.* 2nd ed. London: Academic Press,
1987. 405pp. (Animal Care, Health and Welfare Series.)
A readable account of good practice in managing the welfare for horses. Suitable
for both veterinarians and owners of horses.

720   Hickman, J. (ed.) *Equine surgery and medicine.* London: Academic Press,
1985–6. 2 vols. 398pp + 323pp. (Animal Care, Health and Welfare Series.)
Volume 1 covers anaesthesia, abdominal surgery, ophthalmology, the respiratory
tract, dermatology and parasitic diseases. Volume 2 deals with cardiology, fractures, the foot, haematology, and pulmonary and pleural diseases.

721   Hickman, J. and **Humphrey, M.** *Hickman's Farriery: a complete illustrated
guide.* 2nd ed. London: J. A. Allen, 1988. 245pp.

722   Holmes, J. R. *Equine cardiology.* Langford House, Langford, Bristol BS18
7DT, England: the Author, 1988. 4 vols. 89 + 80 + 89 + 99pp. with
appendices.
Anatomical and physiological aspects and the clinical examination are covered in
volume 1, electrocardiology in volume 2, cardiac murmurs and pathology in
volume 3 and cardiac rhythm in volume 4. Each volume has many illustrations
and volumes 3 and 4 contain detailed case histories.

723   Jacobs, D. E. *A colour atlas of equine parasites.* London: Baillière Tindall and Gower Medical Publishing, 1986. Chapters paginated separately.
Brief informative descriptions and notes on the parasites accompany the many excellent colour plates.

724   Johnston, A. M. *Equine medical disorders.* Oxford: Blackwell, 1986. 195pp. (Library of Veterinary Practice.)

725   Jones, W. E. (ed.) *Equine sports medicine.* Philadelphia: Lea & Febiger, 1988. 329pp.
Deals with equine physiology, scientific training methods, and the nature, diagnosis and treatment of sports injuries.

726   Jones, W. E. *Genetics and horse breeding.* Philadelphia: Lea & Febiger, 1982. 660pp.

727   Kellon, E. M. *The older horse: a complete guide to care and conditioning for horses 10 and up.* PO Box 594, Millwood, New York 10546: Breakthrough Publications, 1988. 212pp.

728   Kiley-Worthington, M. *The behaviour of horses: in relation to management and training.* London: J. A. Allen, 1987. 265pp.
Written for the horse owner to give an insight into equine behaviour but includes references to the original literature.

729   Lewis, L. D. *Feeding and care of the horse.* Philadelphia: Lea & Febiger, 1982. 248pp.

730   McBane, S. *Behaviour problems in horses.* Newton Abbot: David & Charles, 1987. 304pp.

731   McBane, S. *Keeping a horse outdoors.* Newton Abbot: David & Charles, 1984. 128pp.

732   McCarthy, G. *Pasture management for horses and ponies.* London: Collins, 1987, 259pp.

733   McIlwraith, C. W. *Diagnostic and surgical arthroscopy in the horse.* Edwardsville: Veterinary Medicine Publishing, 1984. 137pp.
Comprehensive review of an important diagnostic and surgical procedure.

734   McIlwraith, C. W. and **Turner, A. S.** *Equine surgery: advanced techniques.* Philadelphia: Lea & Febiger, 1987. 391pp.
Describes over fifty of the more complex and difficult procedures in detail with

references to the literature. Also has chapters on aspects of pre- and post-operative care and appendices describing equipment.

735   Madigan, J. E. *Manual of equine neonatal medicine.* PO Box 8329, Woodland, California 95695: Live Oak Publishing, 1987. 363pp.

736   Manolson, F. and **Fraser, A.** *Fraser's horse book.* London: Pitman, 1979. 370pp.
Well-illustrated guide to the care of horses. Much of the book deals with diseases and disorders. Uses an encyclopaedic style with brief articles arranged into appropriate chapters.

737   Mansmann, R. A. and **McAllister, E. S.** (eds) *Equine medicine and surgery.* 3rd ed. Edited by P. W. Pratt. Santa Barbara: American Veterinary Publications, 1982. 2 vols. 1417pp.
A standard American text with over a hundred contributors. Intended as a companion for the veterinary practitioner.

738   Menendhall, A. L. and **Cantwell, H. D.** *Equine radiographic procedures.* Philadelphia: Lea & Febiger, 1988. 175pp.
A complete manual describing basic radiographic technique and specific procedures. Discusses the results obtained.

739   Milne, D. W. and **Turner, A. S.** *An atlas of surgical approaches to the bones of the horse.* Philadelphia: W. B. Saunders, 1979. 210pp.

740   Montes, L. F. and **Vaughan, J. T.** *Atlas of skin diseases of the horse: diagnosis and treatment in equine dermatology.* Copenhagen: Munksgaard, 1983. 202pp.
Excellent colour plates illustrate individual cases. There are notes on the clinical appearance, histopathological investigations used and on treatment.

741   Naviaux, J. L. *Horses in health and disease.* 2nd ed. Philadelphia: Lea & Febiger, 1985. 300pp.
Basic non-technical guide to the care and breeding of horses.

742   Ogbourne, C. P. and **Duncan, J. L.** *Strongylus vulgaris in the horse: its biology and veterinary importance.* 2nd ed. Farnham Royal: CAB, 1985. 68pp. (Commonwealth Institute of Parasitology Miscellaneous Publication, no. 9.)
Comprehensive review of an important nematode parasite.

743   Pasquini, C., Reddy, V. K. and **Ratzlaff, M. H.** *Atlas of equine anatomy.* 2nd ed. 2931 Eureka Street, Eureka, California 95501: Sudz, 1983. 339pp.

744   Pavord, A. and **Fisher, R.** *The equine veterinary manual.* Marlborough: Crowood Press, 1987. 172pp.
An up-to-date discussion for the horse owner.

745   Pilliner, S. *Getting horses fit.* London: Collins, 1986. 236pp.

746   Prince, E. F. and **Collier, G. M.** *Basic horse care.* Garden City, New York: Doubleday, 1986. 314pp.

747   Rooney, J. R. *Autopsy of the horse: technique and interpretation.* Baltimore: Williams & Wilkins, 1970. 148pp.

748   Rossdale, P. D. *Horse breeding.* Newton Abbot: David & Charles, 1981. 320pp.

749   Rossdale, P. D. and **Ricketts, S. W.** *Equine stud farm medicine.* 2nd ed. London: Baillière Tindall, 1980. 564pp.
Describes all the medical problems likely to be encountered at an equine breeding establishment and so is useful to all equine practitioners.

750   Sack, W. O. and **Habel, R. E.** *Rooney's guide to the dissection of the horse.* Ithaca: Veterinary Textbooks, 1982. 248pp.
An illustrated procedural manual. Supplied with microfiches containing 484 colour photographs of the dissected horse (by W. O. Sack and L. Z. Saddler).

751   Schebitz, H. and **Wilkens, H.** *Atlas of radiographic anatomy of the horse.* 4th ed. Berlin: Paul Parey, 1986. 100pp.
The legends and labels to the radiographs and drawings are in English and German.

752   Sevelius, F., Pettersson, H. and **Olsson, L.** *Keeping your horse healthy: the prevention and cure of illness.* Newton Abbot: David & Charles, 1978. 176pp.

753   Snow, D. H. and **Vogel, C. J.** *Equine fitness: the care and training of the athletic horse.* Newton Abbot: David & Charles, 1987. 271pp.
Covers practical aspects of the training and care of horses used for athletic purposes with an emphasis on improving performance.

754   Stashak, T. S. (ed.) *Adams' lameness in horses.* 4th ed. Philadelphia: Lea & Febiger, 1987. 906pp.
The most recent edition of a classic work on the disorders of the musculoskeletal system which cause lameness. Methods of therapy, including corrective trimming and shoeing are described. An abridged version of the third edition, intended for horse owners, is also available.

755   Svendsen, E. D. (compiler). *The professional handbook of the donkey.* Sidmouth: The Donkey Sanctuary, 1986. 248pp.
About a quarter of the book is concerned with the health of donkeys. The remainder covers nutrition, management, housing and the uses of donkeys.

756   Tobin, T. *Drugs and the performance horse.* Springfield: C. C. Thomas, 1981. 463pp.
Covers both drugging and medication in the racehorse.

757   Turner, A. S. (ed.) *Some techniques and procedures in equine surgery.* Edwardsville: Veterinary Medicine Publishing, 1983. 211pp.
A collection of articles originally published in *Veterinary medicine/small animal clinician.*

758   *The TV Vet horse book: recognition and treatment of common horse and pony ailments.* 8th ed. Ipswich: Farming Press, 1987. 199pp.

759   Waring, G. H. *Horse behavior: the behavioral traits and adaptations of domestic and wild horses, including ponies.* Park Ridge: Noyes, 1983. 292pp.
A review of current scientific knowledge on the behaviour of horses.

760   White, N. A. (ed.) *Equine acute abdomen.* Philadelphia: Lea & Febiger. Forthcoming.
Discussion of the causes, diagnosis and treatment of colic.

761   Whitlock, R. H. (ed.) *Equine medicine and surgery in practice.* Lawrenceville: Veterinary Learning Systems, 1984. 256pp.
Collection of articles from the *Compendium on continuing education for the practicing veterinarian.*

762   Wintzer, H-J. (ed.) translated and revised by **A. D. Weaver**. *Equine diseases: a textbook for students and practitioners.* Berlin: Paul Parey, 1986. 439pp.
An up-to-date text dealing with the various body systems in turn and with diseases and toxicology. There are almost 400 illustrations, many in colour.

763   Wyn-Jones, G. *Equine lameness.* Oxford: Blackwell, 1988. 302pp.
Thorough treatment of equine orthopaedics.

Conferences

764   Moore, J. N., White, N. A. and **Becht, J. L.** (eds) *Equine colic research: proceedings of the second symposium at the University of Georgia.* Lawrenceville: Veterinary Learning Systems, 1986. 2 vols.
The first symposium was held in 1982 with the proceedings published by the College of Veterinary Medicine, Athens, Georgia in 1984. The third was held in 1988 and the proceedings will be published as the seventh supplement to the *Equine veterinary journal.*

764a   *Equine infectious diseases V: proceedings of the fifth international conference.* Edited by D. G. Powell. Lexington, Kentucky: University Press of Kentucky, 1988. 293pp.

Journals

765   *The equine athlete.* 1988–. Santa Barbara: Veterinary Practice Publishing. Bimonthly.
Has articles on equine sports medicine and on sports performance studies.

766   *Equine practice.* 1979–. Santa Barbara: Veterinary Practice Publishing: Eleven a year.

767   *Equine veterinary data.* 1980–. PO Box 1127, Wildomar, California 92395: W. E. Jones. Fortnightly.
A topical newsletter for the equine practitioner. Particularly useful for its reports of US meetings.

768   *Equine veterinary journal.* 1968–. London: BVA. Bimonthly.
Journal of the British Equine Veterinary Association. Also appears in a North American edition. Each issue usually has editorials, a review article, a dozen or so general articles, short communications and case reports, book reviews, abstracts and details of forthcoming events. Supplements to the journal are published (1983–): 1. *Tendon injury, healing and treatment*; 2. *Equine ophthalmology*; 3. *Equine embryo transfer*; 4. *Equine radiography: a guide to interpretation*; 5. *Perinatology*; 6. *Equine orthopaedic injury and repair*. The eighth supplement will contain the proceedings of the Second International Conference on Equine Embryo Transfer held in 1989. Some of the issues are devoted to special topics: **19** (1987): (5) *Equine respiratory medicine and surgery*; **18** (1986): (4) *Gastroenterology*; **16** (1984): (4) *Equine perinatal physiology and medicine*.

769   *Journal of equine veterinary science.* 1981–. PO Box 1209, Wildomar, California 92395: W. E. Jones. Bimonthly.
Publishes research papers, case reports and non-refereed short articles. Also contains proceedings from meetings of various equine veterinary associations and societies.

Other Journals

Bulletin of Equine Research Institute
Equine sports medicine news
Equus
Horse digest
Modern horse breeding
Pferdeheilkunde
Pratique vétérinaire équine

11 Small Animals

Most of the texts on 'small animals' deal solely with cats and dogs but some also include brief discussions of other domestic and exotic pets.

GENERAL

Abstracting Services

770 *Quarterly index: information access for the small animal practitioner.* 1983–. 5679 Claribel Road, Oakdale, California 95361: Veterinary Interface. Quarterly with annual cumulation.
Gives abstracts of all the literature dealing with cats, dogs, birds and domestic and exotic pets from nineteen journals.

771 *Small animal abstracts.* 1975–. Wallingford. CAB International. Quarterly.
Covers the core literature on cats, dogs and other pets. Items on laboratory animals are excluded.

Current Awareness List

772 'Small animal literature index'. In: *Journal of small animal practice.* Every two or three months.
A classified list of newly published journal articles.

Review Journals and Book Series

773   *Advances in Small Animal Practice.* 1988–. Edited by E. A. Chandler. Oxford: Blackwell. Annual.
Each volume will contain about ten reviews written for the practising veterinary surgeon. The first volume includes colour plates to support some of the articles.

774   *Contemporary Issues in Small Animal Practice.* 1985–. New York: Churchill Livingstone. Occasional.
Each volume has about a dozen clinically orientated reviews and therefore provides a reasonable overview of current knowledge and practice. The titles and editors are as follows:

1988	9	*Disorders of exotic animals.* E. R. Jacobson and G. V. Kollias Jr. 328pp.
1987	8	*Dermatology.* G. H. Nesbitt. 332pp.
	7	*Cardiology.* J. D. Bonagura. 331pp.
1986	6	*Oncology.* N. T. Gorman. 300pp.
	5	*Neurologic disorders.* J. N. Kornegay. 222pp.
	4	*Nephrology and urology.* E. B. Breitschwerdt. 282pp.
	3	*Infectious diseases.* F. W. Scott. 259pp.
	2	*Surgical emergencies.* R. M. Bright. 202pp.
1985	1	*Medical emergencies.* R. G. Sherding. 388pp.

775   *Manual of small animal . . .* 1986–. New York: Churchill Livingstone. The volumes are designed for quick reference purposes and most are in outline format. Where appropriate algorithms to assist diagnosis and step-by-step therapeutic measures are included.
Manual of small animal anaesthesia. R. R. Paddleford. 1988. 344pp.
Manual of small animal cardiology. L. P. Tilley and J. M. Owens. 1985. 447pp.
Manual of small animal infectious diseases. J. E. Barlough. 1988. 444pp.
Manual of small animal ophthalmology. M. Wyman. 1986. 289pp.
Manual of small animal nephrology and urology. D. J. Chew and S. P. DiBartola. 1986. 340pp.
Manual of small animal surgical therapeutics. C. W. Betts and S. W. Crane. 1986. 426pp.
Manual of small animal emergencies. R. V. Morgan. 1985. 575pp.

776   *Seminars in veterinary medicine and surgery (small animal).* 1986–. Philadelphia: Grune & Stratton. Quarterly.
Most of the issues contain about a dozen articles most of which are reviews. Also published in Spanish.

1988	3	(4)	Emergency medicine and critical care 2
		(3)	Emergency medicine and critical care 1
		(2)	Diagnostic cytology

          (1) Ophthalmology
1987 **2** (4) Gastroenterology
          (3) Dermatology
          (2) Hip dysplasia: perspectives of the eighties
          (1) Current concepts in heartworm disease
1986 **1** (4) Current concepts in pulmonary disease
          (3) Special considerations in anaesthesia
          (2) Diagnostic techniques in radiology
          (1) Advances in the treatment of cancer

Veterinary clinics of North America: small animal practice [73]

Books

777   Ackerman, N. *Radiology of urogenital diseases in dogs and cats.* Ames: Iowa State UP, 1983, 116pp. (Venture Series in Veterinary Medicine.)
Primarily concerned with radiographic evaluation and decision making. An atlas section forms the bulk of the book.

778   Alden, C. L. *Color atlas for small animal necropsy.* Bonner Springs: Veterinary Medicine Publishing, 1981. 82pp.

779   Allen, D. G. and **Kruth, S. A.** *Small animal cardiopulmonary medicine.* Toronto: B. C. Decker, 1988. 233pp.
A handbook on the diagnosis and management of the common clinical disorders. Appendices deal with drugs and their use and give normal ECG values.

780   Archibald, J. and **Catcott, E. J.** (eds) *Canine and feline surgery. Volume 1: Abdomen.* Santa Barbara: American Veterinary Publications, 1984. 551pp.
Gives detailed instructions for many surgical procedures. A revision of the former *Canine surgery.*

781   Baker, K. P. and **Thomsett, L. R.** *Dermatology of the dog and cat.* Oxford: Blackwell. Forthcoming.

782   Bojrab, M. J. (ed.) *Pathophysiology in small animal surgery.* Philadelphia: Lea & Febiger, 1981. 906pp.
Describes normal functioning and how this is altered by disease states. The correction of the disorders using surgical techniques is covered.

783   Bojrab, M. J., Crane, S. W. and **Arnoczky, S. P.** (eds) *Current techniques in small animal surgery.* 2nd ed. Philadelphia: Lea & Febiger, 1983. 811pp.
Over a hundred authors have contributed to this compendium of procedures. The basic organization is by body system. There are sections on soft tissue surgery and orthopaedic surgery.

784   Bojrab, M. J. and **Tholen, M.** *Small animal oral and dental surgery.* Philadelphia: Lea & Febiger. Forthcoming.

785   Brasmer, T. H. *The acutely traumatized small animal patient.* Philadelphia: W. B. Saunders, 1984. 167pp. (Major Problems in Veterinary Medicine, vol. 2.)

786   Braund, K. G. *Clinical syndromes in veterinary neurology.* Baltimore: Williams & Wilkins, 1986. 257pp.
The most important neurological syndromes are described in detail and there is a list, in alphabetical order, of the most important diseases. Primarily a text to assist diagnosis.

787   Brinker, W. O., Hohn, R. B. and **Prieur, W. D.** (eds) *Manual of internal fixation in small animals.* Berlin: Springer-Verlag, 1984. 289pp.
Detailed manual intended for use by veterinary surgeons who have completed a training course in the speciality.

788   Brinker, W. O., Piermattei, D. L. and **Flo, G. L.** *Handbook of small animal orthopedics and fracture treatment.* Philadelphia: W. B. Saunders, 1983. 435pp.
Mostly concerned with the management of fractures, lameness and joint disorders (including joint surgery).

789   Burk, R. L. and **Ackerman, N.** *Small animal radiology: a diagnostic atlas and text.* New York: Churchill Livingstone, 1986. 382pp.
Contains 468 radiographs and deals with basic radiographic principles and differential diagnosis. There are 246 literature references.

790   Burke, T. J. (ed.) *Small animal reproduction and infertility: a clinical approach to diagnosis and treatment.* Philadelphia: Lea & Febiger, 1986. 408pp.
A practical guide to normal and abnormal reproduction including the artificial control of reproduction.

791   Burkholder, C. R. *Emergency care for cats and dogs: first aid for your pet.* New York: M. Kesend, 1987. 174pp.

792   Bush, B. *First aid for pets.* 2nd ed. London: A & C Black, 1984. 168pp.
This and the previous title are the two most recent works. Both are suitable for pet owners and trainee nurses.

793   Campbell, W. E. *Owner's guide to better behavior in dogs and cats.* Goleta: American Veterinary Publications, 1986. 287pp.
Describes how to pre-empt and avoid behavioural problems and how to combat specific traits. Illustrated with 150 drawings by 'RMM'.

794   Caywood, D. D. and **Lipowitz, A. J.** *Atlas of general small animal surgery*. St Louis: C. V. Mosby, 1988. 361pp.
Illustrates 125 techniques in general or soft tissue surgery with accompanying line diagrams and text.

795   Chastain, C. B. and **Ganjam, V. K.** *Clinical endocrinology of companion animals*. Philadelphia: Lea & Febiger, 1986. 568pp.
The normal anatomy and physiology of the endocrine organs are outlined with information on clinical tests of organ function and on organ dysfunction.

796   Chrisman, C. L. *Problems in small animal neurology*. Philadelphia: Lea & Febiger, 1982. 461pp.
Describes the evaluation and management of animals with neurological diseases and then reviews each of the major neurological diseases in turn. Treatment and prognosis is discussed.

797   Christiansen, I. J. *Reproduction in the dog and cat*. London: Baillière Tindall, 1984. 309pp.
The first part of the book is devoted to the dog. The second part deals with the cat and uses the same arrangement of chapters.

798   Crow, S. E. and **Walshaw, S. O.** *Manual of clinical procedures in the dog and cat*. Philadelphia: J. B. Lippincott, 1987. 271pp.
Illustrates the diagnostic and therapeutic procedures commonly used in small animal practice with an accompanying text in outline format.

799   *Current veterinary therapy X: small animal practice*. Edited by R. W. Kirk. Philadelphia: W. B. Saunders, 1989. 1421pp.
An essential guide and reference text for the small animal practitioner. A vast amount of information is presented in the brief chapters and in the appendices. Previous editions are still valuable sources of information and the most recent editions refer to previous volumes.

800   Davis, L. E. (ed.) *Handbook of small animal therapeutics*. New York: Churchill Livingstone, 1985. 718pp.
Written in a concise note form. Most of the chapters deal with the chemotherapy of the diseases affecting a particular organ system. The drug regimes are described in detail.

801   Day, C. *The homeopathic treatment of small animals: principles and practice*. London: Wigmore Publications, 1984. 153pp.

802   Drazner, F. H. (ed.) *Small animal endocrinology*. New York: Churchill Livingstone, 1987. 508pp.
Thorough review of endocrine disorders and their diagnosis and treatment.

803   Edney, A. T. B. (ed.) *The Waltham book of dog and cat nutrition: a handbook for veterinarians and students*. 2nd ed. Oxford: Pergamon, 1988. 143pp.
Comprehensive introduction to the topic from the first principles of nutrition to clinical aspects of small animal nutrition.

804   Edney, A. T. B. and **Hughes, I. B.** *Pet care: a straightforward guide to keeping pet animals*. Oxford: Blackwell, 1986. 230pp. (Library of Veterinary Practice.)
Intended as a guide for pet owners and covers all aspects of pet care. The final chapter gives a list of popular publications on pets and details of societies that may provide further information.

805   Edwards, N. J. *Bolton's handbook of canine and feline electrocardiography*. 2nd ed. Philadelphia: W. B. Saunders, 1987. 381pp.
Explains basic electrocardiographic interpretation.

806   Ettinger, S. J. (ed.) *Textbook of veterinary internal medicine: diseases of the dog and cat*. 2nd ed. Philadelphia: W. B. Saunders, 1983. 2 vols. 2260pp.
Comprehensive textbook for undergraduates. The basic starting point for a search for information on medical disorders.

807   Farrow, C. S. *Emergency radiology in small animal practice*. Toronto: B. C. Decker, 1988. 375pp.
Almost 100 specific problems encountered in the thorax, abdomen and skeleton are dealt with under the following headings: general considerations, major radiographic observations, diagnostic strategy, pitfalls, and alternative diagnosis and suggested findings. Intended as a text for quick reference in emergencies.

808   Feldman, E. C. and **Nelson, R. W.** *Canine and feline endocrinology and reproduction*. Philadelphia: W. B. Saunders, 1987. 564pp.
Most of the book is concerned with endocrinology, with three final chapters on reproduction and reproductive disorders.

809   Fenner, W. R. (ed.) *Quick reference to veterinary medicine*. Philadelphia: J. B. Lippincott, 1982. 592pp.
Similar to Lorenz and Cornelius's work in being based on presenting signs and client complaints. Divided into sections dealing with client complaints or abnormal physical findings, laboratory abnormalities and principles of fluid management and physical and chemical injuries and intoxications.

810   Fogle, B. *Games pets play: or how not to be manipulated by your pet*. London: Michael Joseph, 1986. 218pp.
A humorous popular work with a list of further reading for those interested in human–pet relationships.

811   Ford, R. B. (ed.) *Clinical signs and diagnosis in small animal practice*. New York: Churchill Livingstone, 1988. 760pp.
The chapters are grouped around the type of presenting problem. Each gives a full discussion of diagnostic methods and procedures likely to be of value. Includes discussions of the pathogenic mechanisms leading to the presenting problem.

812   Fox, P. R. (ed.) *Canine and feline cardiology*. New York: Churchill Livingstone, 1988. 676pp.
Comprehensive text with chapters on the normal functioning of the cardiovascular system, clinical examination, abnormalities, diseases, surgery and pathology.

813   Gourley, I. M. and **Vasseur, P. B.** (eds) *General small animal surgery*. Philadelphia: J. B. Lippincott, 1985. 1124pp.
Surgical techniques are not described in detail. The book provides general discussions of the surgery of each organ or body system.

814   Grant, D. I. *Skin diseases in the dog and cat*. Oxford: Blackwell, 1986. 187pp. (Library of Veterinary Practice.)
Written in note-form to allow for quick reference.

815   Greene, C. E. (ed.) *Clinical microbiology and infectious diseases of the dog and cat*. Philadelphia: W. B. Saunders, 1984. 967pp.
There are chapters on each of the major diseases and on the infections of the various organ systems. There are also sections devoted to agent–host–environment interactions, laboratory diagnosis and antimicrobial therapy, immunoprophylaxis and immunotherapy, neurologic diseases and zoonoses. There are appendices giving recommendations for immunization and information on diagnosis and therapy.

816   Hart, B. L. and **Hart, L. A.** *Canine and feline behavioral therapy*. Philadelphia: Lea & Febiger, 1985. 275pp.

817   Hilbery, A. D. R. (ed.) *Manual of anaesthesia for small animal practice*. 2nd ed. Cheltenham: BSAVA, 1984. 108pp.
Intended as a handbook to be used as a reference guide. Two of the sections are devoted to special techniques and anaesthesia for exotic animals.

818   Houlton, J. E. F. and **Taylor, P. M.** *Trauma management in the dog and cat.*
Bristol: Wright, 1987. 159pp. (Veterinary Practitioner Handbook Series.)
Practical guide to the management of injured small animals including the treatment of shock and methods of intensive care. Gives details of the equipment and
techniques used.

819   Hughes, I. *Small animal emergencies.* Oxford: Blackwell. Forthcoming.
(Library of Veterinary Practice.)

820   *In practice: the small animal book.* London: BVA, 1985. 140pp.
A collection of continuing education articles featured in *In practice* from 1981–4.
Most of the items concern dogs or cats. There are also items on cagebirds, first aid
for wild birds and children's pets.

821   Jones, B. D. and **Liska, W. D.** (eds) *Canine and feline gastroenterology.*
Philadelphia: W. B. Saunders, 1986. 531pp.
Has chapters on both medical and surgical topics. Approximately one-fifth of the
book is devoted to a chapter on the radiology of the digestive system.

822   Kay, W. J., Nieburg, H. A., Kutscher, A. H., Grey, R. M. and **Fudin,
C. E.** (eds) *Pet loss and human bereavement.* Ames: Iowa State UP, 1984. 198pp.

823   Kealy, J. K. *Radiology of the dog and cat.* 2nd ed. Philadelphia: W. B.
Saunders, 1987. 547pp.
An established textbook of diagnostic interpretation which discusses both the nor-
mal anatomy and the more commonly encountered abnormalities and anomalies.

824   Keller, P. D. and **Freudiger, U. D.** *Atlas of hematology of the dog and cat.*
Berlin: Paul Parey, 1983. 159pp.
Has over 650 illustrations, nearly 400 of which are in colour, of normal and abnor-
mal blood cells and of blood cell parasites.

825   Kelly, D. F., Lucke, V. M. and **Gaskell, C. J.** *Notes on pathology for small
animal clinicians.* Bristol: Wright, 1982. 118pp. (Veterinary Practitioner Handbook Series.)
Practical approach to pathology/necropsy emphasizing aspects important in small
animal practice.

826   Lane, J. G. *ENT and oral surgery of the dog and cat.* Bristol: Wright, 1982.
288pp. (Veterinary Practitioner Handbook Series.)
Covers both diagnosis and treatment.

827   Leighton, R. L. and **Jones, K.** *A compendium of small animal surgery.* Ames:
Iowa State UP, 1983. 274pp. (Venture Series in Veterinary Medicine.)
Describes and illustrates, using line drawings, 160 surgical procedures.

828 *Leonard's Orthopedic surgery of the dog and cat.* 3rd ed. Edited by J. W. Alexander. Philadelphia: W. B. Saunders, 1985. 242pp.
Basic text on the principles, methods and techniques used in small animal orthopaedics.

829 **Lewis, L. D., Morris, M. L. Jr.** and **Hand, M. S.** *Small animal clinical nutrition.* 3rd ed. 5500 SW 7th Street, Topeka, Kansas 66606: Mark Morris Associates, 1987. 474pp.
Excellent source of basic information on nutrition. Deals with the dietary and medical management of a wide range of disorders. Discusses prescription diets in detail. Available in the UK from Hill's Pet Products.

830 **Lorenz, M. D.** and **Cornelius, L. M.** (eds) *Small animal medical diagnosis.* Philadelphia: J. B. Lippincott, 1987. 654pp.
Organized by the problems which are presented rather than by specific diseases.

831 **Martin, R. J.** *Small animal therapeutics.* London: Wright, 1989. 333pp.
Reviews the principles and practice of drug use with recommendations for the treatment of common conditions.

832 **Michell, A. R.** (ed.) *Renal disease in dogs and cats: comparative and clinical aspects.* Oxford: Blackwell, 1988. 166pp.
Collection of reviews on aspects of renal disease in small animals. There are introductory chapters on renal function and water balance.

833 **Morgan, R. V.** (ed.) *Handbook of small animal practice.* New York: Churchill Livingstone, 1988. 1257pp.
A large book in both detail and weight. Written entirely in outline format. Provides a reference text for all the common small animal ailments and diseases.

834 **Muller, G. H., Kirk, R. W.** and **Scott, D. W.** *Small animal dermatology.* 3rd ed. Philadelphia: W. B. Saunders, 1983. 889pp.
A fourth edition which will contain over 1,000 illustrations is in preparation.

835 **Murdoch, D. B.** *Clinical gastroenterology in the dog and cat.* Oxford: Blackwell, 1985. 180pp. (Library of Veterinary Practice.)

836 **Nesbitt, G. H.** *Canine and feline dermatology: a systematic approach.* Philadelphia: Lea & Febiger, 1983. 224pp.
Has both diagnostic and therapeutic keys supported by a detailed accompanying text with many colour and black and white photographs.

837 **Newton, C. D.** and **Nunamaker, D. M.** (eds.) *Textbook of small animal orthopaedics.* Philadelphia: J. B. Lippincott, 1985. 1140pp.

838   O'Brien, T. R. *Radiographic diagnosis of abdominal disorders in the dog and cat: radiographic interpretation, clinical signs, pathophysiology.* Philadelphia: W. B. Saunders, 1978. 682pp.

839   Olsson, S.-E. *The radiological diagnosis in canine and feline emergencies: an atlas of thoracic and abdominal changes.* Philadelphia: Lea & Febiger, 1973. 213pp.

840   Osborne, C. A., Low, D. G. and **Finco, D. R.** *Canine and feline urology.* Philadelphia: W. B. Saunders, 1972. 417pp.

841   Peiffer. R. L. Jr *Small animal ophthalmology: a problem-oriented approach.* Philadelphia: W. B. Saunders, 1989. 242pp. (A Saunders Veterinary Quick Reference Handbook.)

842   Piermattei, D. L. and **Greeley, R. G.** *An atlas of surgical approaches to the bones of the dog and cat.* 2nd ed. Philadelphia:. W. B. Saunders, 1979. 202pp.

843   Rawlings, C. A. *Heartworm disease in dogs and cats.* Philadelphia: W. B. Saunders, 1986. 329pp.
Reviews the diagnosis, pathology, treatment and prevention of *Dirofilaria immitis* infection.

844   Redding, R. W. and **Knecht, C. D.** *Atlas of electroencephalography in the dog and cat.* New York: Praeger, 1984. 387pp.
There is a brief account of the principles and practice of electroencephalography. Most of the book is a compilation of EEC recordings illustrating typical results which may be obtained from animals in a variety of conditions.

845   Reedy, L. M. and **Miller, W. H. Jr.** *Allergic skin diseases of dogs and cats.* Philadelphia: W. B. Saunders, 1989. 222pp. (Saunders Veterinary Quick Reference Handbook.)

846   Ryan, G. D. *Radiographic positioning of small animals.* Philadelphia: Lea & Febiger, 1981. 147pp.
Describes and illustrates correct positioning techniques.

847   Sawyer, D. C. *The practice of small animal anesthesia.* Philadelphia: W. B. Saunders, 1982. 243pp. (Major Problems in Veterinary Medicine, vol. 1.)

848   Schebitz, H. and **Wilkens, H.** *Atlas of radiographic anatomy of the dog and cat.* 4th ed. Berlin: Paul Parey, 1986. 244pp.

849   Shively, M. J. and **Beaver, B. G.** *Dissection of the dog and cat: a guide.* Ames: Iowa State UP, 1985. 152pp.

850   Slatter, D. H. (ed.) *Textbook of small animal surgery.* 2nd ed. Philadelphia: W. B. Saunders, 1985. 2 vols 2718pp.
A comprehensive reference text with nearly 200 contributors. Each of the chapters has excellent bibliographies.

851   Sodikoff, C. *Laboratory profiles of small animal diseases: a guide to laboratory diagnosis.* Edited by P. W. Pratt. Santa Barbara: American Veterinary Publications, 1981. 215pp.
Describes the results likely to be obtained in twenty-three blood chemistry, twelve haematology and thirteen urinalysis tests in ninety diseases.

852   Suter, P. F. and **Lord, P. F.** *Thoracic radiography: a text atlas of thoracic diseases of the dog and cat.* Wettswil, Switzerland: Peter F. Suter, 1984. 790pp.
Classic text integrating the radiographic picture with clinical and laboratory findings.

853   Swaim, S. F. *Surgery of traumatized skin: management and reconstruction in the dog and cat.* Philadelphia: W. B. Saunders, 1980. 585pp.

854   Tams, T. *Endoscopy in the dog and cat.* St. Louis: C. V. Mosby. Forthcoming.

855   Thomas, W. P. and **Sisson, D. D.** *Canine and feline cardiology.* Philadelphia: W. B. Saunders, 1987. 600pp.
Complete review of diagnostic evaluation, pathophysiology and treatment.

856   Ticer, J. W. *Radiographic technique in small animal practice.* 2nd ed. Philadelphia: W. B. Saunders, 1984. 511pp.

857   Tilley, L. P. (ed.) *Essentials of canine and feline electrocardiography: interpretation and treatment.* 2nd ed. Philadelphia: Lea & Febiger, 1985. 484pp.

858   Webbon, P. M. (ed.) *Guide to diagnostic radiography in small animal practice.* London: BSAVA, 1981. 79pp.
The common clinical conditions are used as the starting point and the indications and relative value of radiography in their diagnosis and management are outlined. There are ten pages of suggested further reading. A video is also available which covers part of the book: *Radiography and radiology of the canine chest.*

859   Wilkinson, G. T. *A colour atlas of small animal dermatology.* London: Wolfe Medical Publications, 1985. 272pp.
Has 513 colour photographs illustrating both the common and the most recently recognized rarer dermatological problems. In most cases several illustrations are used to show different manifestations of the condition. Intended to be used in conjunction with standard textbooks of veterinary dermatology.

860   Wingfield, W. E. and **Rawlings, C. A.** *Small animal surgery: an atlas of operative techniques.* Philadelphia: W. B. Saunders, 1979. 228pp.
Describes and illustrates all the common procedures with space for the user to add their own notes.

861   Yoxall, A. T. and **Hird, J. F. R.** (eds) *Physiological basis of small animal medicine.* Oxford: Blackwell, 1980. 389pp.

862   Yoxall, A. T. and **Hird, J. F. R.** (eds) *Pharmacological basis of small animal medicine.* Oxford: Blackwell, 1979. 318pp.

Conference

863   Anderson, R. S. (ed.) *Nutrition and behaviour in dogs and cats.* Oxford: Pergamon, 1984. 241pp.
Proceedings of the First Nordic Symposium on Small Animal Medicine, Oslo, September 1982. Comprises reviews of many individual aspects of behaviour and nutrition.

Journals

864   *Australian veterinary practitioner.* 1971–. PO Box 243, Bondi, New South Wales 2026, Australia: Australian Small Animal Veterinary Association. Quarterly.

865   *Companion animal practice.* 1987–. Santa Barbara: Veterinary Practice Publishing. Monthly.
Incorporates *Feline practice* (1971–86), *Canine practice* (1974–86) and *Avian/exotic practice* (1984–6). Most issues have two articles in each of these fields.

866   *Journal of the American Animal Hospital Association.* 1965–. Golden: AAHA. Bimonthly.
Most issues have about a dozen or so refereed articles plus case reports and occasional reviews.

867   *Journal of small animal practice.* 1960–. London: BVA. Monthly.
There is a cumulative subject and author index to volumes **1–15** (1960–74). Some of the issues are devoted to special topics e.g. **29** (1988): (7) Ophthalmology. Published on behalf of the British and World Small Animal Veterinary Associations and from 1988 onwards incorporates *BSAVA news.*

868   *Pratique médicale & chirurgicale de l'animal de compagnie.* 1966–. 10 Place Léon Blum, 75011 Paris, France: Conférence Nationale des Vétérinaires Specialistes des Petits Animaux. Bimonthly.

CATS

Bibliography

869 **Berman, E.** and **Liddle, C. G.** (eds) *Bibliography of the cat: revised edition.* Research Triangle Park, North Carolina: US Environmental Protection Agency, Health Effects Research Laboratory, 1976. 632pp.
Over 2300 references with author and subject indexes.

Books

870 **Allan, E., Bonning, L.** and **Rowan Blogg, J.** *Everycat: the complete guide to cat care, behaviour and health.* London: Peter Lowe, 1986. 271pp.
Popular text on feline care and medicine intended for the layman but indicating where veterinary attention is necessary.

871 **Beaver, B. V. G.** *Veterinary aspects of feline behaviour.* St Louis: C. V. Mosby, 1980. 217pp.
General survey with a detailed bibliography.

872 **Bohensky, F.** and **Rickard, J.** *Photo manual and dissection guide of the cat.* 2nd ed. Wayne, New Jersey: Avery Publishing Group, 1977. 154pp.

873 **Booth, E. S.** *Laboratory anatomy of the cat.* 7th ed. Revised by R. B. Chiasson. Dubuque: W. C. Brown, 1982. 106pp. (Booth Laboratory Anatomy Series.)

874 **Chandler, E. A., Hilbery, A. D. R.** and **Gaskell, C. J.** (eds) *Feline medicine and therapeutics.* Oxford: Blackwell, 1985. 405pp.
Prepared for the BSAVA and gives information relevant to UK practice. The various systems of the body are dealt with followed by chapters on the major infectious diseases. Chapters are also devoted to poisoning, feline nutrition and disease, endoparasites, behavioural problems, paediatrics and therapeutics.

875 *The complete book of cat health.* By W. J. Kay, E. Randolph, Animal Medical Center. New York: Macmillan, 1985. 258pp.
The same authors have written *The complete book of dog health* (1985, 253pp.).

876 **Donnersberger, A. B., Lesak, A. E.** and **Timmons, M. J.** *A manual of anatomy and physiology: laboratory animal, the cat.* 3rd ed. Lexington: D. C. Heath, 1985. 455pp.

877 **Evans, J. M.** and **White, K.** *The catlopaedia: a complete guide to cat care.* Guildford: Henston, 1988. 212pp.
Complete guide for the layman to caring for cats. Includes discussions of health problems.

878   Field, H. E. and **Taylor, M. E.** revised by **B. B. Butterworth.** *An atlas of cat anatomy*. 2nd ed. Chicago: University of Chicago Press, 1985. 77pp.
Fifty-seven black and white illustrations of dissections with an explanatory text.

879   Hart, B. L. *Feline behavior: collected columns from Feline practice journal*. Santa Barbara: Veterinary Practice Publishing, 1978. 110pp.

880   Holzworth, J. (ed.) *Diseases of the cat: medicine and surgery. Volume 1.* Philadelphia: W. B. Saunders, 1987. 971pp.
Universally acknowledged as what is to become the definitive textbook on feline medicine and surgery. The first volume of the two volume work deals with nutrition, surgery and anaesthesia, immunology, microbial diseases, tumours and neoplasms, the skin, eye, ear, haematopoietic system, cardiovascular system and with inherited metabolic diseases.

881   Leyhausen, P. *The predatory and social behaviour of domestic and wild cats*. New York: Garland STPM Press, 1979. 340pp. (Garland Series in Ethology).

882   McClure, R. C., Dallman, M. J. and **Garrett, P. D.** *Cat anatomy: an atlas, text and dissection guide*. Philadelphia: Lea & Febiger, 1973. 240pp.

883   Morris, D. *Catwatching*. London: Jonathan Cape, 1986. 106pp.
An elementary explanation of feline behaviour using the technique of answering specific questions. The author has written similar works on the behaviour of dogs (*Dogwatching*, 1986, 106pp.) and horses (*Horsewatching*, 1988, 114pp.).

884   Olsen, R. G. (ed.) *Feline leukemia*. Boca Raton: CRC Press, 1981. 171pp.

885   Povey, R. C. *Infectious diseases of cats: a clinical handbook*. Box 223, Guelph, Ontario, Canada: Centaur Press, 1985. Ringbound with supplements to be issued.
Gives concise summaries of all the common diseases. A companion volume, issued in 1988, is entitled *Infectious diseases of dogs*.

886   Pratt, P. W. (ed.) *Feline medicine*. Santa Barbara: American Veterinary Publications, 1983. 687pp.
Multiauthored American text. Likely to be replaced in general use by Holzworth's work.

887   Robinson, R. *Genetics for cat breeders*. 2nd ed. Oxford: Pergamon, 1977. 202pp.

888   *A standard guide to cat breeds*. Edited by R. H. Gebhardt, G. Pond and I. Raleigh. London: Macmillan, 1982. 318pp.

Gives standards for pedigree breeds recognized in the United States and Britain. Includes many photographs and line drawings and illustrations of coat and eye colours.

889   Taylor, D. *You and your cat.* London: Dorling Kindersley, 1986. 288pp. An owner's guide to the care, health and welfare of cats. The same author has written a similar work on dogs (1986, 288pp.).

890   The TV vet. *Cats . . . their health and care: owner's guide to cat ailments and conditions.* Ipswich: Farming Press, 1977. 128pp.

891   Wilkinson, G. T. (ed.) *Diseases of the cat and their management.* 2nd ed. Oxford: Blackwell, 1984. 602pp.
There are chapters on nutrition, toxicology, on diseases of the various anatomical systems, neoplasia, and on viral, bacterial, mycotic and parasitic diseases. Appendices give physiological values and a posological table.

Conference

892   *The ecology and control of feral cats: proceedings of a symposium held at Royal Holloway College, University of London, 23rd and 24th September, 1980.* Potters Bar: UFAW, 1981. 99pp.

Journal

893   *Feline health topics for veterinarians.* 1986–. Cornell University, College of Veterinary Medicine, Ithaca, New York 14853: Cornell Feline Health Center. Quarterly.

Other Journal

Feline Advisory Bureau bulletin

DOGS

Bibliography

894   Mason, M. M. *Bibliography of the dog.* Ames: Iowa State UP, 1959. 401pp.
There are author and subject indexes.

Historical bibliography

895   Jones, E. G. *A bibliography of the dog: books published in the English language 1570–1965.* London: Library Association, 1971. 431pp.

Has 3,986 entries in subject classified order with indexes to names, titles and subjects. There is a chronological list of works published up to 1850.

Dictionaries

896   Bleby, J. and **Bishop, G.** *The dog's health from A–Z: a canine veterinary dictionary*. Newton Abbot: David & Charles, 1986. 331pp.
Has brief definitions of terms likely to be used by veterinarians.

897   Spira, H. R. *Canine terminology* London: Harper & Row, 1982. 145pp.
An illustrated glossary defining words and phrases used by breeders of dogs.

Books

898   Adam, W. S., Calhoun, M. L., Smith, E. M. and **Stinson, A. W.** *Microscopic anatomy of the dog: a photographic atlas*. Springfield: C. C. Thomas, 1970. 292pp.

899   Adams, D. R. *Canine anatomy: a systematic study*. Ames: Iowa State UP, 1986. 513pp.
Intended as an adjunct to Miller's anatomy of the dog and gives introductory anatomical information on the dog and cat. Details the systematic dissection of non-embalmed canine carcasses.

900   Alcock, J. *A dog of your own*. London: Sheldon, 1981. 102pp.
A brief but amusing book on choosing a dog and caring for it correctly.

901   American Kennel Club. *The complete dog book: the photograph, history, and official standard of every breed admitted to AKC registration, and the selection, training, breeding, care and feeding of pure-bred dogs*. 17th ed. New York: Howell Book House, 1985. 768pp.
The dogs are arranged by group and then alphabetically by breed with each breed described in detail. There is a general section on caring for dogs.

902   Amman, K., Seiferle, E. and **Pelloni, G.** *Atlas of topographical surgical anatomy of the dog*. Berlin: Paul Parey, 1978. 77pp.
Comprises ninety-five coloured anatomical drawings with text in five languages.

903   Andersen, A. C. (ed.) *The Beagle as an experimental dog*. Ames: Iowa State UP, 1970. 616pp.

904   Andersen, A. C. and **Simpson, M. E.** *The ovary and reproductive cycle of the dog*. Los Altos, California: Geron-X Inc., 1973. 290pp.
Gives data recorded in a long-term study of the normal reproductive function in beagles.

905   Archibald, J. (ed.) *Canine surgery: a text and reference work.* 2nd ed. Wheaton, Illinois: American Veterinary Publications, 1974. 1172pp.

906   Beck, A. M. *The ecology of stray dogs: a study of free-ranging urban animals.* Baltimore: York Press, 1973. 98pp.

907   Bedford, P. G. C. (ed.) *An atlas of canine surgical techniques.* Oxford: Blackwell, 1984. 186pp.
The first section covers instruments and equipment, sterilization and disinfection, anaesthesia and fluid therapy and radiography. The second section describes specific surgical procedures.

908   Boreham, P. F. L. and **Atwell, R. B.** (eds) *Dirofilariasis.* Boca Raton: CRC Press, 1988. 249pp.
Review of *Dirofilaria immitis* infection.

909   Bovee, K. C. (ed.) *Canine nephrology.* PO Box 210, RD 1, Malvern, Pennsylvania 19355: the Author, 1984. 818pp.
The most comprehensive work on the canine kidney.

910   Budras, K-D. and **Fricke, W.** *Atlas der Anatomie des Hundes: Lehrbuch für Tierärzte und Studierende.* Hanover: Schlütersche Verlagsanstalt, 1987. 117pp.
The coloured plates are labelled with Latin terms from the *Nominia anatomica veterinaria.*

911   Bush, B. *The dog care question and answer book.* London: Orbis, 1982. 303pp.
A popular work for dog owners. The author has written a similar work on cats (1981, 240pp.)

912   Bush, B. M. *Differential diagnosis in canine practice.* Oxford: Blackwell. Forthcoming. (Library of Veterinary Practice.)
Most of the data will be in tables. These will list the conditions responsible for particular clinical signs, the breeds, age and sex of dogs most commonly affected by particular disorders and the disorders and diseases most likely to occur in different breeds, ages and sexes of dogs.

913   Campbell, W. E. *Behavior problems in dogs.* Santa Barbara: American Veterinary Publications, 1975. 306pp.

914   Catcott, E. J. (ed.) *Canine medicine.* 4th ed. Santa Barbara: American Veterinary Publications, 1979. 2 vols. 1360pp.
The standard American reference work.

915   Chandler, E. A., Sutton, J. B. and **Thompson, D. J.** (eds) *Canine medicine and therapeutics.* 2nd ed. Oxford: Blackwell, 1984. 566pp.

The standard British text. Sponsored by the BSAVA. Deals with each anatomical system in turn and has chapters on other aspects of clinical medicine including endoparasites, poisoning, behavioural problems and canine nutrition and disease.

916   Christoph, H-J. *Diseases of dogs*. Oxford: Pergamon, 1975. 496pp.
Translated from an East German work published in 1962. Mainly concerned with diagnosis and treatment. The same author has also collaborated in a more recent work *Klinik der Hundekrankheiten* (by H-J. Christophe, U. Freudiger, E-G. Grunbaum and E. Schimke, Stuttgart: Gustav Fischer, 1986, 1067pp.).

917   Clarke, R. D., Stainer, J. R., Haynes, H. D., Buckner, R., Mosier, J. E. and **Quinn, A. J.** (eds) *Medical and genetic aspects of purebred dogs*. Edwardsville: Veterinary Medicine Publishing, 1983. 576pp.
Provides information on hereditary diseases in 130 breeds of dogs.

918   Croft, P. G. *The management of epilepsy in dogs*. London: Henston, 1984. 49pp.

919   Darke, P. G. G. *Notes on canine internal medicine*. 2nd ed. Bristol: Wright, 1986. 286pp. (Veterinary Practitioner Handbook Series.)
A handbook providing a step-by-step approach to the investigation of common clinical syndromes and particularly useful as an aid in differential diagnosis.

920   Denny, H. R. *A guide to canine orthopaedic surgery*. 2nd ed. Oxford: Blackwell, 1985. 283pp. (Library of Veterinary Practice.)
Popular work on orthopaedic problems which went into a second edition quickly.

921   Edgson, F. A. and **Gwynne-Jones, O.** *First aid and nursing for your dog*. 9th ed. London: Popular Dogs, 1987. 96pp.

922   Ettinger, S. J. and **Suter, P. F.** *Canine cardiology*. Philadelphia: W. B. Saunders, 1970. 626pp.

923   Evans, H. E. and **Christensen, G. C.** *Miller's anatomy of the dog*. 2nd ed. Philadelphia: W. B. Saunders, 1979. 1181pp.
Complete survey of canine anatomy.

924   Evans, H. E. and **de Lahunta, A.** *Miller's guide to the dissection of the dog*. 3rd ed. Philadelphia: W. B. Saunders, 1988. 361pp.
Gives detailed descriptions of dissections on each body region with accompanying illustrations. At appropriate sections instructions are given for the palpation of structures in live dogs.

925   Evans, J. M. and **White, K.** *The doglopaedia: a complete guide to dog care.* Guildford: Henston, 1985. 251pp.
Comprehensive guide for the layman to the health and well being of dogs. The same authors have written *The book of the bitch* (1988, 230pp.), a guide to the handling and management of breeding from bitches.

926   Fox, M. W. *Canine behavior.* Springfield: C. C. Thomas, 1978. 152pp.

927   Fox, M. W. *The dog: its domestication and behavior.* New York: Garland STPM Press, 1978. 296pp.

928   Fox, M. W. *Canine pediatrics: development, neonatal and congenital diseases.* Springfield: C. C. Thomas, 1966. 148pp.

929   Glover, H. (ed.) *A standard guide to pure-bred dogs.* London: Macmillan, 1977. 472pp.
Describes 350 breeds in detail.

930   Hall, D. E. *Blood coagulation and its disorders in the dog.* London: Baillière Tindall, 1972. 188pp.

931   Hart, B. L. *Canine behavior: collected columns for 'Canine practice journal'.* Santa Barbara: Veterinary Practice Publishing, 1980. 118pp.

932   Hutt, F. B. *Genetics for dog breeders.* San Francisco: W. B. Freeman, 1979. 245pp.

933   Jenkins, T. W. *Functional mammalian neuroanatomy, with emphasis on dog and cat, including an atlas of dog central nervous system.* 2nd ed. Philadelphia: Lea & Febiger, 1978. 480pp.

934   Jones, D. E. and **Joshua, J. O.** *Reproductive clinical problems in the dog.* 2nd ed. Bristol: Wright, 1988. 238pp. (Veterinary Practitioner Handbook Series.)
Describes reproductive anatomy, physiology and endocrinology of the bitch and male dog. Covers reproductive disorders and their treatment.

935   Jones, H. G. and **Collins, B. C.** *A way of life: sheepdog training, handling and trialling.* Ipswich: Farming Press, 1987. 192pp.
Has brief veterinary appendices.

936   Lanting, F. L. *Canine hip dysplasia and other orthopedic problems.* Loveland, Colorado: Alpine Publications, 1980. 212pp.

937   Magrane, W. G. *Canine ophthalmology*. 3rd ed. Philadelphia: Lea & Febiger, 1977. 305pp.
Reviews ophthalmic diseases and covers surgical procedures. A fourth edition is in preparation (edited by L. C. Helper).

938   Morgan, J. P. *Radiology of skeletal disease: principles of diagnosis in the dog.* Ames: Iowa State UP, 1981. 106pp. (Venture Series in Veterinary Medicine.)
Seventy case histories are followed over time using 170 radiographic images and differential and final diagnoses are discussed.

939   Morgan, J. P. and **Stephens, M.** *Radiographic diagnosis and control of canine hip dysplasia.* Ames: Iowa State UP, 1985. 145pp. (Venture Series in Veterinary Medicine.)
Comprehensive discussion of the disease and its control. The bulk of the work is concerned with radiographic techniques and procedures.

940   O'Farrell, V. *Manual of canine behaviour.* Cheltenham: BSAVA, 1986. 130pp.
Reviews the basics of canine psychology and then deals with specific disorders and their prevention.

941   Ritchie, C. I. A. *The British dog: its history from earliest times.* London: Robert Hale, 1981. 192pp.

942   Rolins, A. *All about the greyhound.* Letchworth, Hertfordshire: Ringpress, 1986. 264pp.
Describes the anatomy, physiology and metabolism of the greyhound.

943   Rubin, L. F. *Inherited eye diseases in purebred dogs.* Baltimore: Williams & Wilkins, 1989. 363pp.

944   Sandys-Winsch, G. *Your dog and the law.* London: Shaw & Sons, 1984. 87pp.

945   Shifrine, M. and **Wilson, F. D.** (eds) *The canine as a biomedical research model: immunological, hematological and oncological aspects.* Washington, DC: US Department of Energy, Technical Information Center, 1980. 425pp. (Available as report no. DOC/TIC-10191 from NTIS.)

946   Siegel, E. T. *Endocrine diseases of the dog.* Philadelphia: Lea & Febiger, 1977. 212pp.

947   Sokolowski, J. H. and **Fletcher, A. M.** (eds) *Basic guide to canine nutrition.* 5th ed. PO Box 9003, Chicago, Illinois 60604: Gaines Pet Food Corp., Gaines Professional Services, 1987. 95pp.

948 Sutton, C. G. and **Lampson, S. M.** *The new observer's book of dogs*. London: Frederick Warne, 1983. 192pp.
Inexpensive guide to all the breeds.

949 *The TV Vet dog book: recognition and treatment of common dog ailments*. 3rd ed. Ipswich: Farming Press, 1980 (amended 1983). 208pp.
A fourth edition is shortly to be published under the title *Dog ailments*.

950 Whittick, W. G. (ed.) *Canine orthopedics*. Philadelphia: Lea & Febiger, 1974. 481pp.
A new edition is in preparation.

951 Willis, M. B. *Genetics of the dog*. London: H. F. & G. Witherby, 1989. 417pp.
A complete guide including discussions of inherited defects and diseases.

952 Wolvekamp, W. Th. C. *Enteroclysis: a new radiographic technique for evaluation of the small intestine of the dog*. Ames: Iowa State UP, 1989. 139pp. (Venture Series in Veterinary Medicine.).
Explains and evaluates the use of enteroclysis, small bowel enema, for improving X-ray examinations.

RABBITS

Rabbits are popular domestic pets and are bred as show animals. They are also farmed in many countries for meat, angora wool and fur. Many of the works on laboratory animal science also discuss rabbits.

Books

953 Arrington, L. R. and **Kelley, K. C.** *Domestic rabbit biology and production*. Gainesville: The University Presses of Florida, 1976. 230pp.
A general survey of the biology and husbandry of the rabbit.

954 Barone, R., Pavaux, C., Blin, P. C. and **Cuq, P.** *Atlas d'anatomie du lapin: atlas of rabbit anatomy*. Paris: Masson et Cie, 1973. 219pp.

955 Cheeke, P. R. *Rabbit feeding and nutrition*. London: Academic Press, 1987. 376pp. (Animal Feeding and Nutrition.)
Also covers the nutrition of guinea pigs and the capybara.

956 Cheeke, P. R., Patton, N. M., Lukefahr, S. D. and **McNitt, J. I.** *Rabbit production*. 6th ed. Danville: Interstate Printers and Pubishers, 1987. 472pp.
An established text on the husbandry of rabbits which contains a section on diseases. Has colour illustrations of the major breeds.

957   *Commercial rabbit production.* 11th ed. London: HMSO, 1985. 48pp. (MAFF Bulletin 50.)
A brief review of the technical and economic problems facing producers with sections on marketing, determining production costs and record keeping.

958   Craigie, E. H. *A laboratory guide to the anatomy of the rabbit.* 2nd ed. Toronto: University of Toronto Press, 1966. 115pp.

959   Dubiski, S. (ed.) *The rabbit in contemporary immunological research.* Harlow: Longman, 1987. 206pp. (Monographs and Surveys in the Biosciences.)

960   *The encyclopaedia of pet rabbits.* By D. Robinson. Hong Kong: TFH Publications, 1979. 320pp.

961   Fenner, F. and **Ratcliffe, F. N.** *Myxomatosis.* Cambridge: CUP, 1965. 379pp.

962   Harkness, J. E. and **Wagner, J. E.** *The biology and medicine of rabbits and rodents.* 3rd ed. Philadelphia: Lea & Febiger, 1989. 230pp.
Deals with rabbits, guinea pigs, hamsters, gerbils, mice and rats. Detailed guide to all the significant diseases and conditions.

963   Kaplan, H. M. and **Timmons, E. H.** *The rabbit: a model for the principles of mammalian physiology and surgery.* New York: Academic Press, 1979. 167pp.
Describes the basic principles of rabbit surgery and anaesthesia. Then gives details on forty-four basic physiological and surgical techniques and twenty advanced specialized procedures for which rabbits are suitable subjects.

964   Leverett, B. *Keeping rabbits: a complete manual.* London: Blandford Press, 1987. 160pp.

965   McLaughlin, C. A. and **Chiasson, R. B.** *Laboratory anatomy of the rabbit.* 2nd ed. Dubuque: W. C. Brown, 1979. 68pp. (Booth Laboratory Animal Series.)

966   Okerman, L. *Diseases of domestic rabbits.* Translated by R. Sundahl. Oxford: Blackwell, 1988. 120pp. (Library of Veterinary Practice.)
The only modern text in English. Gives basic zootechnical data and notes on diseases and their treatment. There are twenty-eight colour photographs.

967   Portsmouth, J. I. *Commercial rabbit keeping.* Hindhead: Saiga, 1979. 142pp.

968   Sandford, J. *Rabbits.* Marlborough: Crowood Press, 1988. 128pp.
Popular guide for small-scale breeders. Published in the *A Guide to Management*

Series which also has books on *Sheep* (E. Hart), Poultry (C. Twinch), *Ducks and geese* (T. Bartlett) and *Honey bees* (R. Brown).

969   Sandford, J. C. *The domestic rabbit.* 4th ed. London: Collins, 1986. 272pp.
Intended for rabbit farmers and covers every aspect of production, management and marketing.

970   Shek, J. W., Wen, G. Y. and **Wisniewski, H. M.** *Atlas of the rabbit brain and spinal cord.* Basel: Karger, 1985. 139pp.

971   Weisbroth, S. H., Flatt, R. E. and **Kraus, A. L.** (eds) *The biology of the laboratory rabbit.* New York: Academic Press, 1974. 496pp.
Comprehensive review of the anatomy, biochemistry, physiology, genetics and health of rabbits. Has several chapters on diseases and parasites.

Conference

972   *Proceedings of the 3rd World's rabbit congress. Rome, 4–8 April 1984.* Summaries of the papers appear in *Cuni-sciences* **2** (1984): (2) 1–56.
The Fourth Congress (of the World Rabbit Science Association) was held in Budapest in October 1988 with summaries of the communications published in *Cuni-sciences* **4** (1987/8): (3) 11–37. The Second Congress was held in Barcelona in 1980.

Journals

973   *Cuni-sciences: éditions de synthèses scientifiques.* 1983–. BP 50, 63370 Lempdes, France: Association Française de Cuniculture. Two or three per year.
A classified bibliography on rabbit health, diseases and parasites has been published in **4** 1987/8 (1), (2) and (3).

974   *Journal of applied rabbit research.* 1978–. Oregon State University, Corvallis, Oregon 97331: Rabbit Research Center. Quarterly.

Other Journals

American rabbit journal
Coniglicoltura
Cunicultura
Cuniculture
Journées de la recherche cunicole en France
Rabbits
Rabbits in Canada
Rivista di coniglicoltura

LABORATORY ANIMALS

Many of the small laboratory animals are kept as pets but the main interest is due to the veterinarian's role in ensuring the health and welfare of animals used in research and in industrial laboratories.

Current Awareness Service

975   *Current primate references*. 1964–. SJ-50, Seattle, Washington 98195: University of Washington, Primate Information Center. Monthly.

Bibliography

976   **Cass, J. S.** (ed.) *Laboratory animals: an annotated bibliography of informational resources covering medicine – science (including husbandry) – technology*. New York: Hafner Publishing, 1971. 446pp.

Directory

977   *International index of laboratory animals*. 5th ed. Compiled by M. F. W. Festing. London: Laboratory Animals, 1987. 118pp. (Laboratory Animal Handbooks 10.)
Gives the names and locations of strains and stocks of laboratory animals.

Handbooks and Guides

978   **Biology Databook Editorial Board** and **Altman, P. L.** (ed.) *Pathology of laboratory rats and mice*. Bethesda: Federation of American Societies for Experimental Biology/McLean, Virginia: Pergamon Infoline, 1985. 488pp. (Biology Databook Series.)
Has data on six of the most commonly used strains of mice and rats.

979   **Committee on Care and Use of Laboratory Animals of the Institute of Laboratory Animal Resources.** *Guide for the care and use of laboratory animals*. Bethesda: US Department of Health and Human Services, Public Health Service, National Institutes of Health, 1985. 83pp. (NIH Publication No. 86–23.).
Investigators and institutions in the United States must comply with the recommendations in order for their research to be approved and government funds provided. Contains a detailed bibliography of key works.

980   *Guide to the care and use of experimental animals*. 1105–151 Slater Street, Ottawa, Ontario K1P 5H3: Canadian Council on Animal Care, 1980, 1984. 2 vols. 112 + 208pp.

981   Melby, E. C. Jr and **Altman, N. H.** (eds) *Handbook of laboratory animal science*. Cleveland: CRC Press, 1974, 1974, 1976. 3 vols. 451 + 523 + 943pp.
Each volume reviews a diverse range of topics of interest to laboratory workers.

982   *The UFAW Handbook on the care and management of laboratory animals*. 6th ed. Edited by T. B. Poole. Harlow: Longman, 1987. 933pp.
An authoritative text on all aspects of the humane treatment and care of laboratory animals. Mostly concerned with mammals, the book also covers birds, reptiles, amphibians and fish. Previous editions also dealt with various invertebrates (mainly insects).

Books

983   Andrews, E. J., Ward, B. C. and **Altman, N. H.** (eds) *Spontaneous animal models of human disease*. London: Academic Press, 1979. 2 vols. 322 + 324pp. (American College of Laboratory Animal Medicine Series.)

984   Baker, H. J., Lindsey, J. R. and **Weisbroth, S. H.** (eds) *The laboratory rat*. London: Academic Press, 1979–80. 2 vols. 435 + 276pp. (American College of Laboratory Animal Medicine Series.)
Volume 1 deals with basic biology and diseases, volume 2 with research applications including methodology and experimental technique. Appendices to volume 2 give normative data and details of drugs and dosages.

985   Benirschke, K., Garner, F. M. and **Jones, T. C.** *Pathology of laboratory animals*. New York: Springer-Verlag, 1978. 2 vols. 2171pp.
The first volume is a general discussion of pathology, the second is devoted to laboratory animals.

986   Calabrese, E. J. *Principles of animal extrapolation*. New York: John Wiley, 1983. 603pp.

987   Chiasson, R. B. *Laboratory anatomy of the white rat*. 4th ed. Dubuque: W. C. Brown, 1980. 101pp. (Laboratory Anatomy Series.)

988   Committee on Infectious Diseases of Mice and Rats, National Research Council. *Guide to infectious diseases of mice and rats*. Washington, DC: National Academy Press. Forthcoming.
Will describe the principles of disease prevention in rodents, the diagnosis and control of each infectious agent and contain a tabular index to assist diagnosis.

989   Crispens, C. G. Jr *Handbook on the laboratory mouse*. Springfield: C. C. Thomas, 1975. 267pp.
A compilation of numerical data on every aspect of the mouse. The bibliography consists of nearly 1,000 references.

990   Feldman, D. B. and **Seely, J. C.** *Necropsy guide: rodents and the rabbit.* Boca Raton: CRC Press, 1988. 167pp.
An illustrated guidebook to dissection and the collection of organs and tissues.

991   Flecknell, P. A. *Laboratory animal anaesthesia: an introduction for research workers and technicians.* London: Academic Press, 1987. 156pp.
Introduction to the principles of anaesthesia for non-veterinary qualified personnel. There is a section describing anaesthetic regimes for the common laboratory species. The only large animals discussed in detail are pigs, sheep and primates. Appendices contain a wealth of useful data. C. J. Green's *Animal anaesthesia* (2nd ed. London: Laboratory Animals, 1982, 300pp., Laboratory Animal Handbooks, no. 8) has a slightly broader scope.

992   Flynn, R. J. *Parasites of laboratory animals.* Ames: Iowa State UP, 1973. 884pp.

993   Fogh, J. and **Giovanella, B. C.** (eds) *The nude mouse in experimental clinical research.* London: Academic Press, 1978/82. 2 vols. 502 + 587pp.
Volume 1 discusses the biology and use of the nude mouse and has a section on diseases. Volume 2 updates this work and describes its use in experimental investigations.

994   Foster, H. L., Small, J. D. and **Fox, J. G.** (eds) *The mouse in biomedical research.* London: Academic Press, 1981–3. 4 vols. 306 + 449 + 447 + 561pp. (American College of Laboratory Animal Medicine Series.)
The four volumes are entitled:
1 *History, genetics and wild mice.* 1981
2 *Diseases.* 1982
3 *Normative biology, immunology and husbandry.* 1983
4 *Experimental biology and oncology.* 1982

995   Fox, J. G. *Biology and diseases of the ferret.* Philadelphia: Lea & Febiger, 1988. 345pp.
First work devoted to scientific and veterinary aspects of this animal.

996   Fox, J. G., Cohen, B. J. and **Loew, F. M.** (eds) *Laboratory animal medicine.* Orlando: Academic Press, 1984. 750pp. (American College of Laboratory Animal Medicine Series.)
Chapters deal with all the major species, including ungulates, primates, amphibians, reptiles and fish. Covers both basic biology and diseases and subjects of common interest such as welfare, care, genetic monitoring, anaesthesia, methods of experimentation.

997   Frith, C. H., Pattengale, P. K. and **Ward, J. M.** *A colour atlas of hematopoietic pathology of mice.* 1102 Briar Creek Road, Little Rock, Arkansas 72211: Toxicology Pathology Associates, 1985. 30pp.

998   Frith, C. H. and **Ward, J. M.** *Color atlas of neoplastic and non-neoplastic lesions in aging mice.* Amsterdam: Elsevier, 1988. 109pp.

999   Greaves, P. and **Faccini, J. M.** *Rat histopathology: a glossary for use in toxicity and carcinogenicity studies.* Amsterdam: Elsevier, 1984. 251pp.
Describes typical histopathological findings associated with specific diagnoses.

1000   Gude, W. D., Cosgrove, G. E. and **Hirsch, G. P.** *Histological atlas of the laboratory mouse.* New York: Plenum Press, 1982. 151pp.

1001   Hebel, R. and **Stromberg, M. W.** *Anatomy of the laboratory rat.* Baltimore: Williams & Wilkins, 1976. 173pp.

1002   Hime, J. M. and **O'Donoghue, P. N.** (eds) *Handbook of diseases of laboratory animals: diagnosis and treatment.* London: Heinemann, 1979. 350pp.

1003   Holmes, D. D. *Clinical laboratory animal medicine: an introduction.* Ames: Iowa State UP, 1984. 138pp.
Gives basic data on the biology and care of the usual laboratory species plus ferrets, non-human primates and reptiles. Outlines the diagnosis and treatment of disease. Appendices give drug dosages, normal physiological values and specify the preferred food of selected reptiles.

1004   Huser, H-J. *Atlas of comparative primate hematology.* New York: Academic Press, 1970. 405pp.

1005   Inglis, J. K. *Introduction to laboratory animal science and technology.* Oxford: Pergamon, 1980. 323pp.
A basic text which has a chapter on health and hygiene.

1006   Jones, T. C., Mohr, U. and **Hunt, R. D.** (eds) *Monographs on pathology of laboratory animals.* Berlin: Springer-Verlag, 1983–.
Works in the series deal with the *Respiratory system* (1985, 240pp.), *Endocrine system* (1983, 366pp.), *Digestive system* (1985, 386pp.), *Urinary system* (1986, 405pp.), *Genital system* (1987, 304pp.) and *Nervous system* (1988, 233pp.). The texts are mainly concerned with rats, mice and hamsters and are sponsored by the International Life Sciences Institute.

1007   Lewi, P. J. and **Marsboom, R. P.** *Toxicology reference data, Wistar rat: body and organ weights, biochemical determinations, hematology and urinalysis, compiled at*

Janssen Pharmaceutica. Amsterdam: Elsevier/North Holland, 1981. 358pp. (Janssen Research Foundation Series, vol. 4)

1008   Loeb, W. F. and **Quimby, F. W.** (eds) *The clinical chemistry of laboratory animals.* Oxford: Pergamon, 1989. 519pp.
Discusses the collection of specimens, differences among species or strains and makes evaluations according to classes of analytes.

1009   Needham, J. R. *Handbook of microbiological investigations for laboratory animal health.* London: Academic Press, 1979. 174pp.

1010   Olds, R. J. and **Olds, J. R.** *A colour atlas of the rat: dissection guide.* London: Wolfe Medical Publications, 1979. 112pp.

1011   Petty, C. *Research techniques in the rat.* Springfield: C. C. Thomas, 1982. 368pp.

1012   Reznik, G., Reznik-Schuller, H. and **Mohr, U.** *Clinical anatomy of the European hamster* (Cricetus cricetus L.). Tunbridge Wells: Castle House Publications, 1981. 247pp.
Has many colour and black and white illustrations plus tables of organ and gland weights.

1013   Sanderson, J. H. and **Phillips, C. E.** *An atlas of laboratory animal haematology.* Oxford: Clarendon Press, 1981. 473pp.

1014   Schmidt, R. E. (ed.) *Pathology of aging Syrian hamsters.* Boca Raton: CRC Press, 1983. 242pp.

1015   Seaman, W. J. *Postmortem change in the rat: a histologic characterization.* Ames: Iowa State UP, 1987. 120pp.
Aids the recognition of histologic changes, occurring during time intervals from 20 minutes to 16 hours, solely as the result of death.

1016   Simmons, M. L. and **Brick, J. O.** *The laboratory mouse: selection and management.* Englewood Cliffs: Prentice-Hall, 1970. 184pp. (Biological Techniques Series.)

1017   Tuffery, A. A. (ed.) *Laboratory animals: an introduction for new experimenters.* New York: John Wiley, 1987. 342pp.
Covers the practical use and handling of laboratory animals. Ethical and legal issues are discussed with reference to the UK and USA.

1018   Turusov, V. S. (ed.) *Pathology of tumours in laboratory animals.* Lyon: International Agency for Research on Cancer.

The volumes in the series are: *Volume I: Tumours of the rat. Parts 1 and 2* (1987, 319pp., IARC Scientific Publications 5 and 6), a reprint of works originally published in 1973 (Part 1) and 1976 (Part 2), *Volume II: Tumours of the mouse* (1979, 661pp., IARC Scientific Publication 23) and *Volume III: Tumours of the hamster* (1982, 455pp., IARC Scientific Publication 34).

1019   Van Hoosier, G. L. Jr and **McPherson, C. W.** (eds) *Laboratory hamsters.* Orlando: Academic Press, 1987. 400pp. (American College of Laboratory and Animal Medicine Series.)
Mainly concerned with the Syrian or golden hamster but also has chapters on the Chinese (striped), European and five other lesser-known species.

1020   Wagner, J. E. and **Manning, P. J.** (eds) *The biology of the guinea pig.* 2nd ed. New York: Academic Press, 1987. 317pp. (American College of Laboratory and Animal Medicine Series.)
A comprehensive review of the basic care, biology and science of the guinea pig. About half the chapters are concerned with diseases and parasites.

1021   Waynforth, H. B. *Experimental and surgical technique in the rat.* London: Academic Press, 1980. 269pp.

1022   Whitney, R. A. Jr, Johnson, D. J. and **Cole, W. C.** *Laboratory primate handbook.* New York: Academic Press, 1973. 169pp.

Conferences

1023   Chivers, D. J. and **Ford, E. H. R.** (eds) *Recent advances in primatology: volume 4, Medicine.* London: Academic Press, 1978. 227pp.

1024   Hamm, T. E. Jr *Complications of viral and mycoplasmal infections in rodents to toxicology research and testing.* 75 Madison Avenue, New York 10016: Hemisphere Publishing, 1986. 191pp.

1025   Harris, R. S. (ed.) *Feeding and nutrition of nonhuman primates.* London: Academic Press, 1970. 310pp.

1026   Melby, E. C. Jr and **Balk, M. W.** (eds) *The importance of laboratory animal genetics, health and environment in biomedical research.* Orlando: Academic Press, 1983. 284pp.

1027   Roe, F. J. C. (ed.) *Microbiological standardisation of laboratory animals.* Chichester: Ellis Horwood, 1983. 116pp.

1028   *Standards in laboratory animal management.* Potters Bar: UFAW, 1984. 280pp.

1029   *Viral and mycoplasmal infections of laboratory rodents: effects on biomedical research.*
Edited by P. N. Bhatt, R. O. Jacoby, H. C. Morse III and A. E. New. London:
Academic Press, 1986. 844pp.
Papers deal with the diseases themselves, their effects in research complications
and on their detection, prevention and control.

Journals

1030   *Animal technology.* 1949–. c/o Journal Subscribers Secretary – J. A.
Gregory, Zoology Department, Royal Postgraduate Medical School, Ducane
Road, London W12 0HS, England: Institute of Animal Technology. Three a
year.
Has an events calendar, a section listing the contents of related journals and many
advertisements. Previously known as the *Journal of the Institute of Animal Technicians*.

1031   *The ferret.* 1988–. 1014 Williamson Street, Madison, Wisconsin 53703:
The Ferret. Quarterly.

1032   *ILAR news.* 1959–. Washington, DC: Institute of Laboratory Animal
Resources. Quarterly.
Issued free to individuals working with laboratory animals and requiring information and guidelines on their care and use. *Animals for research – a directory of sources*
(11th ed) will appear in the journal in 1988/89.

1033   *Laboratory animals.* 1967–. 1 Thrifts Mead, Theydon Bois, Essex CM16
7NF, England: Laboratory Animals Ltd. Quarterly.
Published by the Laboratory Animal Science Association. Subscribers also receive
a *Buyer's guide* (5th ed., 1988) to sources of animals, animal supplies and equipment and services.

1034   *Laboratory animal science.* 1950–. 210 N. Hammes Avenue, Suite 205, Joliet,
Illinois 60435: American Association for Laboratory Animal Science. Monthly.

Other Journals

ATLA (Alternatives to laboratory animals) (formerly *ATLA abstracts*)
Charles River digest
Experimental animals
FRAME news
ILAR news
Journal of medical primatology
Mouse, Rat and *Primate newsletter*
STAL (Sciences et techniques de l'animal de laboratoire)
Zeitschrift für Versuchstierkunde/Journal of experimental animal science

POULTRY AND CAGE BIRDS

Wild birds and raptors are discussed in the section on zoo and wild animals.

Abstracting Service

1035 *Poultry abstracts*. 1975–. Wallingford: CAB International. Monthly.

Nomenclature Guide

1036 *Nomina anatomica avium: an annotated anatomical dictionary of birds*. Edited by
J. J. Baumel *et al*. London: Academic Press, 1979. 637pp.
A list of official Latin terms with annotations and explanatory diagrams. There is
an extensive bibliography of literature on avian morphology.

Multivolume Works

1037 *Avian biology*. Edited by D. S. Farner, J. R. King and K. C. Parkes. New
York: Academic Press, 1971–. Continuing series.

1038 **King, A. S.** and **McLelland, J.** (eds) *Form and function in birds*. London:
Academic Press, 1979, 1981, 1985, 1989. 459 + 496 + 522 + 591pp.

1039 *Physiology and biochemistry of the domestic fowl*. Edited by D. J. Bell and B. M.
Freeman. London: Academic Press. 1971, 1971, 1971, 1983, 1984. 5 vols.
Volumes 4 and 5, edited by B. M. Freeman, update the original work. An
appendix in volume 5 gives quantitative biochemical and physiological
data.

Books

1040 **Abs, M.** (ed.) *Physiology and behaviour of the pigeon*. London: Academic
Press, 1983. 360pp.

1041 **Burr, E. W.** (ed.) *Companion bird medicine*. Ames: Iowa State UP, 1987.
247pp.
Covers aspects of general avian management such as sexing, breeding and
quarantine as well as preventive veterinary medicine and the diagnosis and
treatment of disease.

1042 **Burr, E. W.** *Diseases of parrots*. Neptune City: TFH Publications, 1982.
318pp.

1043 **Campbell, T. W.** *Avian hematology and cytology*. Ames: Iowa State UP,
1988. 101pp.

A reference work for cell identification and the interpretation of cellular responses to disease. There are many colour illustrations of the procedures used and of the appearance of normal and abnormal cells.

1044   Coles, B. H. *Avian medicine and surgery*. Oxford: Blackwell, 1985. 288pp. (Library of Veterinary Practice.)
A guide for the practitioner dealing with birds other than poultry. Clinical and surgical procedures are outlined.

1045   Coutts, G. S. *Poultry diseases under modern management*. 3rd ed. Alton, Hampshire: Nimrod Press, 1987. 245pp.
An introduction to poultry diseases for the non-specialist.

1046   Curtis, P. *Poultry diseases: short notes containing strategic information for veterinary students*. 2nd ed. Liverpool: LUP, 1987. 64pp.

1047 *Ducks and geese*. 6th ed. London: HMSO, 1980. 85pp. (MAFF Reference Book 70.)
Describes the husbandry of the birds and has a section on diseases and their prevention.

1048   Eklund, M. W. and **Dowell, V. R. Jr** (eds) *Avian botulism: an international perspective*. Springfield: C. C. Thomas, 1987. 405pp. (American Lecture Series, no. 1068.)
Has reviews on general considerations, articles on epidemiology in different geographical regions and on laboratory investigations and prevention/control.

1049   Ensminger, M. E. *Poultry science*. 2nd ed. Danville: Interstate Printers and Publishers, 1980. 502pp.

1050   Gordon, R. F. and **Jordan, F. T. W.** (eds.) *Poultry diseases*. 2nd ed. London: Baillière Tindall, 1982. 401pp.
Has sections on each of the major diseases and chapters on the diseases of turkey and ducks, field investigation technique, hygiene and pathogen-free flocks, artificial insemination, and on stress/welfare.

1051   Gylstorff, I. and **Grimm, F.** *Vogelkrankheiten*. Stuttgart: Verlag Eugen Ulmer, 1987. 609pp.
Covers the diseases of captive, cage and wild birds other than poultry. Deals with diagnosis, treatment and surgery.

1052   Harrison, G. J. and **Harrison, L. R.** (eds) *Clinical avian medicine and surgery including aviculture*. Philadelphia: W. B. Saunders, 1986. 717pp.

The most recent and complete work devoted to cage birds. The book is divided into eight broad sections: general considerations, the normal bird, a clinical approach, diagnostic procedures, therapy considerations, diseases, surgery and aviculture. Each of the fifty-three chapters has extensive reading lists.

1053 Hodges, R. D. *The histology of the fowl.* London: Academic Press, 1974. 648pp.
Describes each of the major anatomical systems with comprehensive reviews of the literature.

1054 Hofstad, M. S., Barnes, H. J., Calnek, B. W., Reid, W. M. and **Yoder, H. W. Jr** (eds). *Diseases of poultry.* 8th ed. Ames: Iowa State UP, 1984. 831pp.
An encyclopaedic work summarizing current knowledge on all aspects of poultry disease. Each of the thirty-four chapters has a comprehensive list of references. There are many colour and black and white illustrations. Previous editions are still valuable for their reviews of the early literature.

1055 King, A. S. and **McLelland, J.** *Birds: their structure and function.* 2nd ed. London: Baillière Tindall, 1984. 334pp.
A general survey of avian anatomy and physiology, topics which are discussed in greater depth in [1037–1039].

1056 Levi, W. M. *The pigeon.* Sumter, South Carolina: Levi Publishing, 1974 (reprinted 1981). 667pp.
Complete discussion of the breeds, biology and husbandry of this bird.

1057 Low, R. *Parrots: their care and breeding.* Revised ed. Poole: Blandford Press, 1986. 400pp.

1058 *Manual of poultry production in the tropics.* Translated by R. R. Say. Wallingford: CAB International, 1987. 119pp.
A basic introductory text. Translated from *Manuel d'aviculture en zone tropicale* (IEMVT, 1983).

1059 May, C. G. (ed.) and **D. Hawksworth** (reviser) *British poultry standards.* 4th ed. London: Butterworth, 1982. 375pp.
Handbook giving specifications and judging points of breeds of fowl, turkeys, ducks and geese.

1060 Moreng, R. E. and **Avens, J. S.** *Poultry science and production.* Reston, Virginia: Reston Publishing, 1985. 438pp.
Comprehensive guide to the production of chickens, turkeys, ducks and geese written for agricultural students and poultry farmers.

1061   North, M. O. *Commercial chicken production manual.* 3rd ed. Westport: AVI Publishing, 1984. 710pp.
An overview of the husbandry of chickens for the farmer and student.

1062   Petrak, M. L. (ed.) *Diseases of cage and aviary birds.* 2nd ed. Philadelphia: Lea & Febiger, 1982. 679pp.

1063   Portsmouth, J. I. *Practical poultry keeping.* 7th ed. Hindhead: Saiga, 1978. 207pp.

1064   Price, C. J. (ed.) *Manual of parrots, budgerigars and other psittacine birds.* Cheltenham: BSAVA, 1988. 208pp.
Covers the management, handling, diagnosis and treatment of these birds. There is an extensive colour section illustrating a variety of conditions.

1065   Randall, C. J. *A colour atlas of diseases of the domestic fowl and turkey.* London: Wolfe Medical Publications, 1985. 116pp.
Provides the diagnostician with 311 photographs of the main post-mortem and histopathological features of the common diseases.

1066   Robinson, M. C. *Laboratory anatomy of the domestic chicken.* Dubuque: W. C. Brown, 1970. 107pp. (Booth Laboratory Anatomy Series.)

1067   Sainsbury, D. *Poultry health and management.* 2nd ed. London: Granada, 1984. 186pp.
Concise review of poultry production in temperate and hot climates. Has a chapter on welfare and alternative production systems.

1068   Schrag, J., Enz, H., Klette, H. and **Messinger, H.** *Healthy pigeons: recognition, prevention and treatment of the major pigeon diseases.* 5th ed. Hengersberg: Ludwig Schober, 1985. 108pp.
The same publishers have also issued *Fancy pigeons: a handbook of the history, care and breeding of exhibition pigeons with illustrations of 229 breeds* (E. Muller and L. Schrag, translated by W. Mehlig and C. J. Morley, 1985, 252pp.).

1069   Scott, M. L., Nesheim, M. C. and **Young, R. J.** *Nutrition of the chicken.* 2nd ed. Ithaca: M. L. Scott and Associates, 1976. 555pp.

1070   Seller, T. J. (ed.) *Bird respiration.* Boca Raton: CRC Press, 1987. 2 vols. 176 + 208pp.

1071   Steiner, C. V. Jr and **Davis, R. B.** *Caged bird medicine: selected topics.* Ames: Iowa State UP, 1981. 176pp.
A concise compendium covering the diagnosis and therapy of disease and the general principles of care and handling.

1072   Stunkard, J. A. *Diagnosis, treatment and husbandry of pet birds.* Edgewater, Maryland: Stunkard Publishing, 1984. 234pp.
Practical handbook covering the biology and handling of birds with sections on infectious and noninfectious diseases and on vaccination programmes.

1073   Sturkie, P. D. (ed.) *Avian physiology.* 4th ed. New York: Springer-Verlag, 1986. 516pp.
The standard textbook on the topic.

1074   Thear, K. *Keeping quail: a guide to domestic and commercial management.* Saffron Walden: Broad Leys Publishing, 1987. 96pp.

1075   Toivanen, A. and **Toivanen, P.** (eds) *Avian immunology: basis and practice.* Boca Raton: CRC Press, 1987. 2 vols. 236 + 210pp.
Multiauthored overview of current knowledge with special coverage of applied and clinical aspects.

1076   *Turkey production: health.* London: HMSO, 1983. 84pp. (MAFF Reference Book 243.)

1077   *Turkey production: breeding and husbandry.* London: HMSO, 1985. 123pp. (MAFF Reference Book 242.)
Covers housing, nutritional needs and ration formulation and husbandry methods and equipment.

1078   Zayan, R. and **Duncan, I. J. H.** (eds) *Cognitive aspects of social behaviour in the domestic fowl.* Amsterdam: Elsevier, 1987. 492pp.

Conferences

1079   *Avian immunology: proceedings of the second international conference on avian immunology held in Philadelphia, Pennsylvania, July 13–15, 1986.* Edited by W. T. Weber and D. L. Ewert. New York: Alan R. Liss, 1987. 351pp. (Progress in Clinical and Biological Research, vol. 238.)

1080   Metcalfe, J., Stock, M. K. and **Ingermann, R. L.** (eds) *Development of the avian embryo.* New York: Alan R. Liss, 1987. 376pp.
Forty contributions on physiological aspects of avian embryology.

1081   *Poultry Science Symposium Series.* 1964– . London: Butterworths. Annual.
The proceedings are of symposia organized by the UK Branch of the World's Poultry Science Association and originally were published as supplements to *British poultry science.* The volumes contain review articles and research papers. Recent titles are:

21 *Recent advances in turkey science.* C. Nixey and T. C. Grey. 1989. 373pp.

20 *Egg quality: current problems and recent advances.* R. G. Wells and C. G. Belyavin. 1987. 302pp.

19 *Nutrient requirements of poultry and nutritional research.* C. Fisher and K. N. Boorman. 1986. 224pp.

Other volumes have covered many important topics, including genetics and breeding (**18**), reproductive biology (**17**) and immunology (**16**).

1082 *Research in avian coccidiosis: proceedings of the Georgia Coccidiosis Conference, November 19–21, 1985.* Edited by L. R. McDougald, L. P. Joyner and P. L. Long. Athens, Georgia 30602: University of Georgia, Department of Poultry Science, 1986. 642pp.

Journals

1083 *AAV today.* 1987–. 5770 Lake Worth Road, Lake Worth, Florida 33463: Association of Avian Veterinarians. Quarterly.

1084 *Avian diseases.* 1957–. Pennsylvania: American Association of Avian Pathologists. Quarterly.

Each issue has over two dozen research articles. Case reports and research notes are also included. Includes the annual AAAP summaries of disease reports for commercial poultry and for pet, zoo and wild birds.

1085 *Avian pathology.* 1972–. AFRC Institute for Animal Health, Houghton Laboratory, Huntingdon, Cambridgeshire PE17 2DA, England: Avian Pathology. Quarterly.

Journal of the World Veterinary Poultry Association.

1086 *British poultry science.* 1960–. PO Box 25, Abingdon, Oxfordshire OX14 3UE, England: Carfax Publishing. Quarterly.

Over 60 percent of the papers originate outside the UK. Each issue has about thirty articles and short communications on experimental aspects of poultry science. Also publishes the abstracts of papers presented at the spring meeting of the UK Branch of the World's Poultry Science Association.

1087 *Poultry.* 1985–. Doetinchem: Misset International. Bimonthly.

1088 *Poultry science.* 1908–. 309 West Clark Street, Champaign, Illinois 61820: Poultry Science Association. Monthly (semi-monthly in July).

An annual supplement has abstracts of papers from meetings of the PSA and of the Southern Poultry Science Society.

1089 *World's poultry science journal.* 1945–. London: Butterworth. Three a year.

Journal of the World's Poultry Science Association.

Other Journals

Archiv für Geflügelkunde
Broiler industry
Industria avicola
Poultry digest
Poultry international (publish an annual *Who's who international in the egg and poultry industries*)
Poultry times
Poultry tribune
Poultry world
Selections avicoles: aviculture, colombiculture, cuniculture
Turkey world
Zootecnia international

AMPHIBIANS AND REPTILES

Books

1090   *Biology of the Reptilia.* Edited by G. Gans. London: Academic Press, 1969–.
16 vols thus far.
Volumes 14–15 published in New York (Wiley) and volume 16 New York (A. R. Liss).

1091   Cooper, J. E. and **Jackson, O. F.** (eds) *Diseases of the Reptilia.* London: Academic Press, 1981. 2 vols. 584pp.
Volume 1 provides background information and has a series of chapters reviewing the infectious diseases including parasites. Volume 2 covers the non-infectious diseases and also deals with clinical aspects such as diagnosis, anaesthesia and surgery, treatment and the use of drugs.

1092   Frye, F. L. *Biological and surgical aspects of captive reptile husbandry.* Edwardsville: Veterinary Medicine Publishing, 1981. 456pp.
A detailed guide for the practising veterinary surgeon.

1093   Hoff, G. L., Frye, F. L. and **Jacobson, E. R.** (eds) *Diseases of amphibians and reptiles.* New York: Plenum Press, 1984. 784pp.
Deals with both free-living and captive animals and covers both infectious diseases and non-infectious disorders. Immunology, euthanasia, post-mortem examination and comparative histology are also covered.

1094   Hvass, H. *Reptiles and amphibians of the world.* Translated by G. Vevers. London: Eyre Methuen, 1978. 216pp.

1095 'Maintenance and reproduction of reptiles in captivity. Volume I: Maintenance and reproduction. Volume II: Diseases'. Edited by V. L. Bels and A. P. van den Sande. *Acta zoologica et pathologica Antwerpiensia* no. **78** (1984) and no. **79** (1986).

1096 Marcus, L. C. *Veterinary biology and medicine of captive amphibians and reptiles.* Philadelphia: Lea & Febiger, 1981. 239pp.
Practical guide for the veterinary surgeon. Reviews the basic biology of reptiles and amphibians and general aspects of veterinary care such as anaesthesia, surgery and drug administration as well as discussing specific diseases. A German translation was published by Ferdinand Enke Verlag in 1983.

1097 Mattison, C. *The care of reptiles and amphibians in captivity.* 2nd ed. Poole: Blandford Press, 1987. 317pp.
Comprehensive guide to the topic. Discusses general aspects of care and has descriptions of the species and gives practical instructions on their maintenance. The same author has also written *Keeping and breeding snakes* (London, Blandford Press, 1988, 184pp.).

1098 *Physiology of the Amphibia.* Edited by J. A. Moore (volume 1) and B. Lofts (volumes 2 and 3). London: Academic Press, 1964, 1974, 1976. 654 + 592 + 644pp.

1099 Reichenbach-Klinke, H. and **Elkan, E.** *The principal diseases of the lower vertebrates.* London: Academic Press, 1965. 600pp.
Deals with the diseases of fish, amphibia and reptiles.

1100 Ross, R. A. and **Marzec, G.** *The bacterial diseases of reptiles: their epidemiology, control, diagnosis and treatment.* PO Box 2227, Stanford, California 94305: Institute for Herpetological Research, 1984. 114pp.

1101 Welch, K. R. G. *Handbook on the maintenance of reptiles in captivity.* Malabar, Florida: R. E. Krieger, 1987. 156pp.

Conference

1102 Townson, S. and **Lawrence, K.** (eds) *Reptiles: breeding, behaviour and veterinary aspects.* London: British Herpetological Society, 1985. 124pp.

Journals

1103 *Herpetological journal.* 1948–. c/o Zoological Society of London, Regent's Park, London NW1 4RY, England: British Herpetological Society. Biannual. Formerly (until 1985) *British journal of herpetology.* The society also publish a *Bulletin* (1980–).

Other Journals

Herpetologica
Herpetological review
Journal of herpetology
Salamandra

EXOTIC PETS, ZOO AND WILD ANIMALS

Abstracting Services

1104   *Key-word index of wildlife research.* Edited by R. Anderegg. 1974–. Zurich: Swiss Wildlife Information Service. Occasional.
Almost exclusively concerned with European wildlife literature. The full texts of the documents included are available from the service.

1105   *Wildlife disease review: a taxonomic guide to the literature of disease in captive and free-ranging wildlife.* 1983–. PO Box 8938, Fort Collins, Colorado 80525: Wildlife Disease Review. Monthly.
Each issue lists abstracts in four sections: mammals, birds, fish and reptiles. There are subject, taxonomic, geographic and author indexes in each issue, six-monthly author indexes and annual cumulative indexes.

1106   *Wildlife review.* 1935–. 1025 Pennock Place, Fort Collins, Colorado 80524: US Fish and Wildlife Service, Office of Information Transfer. Quarterly.
Index to world-wide wildlife management and conservation literature. Has lists of citations by subject and author, geographic and taxonomic indexes. Since 1981 annual cumulative indexes have been produced. *Wildlife abstracts* is a periodic annotated bibliography of the citations in *Wildlife review* with author and subject indexes. Currently six issues have appeared covering the period 1935–80.

Bibliography

1107   **Karstad, L.** *A partly annotated bibliography on infections, parasites, and diseases of African wild animals.* Ottawa: International Development Research Centre, 1979. 111pp.
1,068 references published up to the end of 1978. There is a subject index.

Directory

1108   *International zoo yearbook.* 1959–. London: Zoological Society of London. Annual.
Contains many articles of interest to those dealing with zoo animals. The first half of each volume is devoted to papers on a special topic, the rest of the volume has

general papers. Lists the species of wild animals bred in captivity, includes a census of rare animals in captivity and lists stud books and world registers for rare species. Has a *List of zoos and aquaria of the world*.

Multivolume Works

1109 *Diseases of marine animals*. Edited by O. Kinne. Notkestr. 31, D-2000 Hamburg 52, Federal Republic of Germany: Biologische Anstalt Helgoland.
The volumes cover all the biotic diseases, proliferative disorders and structural abnormalities of marine animals. The titles in the series are:
- **I** *General aspects, Protozoa to Gastropoda*. 1980. 466pp. (published by John Wiley)
- **II** *Introduction – Bivalvia to Scaphopoda*. 1983. 467–1038pp.
- **III** *Cephalopoda, Crustacea etc. to Urochordata*. Forthcoming.
- **IV** *Part I Introduction – Pisces*. 1984. 541pp.
- **IV** *Part II Introduction – Reptilia, Aves, Mammalia*. 1985. 543–884pp.

1110 *Handbuch der Zootierkrankheiten*. Edited by R. Ippen, H-D. Schroder and K. Elze. Berlin: Akademie-Verlag. 1985–. 7 volumes planned.
The volumes will be devoted to: **1** *Reptiles* (1985, 432pp.), **2** and **3** *Birds*, **4** *Carnivora*, **5** and **6** *Artiodactyla* and **7** *Perissodactyla*.

1111 *Wildbiologische Informationen für den Jäger*. Volumes edited by R. R. Hofmann or F. Muller. Stuttgart: Ferdinand Enke Verlag, 1978–85. 8 vols.
Concerned with the biology of game mammals and birds in Europe.

Books

1112 **Beer, J. V.** *Diseases of gamebirds and wildfowl*. 2nd ed. Fordingbridge: The Game Conservancy, 1988. 112pp.
Illustrated with many colour plates. Describes the signs and symptoms of the diseases and outlines correct husbandry techniques.

1113 **Boch, J.** and **Schneidawind, H.** *Krankheiten des jagbaren Wildes*. Hamburg: Paul Parey, 1988. 398pp.
Survey of the diseases and parasites of European game animals and birds.

1114 **Bosset, R.** (ed.) *Faune sauvage d'Europe: surveillance sanitaire et pathologie des mammifères et des oiseaux*. 175 Rue de Chevaleret, 75646 Paris: Syndicat National des Vétérinaires Inspecteurs, 1987. 407pp. (Informations Techniques des Services Vétérinaires 96–99.)
Describes and illustrates, using over 150 colour photographs, the diseases likely to be seen in the principal wild animals and birds in Europe.

1115   Cooper, J. E. *Veterinary aspects of captive birds of prey.* 2nd ed. Saul, Gloucestershire: Standfast Press, 1985. 256pp.
Authoritative text. New information since the first (1978) edition is presented in a thirty-two page supplement.

1116   Cooper, J. E. and **Eley, J. T.** (eds) *First aid and care of wild birds.* Newton Abbot: David & Charles, 1979. 288pp.
Complete review of the methods of dealing with and treating sick and injured birds.

1117   Cooper, J. E. and **Hutchison, M. F.** assisted by **Jackson, O. F.** and **Maurice, R. J.** *Manual of exotic pets.* 2nd ed. Cheltenham: BSAVA Publications, 1985. 224pp.
Covers all the exotic animals likely to be seen in a veterinary practice. Has chapters devoted to the usual children's pets and to the less common species such as hedgehogs, deer, primates, pigeons, water birds, crocodiles, snakes, amphibians etc.

1118   Crandall, L. S. *The management of wild animals in captivity.* Chicago: University of Chicago Press, 1964. 761pp.

1119   Davis, J. W. and **Anderson, R. C.** (eds) *Parasitic diseases of wild mammals.* Ames: Iowa State UP, 1971. 364pp.

1120   Davis, J. W., Anderson, R. C., Karstad, L. H. and **Trainer, D. O.** (eds) *Infectious and parasitic diseases of wild birds.* Ames: Iowa State UP, 1971. 344pp.

1121   Davis, J. W., Karstad, L. H. and **Trainer, D.O.** (eds) *Infectious diseases of wild mammals.* 2nd ed. Ames: Iowa State UP, 1981. 446pp.
Forty-seven chapters each devoted to a major disease.

1122   Fiennes, R. N. T-W- (ed.) *Pathology of simian primates.* Basel: Karger, 1972. 2 vols. 929 + 770pp.
Part 1 deals with general pathology, Part II with infectious and parasitic diseases.

1123   *Field guide to wildlife diseases. Volume 1: General field procedures and diseases of migratory birds.* Edited by M. Friend. Washington, DC: US Department of the Interior, 1987. 224pp. (Resource Publication 167.)
A general reference work on wildlife diseases with many colour plates and tables. The first section gives information on recording data, collecting, preserving and shipping specimens, disease control and euthanasia.

1124 Fowler, M. E. (ed.) *Zoo and wild animal medicine.* 2nd ed. Philadelphia: W. B. Saunders, 1986. 1127pp.
An essential reference text for zoo veterinarians. A preliminary section covers topics of general relevance and there are sections on amphibians and reptiles, birds, mammals and the care and feeding of invertebrates.

1125 Gabrisch, K. and **Zwart, P.** (eds) *Krankheiten der Wildtiere: exotische und heimische Tiere in der Tierarztpraxis.* Hanover: Schlütersche Verlagsanstalt, 1987. 606pp.
Extensive review with many colour illustrations of the care and diseases of wild European animals and exotic species which may be presented to the veterinarian.

1126 Gabrisch, K. and **Zwart, P.** (eds) *Krankheiten der Heimtiere.* Hanover: Schlütersche Verlagsanstalt, 1985. 402pp.
Has chapters devoted to all the pet animals, other than cats and dogs, and including parrots, pigeons, cage birds, fancy poultry and aquarium fish, likely to be seen in veterinary practice. W. Isenbugel and W. Frank's *Heimtierkrankheiten–Kleinsauger, Amphibien und Reptilien* (Stuttgart: Verlag Eugen Ulmer, 1985, 402pp., Erkrankungen der Haustiere) is a similar work but which only covers small mammals, amphibia and reptiles.

1127 Griner, L. A. *Pathology of zoo animals: a review of necropsies conducted over a fourteen-year period at the San Diego Zoo and San Diego Wild Animal Park.* PO Box 551, San Diego, California 92112: Zoological Society of San Diego, 1983. 608pp.
Describes the post-mortem findings in over 12,000 cases from more than 2,000 species and subspecies which died during the period 1964–78.

1128 Hill, D. A. and **Robertson, P.** *The pheasant: ecology, management and conservation.* Oxford: Blackwell, 1988. 281pp.

1129 Hoff, G. L. and **Davis, J. W.** (eds) *Noninfectious diseases of wildlife.* Ames: Iowa State UP, 1982. 174pp.
Mostly concerned with poisoning of wild animals and birds and with nutritional and metabolic disorders. Also covers stress, shock, physical injury, capture myopathy, amyloidosis, mammalian dental anomalies and soybean impaction of waterfowl.

1130 Howard, E. B. (ed.) *Pathobiology of marine mammal diseases.* Boca Raton: CRC Press, 1983. 2 vols.

1131 Hudson, P. J. and **Rands, M. R. W.** (eds) *The ecology and management of gamebirds.* Oxford: Blackwell, 1988. 263pp.
Has a chapter on the ecology and control of parasites in gamebird populations.

1132   Kavanagh, M. *A complete guide to monkeys, apes and other primates.* London: Jonathan Cape, 1983. 224pp.

1133   Klös, H-G. and **Lang, E. M.** (eds) *Handbook of zoo medicine: diseases and treatment of wild animals in zoos, game parks, circuses and private collections.* Translated by G. Speckmann. New York: Van Nostrand Reinhold, 1982. 453pp.
Concise handbook of treatment dealing with each group of animals in turn.

1134   Lyubashenko, S. Ya. (ed.) *Diseases of fur-bearing animals.* New Delhi: Oxonian Press, 1983. 402pp.

1135   McKeever, K. *Care and rehabilitation of injured owls: a user's guide to medical treatment of raptorial birds – and the housing, release, training and captive breeding of native owls.* 3rd ed. Lincoln, Ontario: W. F. Rannie, 1979. 112pp.

1136   Martin, R. M., Nute, J. and **Nute, G.** *First aid and care of wildlife.* Newton Abbot: David & Charles, 1984. 272pp.

1137   *Raptor management techniques manual.* Edited by B. A. G. Pendleton *et al.* 1412 Sixteenth Street, NW, Washington, DC 20036: Institute for Wildlife Research, National Wildlife Federation, 1987. 394pp. (Ringbound with supplements to be issued). (Scientific and Technical Series, no. 10.)
Describes field research techniques, the technology of raptor management, and methods used in laboratory studies. Has a chapter on literature resources on raptors.

1138   Ridgway, S. H. (ed.) *Mammals of the sea: biology and medicine.* Springfield: C. C. Thomas, 1972. 812pp.

1139   Ridgway, S. H. and **Harrison, R. J.** (eds) *Handbook of marine mammals.* London: Academic Press, 1981, 1981, 1985. 3 vols. 235 + 359 + 362pp.
Volume 1 covers the walrus, sea lions, fur seals and sea otter, 2 seals and 3 the sirenians and baleen whales.

1140   Robbins, C. T. *Wildlife feeding and nutrition.* New York: Academic Press, 1983. 343pp. (Animal Feeding and Nutrition.)

1141   Schmidt, R. E. and **Hubbard, G. B.** *Atlas of zoo animal pathology.* Boca Raton: CRC Press, 1987. 2 vols. 241 + 192pp.
The atlas is arranged by the organ systems. It has over 700 illustrations and these are supported by a review of the literature and an extensive bibliography on each system. Volume 1 deals with mammals and volume 2 with avian, reptile and other species.

1142   Shaw, J. H. *Introduction to wildlife management.* New York: McGraw-Hill, 1985. 316pp.

1143   Wallach, J. D. and **Boever, W. J.** *Diseases of exotic animals: medical and surgical management.* Philadelphia: W. B. Saunders, 1983. 1159pp.
Deals with mammals, birds, reptiles, amphibians and tropical fish. A useful source of normal blood values. An appendix lists feeds available in the USA. Chemical restraint is well covered.

1144   'Wildlife diseases'. *Revue scientifique et technique de l'OIE.* **7** (1988): (4).
Special issue containing papers on aspects of wildlife diseases including reviews of the disease situation in a number of countries.

1145   Wobeser, G. A. *Diseases of wild waterfowl.* New York: Plenum Press, 1981. 300pp.

Conferences

1146   *Breeding and management in birds of prey. Proceedings of the conference held at University of Bristol, January 24–26, 1987.* Edited by D. J. Hill. Bristol: University of Bristol, 1987. 187pp.

1147   Cooper, J. E. and **Greenwood, A. G.** (eds) *Recent advances in the study of raptor diseases.* Keighley: Chiron Publications, 1981. 178pp.

1148   *Diseases of zoo animals. Proceedings of the 30th international symposium on diseases of zoo animals held on 11–15 May 1988, Sofia.* Edited by R. Ippen and H. D. Schroder. Berlin: Akademie-Verlag, 1988. 423pp.
The symposia have been held annually since 1959.

1149   Montali, R. J. (ed.) *Mycobacterial infections of zoo animals.* Washington, DC: Smithsonian Institution Press, 1978. 275pp. (Symposia of the National Zoological Park Series, no. 1.)

1150   Montali, R. J. and **Migaki, G.** (eds) *The comparative pathology of zoo animals.* Washington, DC: Smithsonian Institution Press, 1980. 684pp. (Symposia of the National Zoological Park Series, no. 6.)

1151   *Proceedings: first international conference on zoological and avian medicine: sponsored by Association of Avian Veterinarians and American Association of Zoo Veterinarians, September 6–11 1987, Oahu, Hawaii.* Atlanta: American Association of Zoo Veterinarians, 1987. 586pp.

1152   *Symposia of the Zoological Society of London.* 1960–. Oxford: Clarendon Press, Two or three a year.

The symposia are often concerned with aspects of comparative physiology of interest to veterinarians. A typical example is the most recent (no. 60) *Reproduction and disease in captive and wild animals* (edited by G. R. Smith and J. P. Hearn). This symposium was held to mark the fiftieth anniversary of the Wellcome Trust.

Journals

1153 *Journal of wildlife diseases.* 1965–. Ames: Wildlife Disease Association. Quarterly.

1154 *Journal of zoo animal medicine.* 1970–. c/o M. Fowler, Emory University, Atlanta, Georgia 30322: American Association of Zoo Veterinarians. Quarterly.

Other Journals

Aquatic mammals
International wildlife
International zoo news
Journal of raptor research (formerly *Raptor research*)
Journal of wildlife management (supplements published as *Wildlife monographs*, 1958–)
Journal of zoology
Marine mammal science
Wildlife management
Wildlife research report
Wildlife society bulletin
Zoobiology

FISH

Book Series and Multivolume Works

1155 *Diseases of fishes.* General editors S. F. Snieszko and H. R. Axelrod. Neptune City: TFH Publications, 1970–80. 6 vols.
The emphasis is on farmed fish. The volumes deal with the following topics:
Book 1: *Crustacea as enemies of fishes.* 1970. Z. Kabata. 171pp.
Book 2A: *Bacterial diseases of fishes.* 1971. G. L. Bullock, D. A. Conroy and S. F. Snieszko. 139pp.
Book 2B: *The identification of fish pathogenic bacteria.* 1971. G. L. Bullock. 41pp.
Book 3: *The prevention and treatment of diseases of warmwater fishes under subtropical conditions, with special emphasis on intensive fish farming.* 1971. S. Sarig. 127pp.
Book 4: *Fish immunology.* 1974. D. P. Anderson. 239pp.
Book 5: *Environmental stress and fish diseases.* 1976. G. A. Wedemeyer, F. P. Meyer and L. Smith. 192pp.

1156 *Fish physiology.* Edited by W. S. Hoar and D. J. Randall. Orlando: Academic Press, 1969–84. 10 vols.

1157 *Recent advances in aquaculture.* Edited by J. F. Muir and R. J. Roberts. London: Chapman & Hall, 1982, 1985, 1988. 464 + 320 + 420pp.

Books

1158 **Amlacher, E.** *Taschenbuch der Fischkrankheiten: Grundlagen der Fischpathologie.* 5th ed. Jena: VEB Gustav Fischer Verlag, 1986. 478pp.
Gives information on the diagnosis and pathology of disease in aquarium and farmed fish. A translated version of an earlier edition was published by TFH Publications in 1970 (*Textbook of fish diseases*, translated by D. A. Conroy and R. L. Herman, 302pp.)

1159 **Austin, B.** and **Austin, D. A.** *Bacterial fish pathogens: disease in farmed and wild fish.* Chichester: Ellis Horwood, 1987. 364pp. (Ellis Horwood Series in Aquaculture and Fisheries Support.)
Comprehensive survey of the importance, diagnosis and control of bacterial disease with sections on each of the major pathogens.

1160 **Austin, B.** and **Austin, D. A.** *Microbiological methods for fish and shellfish: a practical manual for use in aquaculture.* Chichester: Ellis Horwood, forthcoming. (Ellis Horwood Series in Aquaculture and Fisheries Support.)
Mostly concerned with methods applicable to the isolation and identification/diagnosis of bacterial pathogens of freshwater and marine fish and shellfish.

1161 **Beveridge, M. C. M.** *Cage aquaculture.* Farnham: Fishing News Books, 1987. 351pp.

1162 **Dulin, M. P.** *Diseases of marine aquarium fishes.* Neptune City: TFH Publications, 1976. 128pp.

1163 **Elkan, E.** and **Reichenbach-Klinke, H-H.** (eds.) *Color atlas of the diseases of fishes, amphibians and reptiles.* Neptune City: TFH Publications, 1974. 256pp.
Comprises 253 colour photographs. There is no text, merely brief legends to the plates.

1164 **Ellis, A. E.** (ed.) *Fish vaccination.* London: Academic Press, 1988. 255pp.
Covers the theory of vaccination, discusses the practical uses of vaccines on fish farms and has chapters on vaccination against the more important and common diseases.

1165   Frerichs, G. N. (ed.) *Isolation and identification of fish bacterial pathogens.* Stirling: Institute of Aquaculture, 1984. 54pp.

1166   Halver, J. E. (ed.) *Fish nutrition.* San Diego: Academic Press, 1989. 2nd ed. 798pp.
A comprehensive monograph with chapters on nutritional pathology and nutrition and fish diseases.

1167   Herwig, N. *Handbook of drugs and chemicals used in the treatment of fish diseases: a manual of fish pharmacology and materia medica.* Springfield: C. C. Thomas, 1979. 272pp.

1168   Hoffman, G. L. and **Meyer, F. P.** *Parasites of freshwater fishes: a review of their treatment and control.* Neptune City: TFH Publications, 1974. 224pp.

1169   Huet, M. translated by **J. Timmermans.** *Textbook of fish culture: breeding and cultivation of fish.* 2nd ed. Farnham: Fishing News Books, 1986. 438pp.
Thorough review of fish farming.

1170   Kabata, Z. *Parasites and diseases of fish cultured in the tropics.* London: Taylor & Francis, 1985. 318pp.
Particularly relevant to those working in aquaculture in South East Asia but provides an overview of parasite diseases and infections found in the tropics.

1171   Kinkelin, P. de, Michel, C. and **Ghittino, P.** *Précis de pathologie des poissons.* Paris: OIE, 1986. 348pp.
A modern survey of diseases of fish and their control. English and Spanish translations will also be published.

1172   Kubota, S. S., Miyazaki, T. and **Egusa, S.** *Color atlas of fish histopathology. Volume 1.* Tokyo: Shin-Suisan Shinbun-Sha, 1982. 213pp.
Contains 800 colour illustrations. The text is bilingual in English and Japanese.

1173   Laird, L. M. and **Needham, T.** (eds) *Salmon and trout farming.* Chichester: Ellis Horwood, 1988. 271pp. (Ellis Horwood Series in Aquaculture and Fisheries Support.)
A review of the science and technology of farming of salmon and trout, includes a chapter on marketing, but veterinary aspects are not discussed.

1174   Lovell, T. *Nutrition and feeding of fish.* New York: Van Nostrand Reinhold, 1988. 224pp.
Provides practical feeding information for various important fish types and discusses the design of experiments in the field.

1175   Mills, R. *You and your aquarium*. London: Dorling Kindersley, 1989. 288pp.
Guide to collecting and keeping aquarium fish.

1176   Moller, H. and **Anders, K.** *Diseases and parasites of marine fishes*. Kiel: Verlag Moller, 1986. 365pp.
Well-illustrated text on the disorders of wild marine fish.

1177   Murty, A. S. *Toxicity of pesticides to fish*. Boca Raton: CRC Press, 1986. 2 vols. 178 + 143pp.

1178   Post, G. W. *Textbook of fish health*. Neptune City: TFH Publications, 1983. 256pp.
Undergraduate textbook with 172 colour plates and many references to the literature.

1179   Ribelin, W. E. and **Migaki, G.** (eds) *The pathology of fishes*. Madison: University of Wisconsin Press, 1975. 1004pp.

1180   Roberts, R. J. (ed.) *Fish pathology*. 2nd ed. London: Baillière Tindall, 1989. 467pp.
Comprehensive text on fish diseases with a section on laboratory methods and chapters on the anatomy, physiology and pathology of fish.

1181   Roberts, R. J. and **Shepherd, C. J.** *Handbook of trout and salmon diseases*. 2nd ed. Farnham: Fishing News Books, 1986. 224pp.
A compact summary which also covers nutritional disorders and contains chapters on anatomy and farming of salmonids.

1182   Ross, L. G. and **Ross, B.** *Anaesthetic and sedative techniques for fish*. Stirling: Institute of Aquaculture, 1984. 37pp.
Describes methods for both fresh water and marine fish.

1183   Schubert, G. *A complete guide to fish diseases*. Ascot: TFH Publications, 1987. 125pp.
Guide with colour illustrations for those keeping tropical fish.

1184   Sedgwick, S. D. *Salmon farming handbook*. Farnham: Fishing News Books, 1988. 208pp.

1185   Sedgwick, S. D. *Trout farming handbook*. 4th ed. Farnham: Fishing News Books, 1985. 160pp.

1186   Shepherd, C. J. and **Bromage, N. R.** (eds) *Intensive fish farming*. Oxford: Blackwell, 1988. 404pp.
Reviews the concept of intensive fish culture and has one chapter devoted to fish health and disease. An appendix lists aquaculture journals and related periodicals.

1187   Sindermann, C. J. and **Lightner, D. V.** (eds) *Disease diagnosis and control in North-American marine aquaculture*. 2nd ed. Amsterdam: Elsevier, 1988. 431pp. (Developments in Aquaculture and Fisheries Science 17.)
Has chapters on diseases of crustacea, molluscs, fish and marine turtles plus information on the control and prophylaxis of disease.

1188   Smith, L. S. *Introduction to fish pathology*. Reigate: TFH Publications, 1982. 352pp.

1189   Stevenson, J. P. *Trout farming manual*. 2nd ed. Farnham: Fishing News Books, 1987. 259pp.
Complete guide to the techniques of farming brown and rainbow trout. Includes sections on parasites and diseases.

1190   Stickney, R. R. (ed.) *Culture of nonsalmonid freshwater fishes*. Boca Raton: CRC Press, 1986. 201pp.
Describes the methodology for producing warm-water and cold-water (North American) species. The diseases of each species are discussed.

1191   Tucker, C. S. (ed.) *Channel catfish culture*. Amsterdam: Elsevier, 1985, 657pp. (Developments in Aquaculture and Fisheries Science 15.)
Has chapters on infectious and·non-infectious diseases.

1192   van Duijn, C. *Diseases of fish*. 3rd ed. London: Iliffe Books, 1973. 372pp.
Mostly concerned with diagnosis and treatment.

1193   *Veterinary aspects of fish farming*. London: BVA, 1983. 20pp.
Compilation of six brief review articles from the *Veterinary record*. Contains a reading list on fish farming.

1194   Weatherley, A. H. and **Gill, H. S.** *The biology of fish growth*. London: Academic Press, 1987. 443pp.
Reviews all the controlling influences on fish growth and interprets their significance for fisheries management.

1195   Wolf, K. *Fish viruses and fish viral diseases*. Ithaca: Cornell University Press, 1988. 476pp.
Includes descriptions of sixty-three diseases and agents of virus, viruslike or of mistaken viral nature.

Conferences

1196 Cowey, C. B., Mackie, A. M. and **Bull, J. G.** (eds) *Nutrition and feeding in fish*. London: Academic Press, 1985. 489pp.

1197 Ellis, A. E. (ed.) *Fish and shellfish pathology*. London: Academic Press, 1985. 412pp.
Proceedings of the first international conference of the European Association of Fish Pathologists.

1198 Manning, M. J. and **Tatner, M. F.** (eds) *Fish immunology*. London: Academic Press, 1985. 374pp.
Proceedings of a symposium held in Plymouth, England in 1983, organized by the Fisheries Society of the British Isles.

1199 Pickering, A. D. (ed.) *Stress and fish*. London: Academic Press, 1981. 367pp.

1200 Roberts, R. J. (ed.) *Microbial diseases of fish*. London: Academic Press, 1982. 305pp. (Society for General Microbiology: Special Publications.)

1201 Stolen, J. S., Anderson, D. P. and **Van Muiswinkel, W. B.** (eds) *Fish immunology: papers presented at an international meeting held at Sandy Hook, New Jersey, USA, 8–12 September 1985*. Amsterdam: Elsevier, 1986. 443pp.

1202 Summerfelt, R. C. and **Hall, G. E.** (eds) *Age and growth of fish*. Ames: Iowa State UP, 1987. 544pp.
Papers describe the methodology for the determination of the age and growth of fish. The implications of these studies for the management of fish populations is discussed.

Journals

1203 *Diseases of aquatic organisms*. 1985/86–. PO Box 1120, D-2124 Amerlinghausen, Federal Republic of Germany: Inter-Research. Bimonthly.

1204 *Fish pathology*. 1966–. c/o Department of Fisheries, Faculty of Agriculture, University of Tokyo, Yayoi-1-1-1, Bukyo-ku, Tokyo 113, Japan: Japanese Society of Fish Pathology. Quarterly.

1205 *Journal of fish diseasaes*. 1978–. Oxford. Blackwell. Bimonthly.

Other Journals

Fish physiology and biochemistry
Some of the most important of the many journals on aquaculture are:
Aquaculture
Aquaculture and fisheries management
Aquaculture magazine
Fish farmer
Fish farming international
Journal of fish biology
Progressive fish culturist

INVERTEBRATES

Abstracting Service

1206 *Apicultural abstracts.* 1950–. Cardiff: International Bee Research Association. Quarterly with separate annual indexes.

Bibliography

1207 **Johnson, P. T.** *An annotated bibliography of pathology in invertebrates other than insects.* Minneapolis: Burgess Publishing, 1968. 322pp.
Lists over 2,000 publications according to the host phylum. There are indexes to general subjects and to scientific names of the hosts.

Books

1208 **Bailey, L.** *Honeybee pathology.* London: Academic Press, 1981. 124pp.
Has chapters on each of the groups of pathogens and parasites and also on the treatment of diseases.

1209 **Bliss, D. E.** and **Provenzano, A. J. Jr** (eds) *The biology of Crustacea. Volume 6: Pathobiology.* New York: Academic Press, 1983. 290pp.
Covers the diseases of Crustacea and crustaceans as parasites of other organisms.

1210 **Cantwell, G. E.** (ed.) *Insect diseases.* New York: Marcel Dekker, 1974. 2 vols. 595pp.
An earlier comprehensive text is E. A. Steinhaus's (ed.) *Insect pathology: an advanced treatise* (New York: Academic Press, 1963, 2 vols. 661 + 689pp.).

1211 **Morse, R. A.** (ed.) *Honey bee pests, predators and diseases.* Ithaca: Cornell University Press, 1978. 430pp.
Complete review of all the organisms affecting honey bees.

1212   Poinar, G. O. Jr and **Thomas, G. M.** *Laboratory guide to insect pathogens and parasites*. Revised ed. New York: Plenum Press, 1984, 392pp.

1213   Sparks, A. K. *Synopsis of invertebrate pathology: exclusive of insects*. Amsterdam: Elsevier, 1985. 423pp.

Journal

1214 *Journal of invertebrate pathology*. 1959–. San Diego: Academic Press. Bimonthly.
Most of the articles deal with pathogens and diseases of insects. Journal of the Society for Invertebrate Pathology. The Society's annual meetings are published in the Comparative Pathobiology series (1976–) by Plenum Press.

12 Specialities

ANAESTHESIA

Anaesthesia is primarily used during surgery so textbooks of surgery discuss anaesthesia. Pharmacology texts review the compounds in current use.

Current Awareness Service

1215 'Anaesthetic literature'. In: *Anaesthesia*. Monthly.
Compiled from *Current contents: life sciences*. A useful summary of new publications on medical, physiological and pharmacological aspects of anaesthesia.

Review

1216 '1986 Report of the AVMA Panel on Euthanasia'. *Journal of the American Veterinary Medical Association* **188** (1986): 252–68.
Summarizes the scientific evidence supporting the use of different methods of euthanasia.

Books

1217 **Fowler, M. E.** *The restraint and handling of wild and domestic animals*. Ames: Iowa State UP, 1978. 332pp.

1218 **Hall, L. W.** and **Clarke, K. W.** *Veterinary anaesthesia*. 8th ed. London: Baillière Tindall, 1983. 417pp.

The standard British text giving a comprehensive introduction for the student and a clinical guide for the veterinary practitioner. Primarily concerned with horses, farm animals, dogs and cats although anaesthesia for birds and wild animals is also covered.

1219   Harthoorn, A. M. *The chemical capture of animals.* London: Baillière Tindall, 1976. 416pp.

1220   Lumb, W. V. and **Jones, E. W.** *Veterinary anesthesia.* 2nd ed. Philadelphia: Lea & Febiger, 1984. 693pp.
A thorough review of current knowledge covering inhalation anaesthesia and other methods. Domestic, laboratory, wild and exotic species are covered. Includes a chapter on euthanasia. Appendix A lists the drugs and equipment mentioned in the text and the addresses of suppliers in the United States. Appendix B lists standard values and equivalents, symbols and abbreviations.

1221   Muir, W. W. and **Hubbell, J. A. E.** (eds) *Handbook of veterinary anesthesia.* St Louis: C. V. Mosby, 1989. 340pp.
Intended to be a reference text on commonly used drugs and techniques. Written in note form.

1222   Short, C. E. (ed.) *Principles and practice of veterinary anesthesia.* Baltimore: Williams & Wilkins, 1987. 669pp.
The most modern and complete survey of anaesthesia. There are chapters on the horse, ruminants, pigs, dog, cat, birds, wild animals, young animals and old animals.

Journals

1223   *Anaesthesia.* 1945–. London: Academic Press. Monthly.
Journal of the Association of Anaesthetists of Great Britain and Ireland. Many of the other journals on anaesthesia in medicine will be of value to those working in the veterinary field.

1224   *Journal of the Association of Veterinary Anaesthetists.* 1973–. c/o Mrs J. C. Brearley, University Department of Anaesthesia, Royal Liverpool Hospital, Prescot Street, PO Box 147, Liverpool L69 3BX, England: the Association. Annual.
Formerly published as the *Proceedings of the Association of Veterinary Anaesthetists of Great Britain and Ireland.*

1225   *Veterinary anesthesia.* 1974–80. **1–7**. Fort Collins: American Society of Veterinary Anesthesiology.

Other Journal

Veterinary surgery [1674]

ANATOMY AND HISTOLOGY

Nomenclature Guide

1226 *Nomina anatomica veterinaria, third edition, together with Nomina histologica, second edition.* Department of Veterinary Anatomy, Cornell University, Ithaca, New York 14853: International Committee on Veterinary Gross Anatomical Nomenclature, 1983. 209 + 60pp.
A list of recommended anatomical names given in hierarchical order but in Latin only. There are alphabetical indexes to the terms given in each of the two works. The *Nomina histologica* is taken from the (human) *Nomina anatomica* (5th ed., 1983).

Multivolume Works

1227 *The anatomy of the domestic animals.* Berlin: Paul Parey.
Four of the five volumes of the *Lehrbuch der Anatomie der Haustiere* originally by R. Nickel, A. Schummer and E. Seiferle have now appeared in English:

1 *The locomotor system of domestic mammals.* R. Nickel, A. Schummer, E. Seiferle, J. Frewein, K-H. Wille and H. Wilkens. Translated by W. G. Siller and W. Stockoe. 1986, 499pp.
2 *The viscera of domestic mammals.* A. Schummer and R. Nickel. Translated by W. O. Sack. 1979, 401pp.
3 *The circulatory system, the skin and the cutaneous organs of the domestic mammals.* A. Schummer, H. Wilkens, B. Vollmerhaus and K-H. Habermehl. Translated by W. G. Siller and P. A. L. Wight. 1981, 610pp.
5 *Anatomy of the domestic birds.* R. Nickel, A. Schummer and E. Seiferle. Translated by W. G. Siller and P. A. L. Wight. 1977, 202pp.

More recent editions of volumes 2 and 3, and volume 4 are available only in German:

4 *Nervensystem, Sinnesorgane, endokrine Drüsen.* 2nd ed. E. Seiferle and G. Böhme. 1984, 425pp.

1228 *Sisson and Grossman's The anatomy of the domestic animals.* 5th ed. Edited by R. Getty. Philadelphia: W. B. Saunders, 1975. 2 vols. 2095pp.
Contains sections devoted to the horse, carnivores, ruminants, pigs and birds. *Nomina anatomica veterinaria* and *Anatomia avium* nomenclature is used. For many years the standard work but now overtaken by the English version of the *Lehrbuch der Anatomie der Haustiere.*

Books

1229   Banks, W. J. *Applied veterinary histology*. 2nd ed. Baltimore: Williams & Wilkins, 1986. 583pp.

1230   de Lahunta, A. and **Habel, R. E.** *Applied veterinary anatomy*. Philadelphia: W. B. Saunders, 1986. 330pp.
Concise textbook for students. Originally derived from lecture notes and supplemented by many illustrations.

1231   Dellmann, H-D. and **Brown, E. M.** (eds) *Textbook of veterinary histology*. 3rd ed. Philadelphia: Lea & Febiger, 1987. 468pp.
Describes the structure of each major body system at light and electron microscope levels.

1232   Dyce, K. M., Sack, W. O. and **Wensing, C. J. G.** *Textbook of veterinary anatomy*. Philadelphia: W. B. Saunders, 1987. 820pp.
The dog is used as the type species for the discussions of individual body systems with specific chapters on the regional anatomy of the carnivores, horse, ruminants and pig. There is a section on avian anatomy. Anglicized anatomical nomenclature is used throughout.

1233   Frandson, R. D. *Anatomy and physiology of farm animals*. 4th ed. Philadelphia: Lea & Febiger, 1986. 560pp.
A useful single volume compilation of information on farm animals.

1234   Ghoshal, N. G., Koch, T. and **Popesko, P.** *The venous drainage of the domestic animals*. Philadelphia: W. B. Saunders, 1981. 268pp.

1235   Habel, R. E. *Guide to the dissection of domestic ruminants*. 3rd ed. 1529 Ellis Hollow Road, RD2, Ithaca, New York 14850: the Author, 1983. 165pp.
A fourth edition is in preparation.

1236   King, A. S. *A guide to the physiological and clinical anatomy of the thorax*. 5th ed. Liverpool: LUP, 1984. 216pp.

1237   King, A. S. and **Cox, J. E.** (eds) *Notes on the abdominal and pelvic anatomy of domestic mammals*. 2nd ed. Liverpool: LUP, 1982. 117pp.

1238   King, A. S. and **Riley, V. A.** *A guide to the physiological and clinical anatomy of the head*. 4th ed. Liverpool: LUP, 1980. 234pp.

1239   Latshaw, W. K. *Veterinary developmental anatomy: a clinically oriented approach*. Toronto: B. C. Decker, 1987. 283pp.
Deals with embryology with an emphasis on organogenesis and on disorders in foetal development in domestic animals.

1240   Noden, D. M. and **de Lahunta, A.** *The embryology of domestic animals: developmental mechanisms and malformations.* Baltimore: Williams & Wilkins, 1985. 367pp.
Gives an applied and clinically oriented approach to prenatal development.

1241   Popesko, P. *Atlas of topographical anatomy of the domestic animals.* 2nd ed. Philadelphia: W. B. Saunders, 1977. 3 vols in one.
Atlas of mostly coloured illustrations of the anatomy of farm animals, cats, dogs, horses and rabbits.

1242   Shively, M. J. *Veterinary anatomy: basic, comparative and clinical.* College Station: Texas A & M University Press, 1985. 582pp.
A well-illustrated text useful for its discussion of anatomy in relation to clinical procedures.

1243   Skerritt, G. C. and **McLelland, J.** *An introduction to the functional anatomy of the limbs of the domestic animals.* Bristol: Wright, 1984. 251pp.
Mostly concerned with dogs, cattle and horses.

Journal

Anatomia, histologia, embryologia [118]

ANIMAL HUSBANDRY AND PRODUCTION

(see also *Reproduction and Genetics)*

Books

1244   Acker, D. *Animal science and industry.* 3rd ed. Englewood Cliffs: Prentice-Hall, 1983. 658pp.
Review of the biological, business and management principles relating to livestock production.

1245   Barnes, M. and **Mander, C.** *Farm building construction: the farmer's guide.* Ipswich: Farming Press, 1986. 219pp.
Describes building techniques for new constructions and improvements.

1246   Blake, P. W. (ed.) *Livestock production.* London: Heinemann, 1985. 376pp.
Basic textbook on livestock husbandry and production in temperate areas.

1247   Blakely, J. and **Bade, D. H.** *The science of animal husbandry.* 4th ed. Reston, Virginia: Reston Publishing, 1985. 683pp.

1248   Campbell, J. R. and **Lasley, J. F.** *The science of animals that serve humanity.* 3rd ed. New York: McGraw-Hill, 1985. 834pp.

1249   Curtis, S. E. *Environmental management in animal agriculture.* Ames: Iowa State UP, 1983. 409pp.
Reviews the effect the environment has on animal function and performance. Covers the effects of thermal and electromagnetic factors and discusses the environment in relation to animal behaviour, management, animal health and housing.

1250   Ensminger, M. E. *Animal science.* 8th ed. Danville: Interstate Printers and Publishers, 1983. 1049pp.
An overview of farming of livestock, including poultry, with particular reference to conditions in the USA.

1251   Ensminger, M. E. *The stockman's handbook.* 6th ed. Danville: Interstate Printers and Publishers, 1983. 1192pp.
Reference work for students and those dealing with meat animals and horses. Much of the information is in tabular form.

1252   Ewer, T. K. *Practical animal husbandry.* Bristol: Wright/Scientechnica, 1982. 257pp.
Covers the handling of animals, and their breeding, development, reproduction, feeding and housing. There are chapters on preventive medicine and welfare.

1253   *Hammond's Farm animals.* 5th ed. Revised by J. Hammond Jr, J. C. Bowman and T. J. Robinson. London: Edward Arnold, 1983. 305pp.
Introductory text on the reproduction, growth and breeding of livestock and poultry.

1254   McNitt, J. I. *Livestock husbandry techniques.* London: Granada, 1983. 280pp.
Practical guide on the management of cattle and calves, pigs and poultry.

1255   Maton, A., Daelemans, J. and **Lambrecht, J.** *Housing of animals: construction and equipment of animal houses.* Amsterdam: Elsevier, 1985. 458pp. (Developments in Agricultural Engineering, vol. 6.)

1256   *Primrose McConnell's The agricultural notebook.* 18th ed. Edited by R. J. Halley and R. J. Soffe. London: Butterworths, 1988. 689pp.
Standard reference work on farm management. Includes sections on farm buildings and animal production (including a brief review of animal health).

1257   Starr, J. R. *Weather and climate and animal performance.* Geneva: World Meteorological Organization, Commission for Agricultural Meteorology, 1986. 139pp.
A related text is T. E. Gibson's (ed.) *Weather and parasitic animal disease* (Geneva: World Meteorological Organization, 1978, 174pp., Technical Note, no. 159.).

1258   Swatland, H. J. *Structure and development of meat animals.* Englewood Cliffs: Prentice-Hall, 1984. 436pp.
Describes the anatomy of meat animals and follows all the processes from livestock production, through slaughtering and meat cutting, to grading and presentation.

1259   Thomas, D. G. M. with **Beynon, D. G., Herbert, T. G. G.** and **Lloyd Jones, J.** *Animal husbandry.* 3rd ed. London: Baillière Tindall, 1983. 257pp.
A general text for students covering breeding, feeding, management and health and disease of farm livestock.

1260   Wilkinson, J. M. *Meat and milk from grass.* London: Granada, 1984. 149pp.
Introduction to grass production, the management of grazing and the storage and use of forage.

Journals

Animal production [92]

1261   *Farmers weekly.* 1934–. Carew House, Wallington, Surrey SM6 0DX, England: Reed Business Publishing. Weekly.
The main magazine for the British farming community. Has an extensive section devoted to livestock each week. Each country has many farming magazines which include material on animal health. UK examples are *Big farm weekly, British farmer and stockbreeder, Farming news, Farmstock, Livestock farming* and *Stock.*

Journal of animal science [113]

1262   *Livestock production science.* 1974–. Amsterdam: Elsevier. Monthly.

Other Journals

Journal of agricultural science
Proceedings of the Australian Society of Animal Production
Proceedings of the New Zealand Society of Animal Production
Productions animales

BACTERIOLOGY

(see also *Microbiology*)

Books

1263 *Bergey's Manual of systematic bacteriology.* Editor-in-chief J. G. Holt. Baltimore: Williams & Wilkins, 1984–.
The definitive reference texts on the classification, nomenclature and identification of bacteria. Four subvolumes are planned although thus far only the first two dealing with Gram-negatives and Gram-positives other than actinomycetes have been published. The editors are:

1   N. R. Krieg. 1984. 964pp.
2   P. H. A. Smeath, N. S. Mair and M. E. Sharpe. 1986. 965–1599pp.
3   J. T. Saley, forthcoming.
4   S. T. Williams, forthcoming.

Volume 3 will deal with the archaeobacteria, cyanobacteria and remaining Gram-negatives and volume 4 with the actinomycetes. The volumes contain determinative material such as keys and tables useful for identification plus detailed descriptive information and taxonomic comments. Purely determinative information will eventually be published in a separate *Bergey's manual of determinative bacteriology*. The history of names can be traced in previous editions of *Bergey's manual of determinative bacteriology* (8th, 1974, 1246pp.) or the *Index Bergeyana* (1966, 1472pp) and its *Supplement* (1981, 442pp).

1264   Bisping, W. and **Amtsberg, G.** *Colour atlas for the diagnosis of bacterial pathogens in animals.* Berlin: Paul Parey, 1988. 339pp.
A bilingual English/German text with many colour photographs illustrating the routine procedures used to identify the more important species and genera.

1265 *Brucellosis diagnosis: standard laboratory techniques.* 2nd ed. Alnwick: MAFF, 1978. 53pp. (MAFF Booklet 2084).
Related works are *Methods for the identification of Brucella* (Alnwick: MAFF, 1983, 65pp., MAFF Booklet 2085) and *Brucella antigen and production* (Alnwick: MAFF, 1985, 96pp., MAFF Booklet 2499) and *Brucellosis: a history of the disease and its eradication from cattle in Great Britain* (Alnwick: MAFF, 1983, 82pp.). A comprehensive text has now been published: *Brucellosis* (M. Monir Madkour (ed.), London: Butterworths, 1989, 294pp.). Another recent text on an important pathogen is *Pasteurella and pasteurellosis* (edited by C. Adlam and J. M. Rutter, London: Academic Press, 1989, 341pp.).

1266   Camus, E. and **Barré, N.** *Heartwater: a review.* Paris: OIE/IEMVT, 1988. 147pp.

Thorough review of *Cowdria ruminantium* infection. Gaps in current knowledge are indicated and there is a bibliography of 400 items. First published in French in 1982.

1267   Gyles, C. L. and **Thoen, C. O.** (eds) *Pathogenesis of bacterial infections in animals*. Ames: Iowa State UP, 1986. 227pp.
Each of the twenty-five chapters is concerned with a specific bacterial genus and describes the diseases caused by the organisms, pathogenesis, virulence factors, host resistance, immunity and control.

1268   Scanlan, C. M. *Introduction to veterinary bacteriology*. Ames: Iowa State UP, 1988. 457pp.
An outline format gives the basic principles of the subject. Important information on organisms and diseases is presented in detail. Has a glossary of microbial terminology.

Conferences

1269   *Virulence mechanisms of bacterial pathogens*. Edited by J. A. Roth. 1913 I St NW, Washington, DC 20006: American Society for Microbiology, 1988. 390pp.
Derived from the International Symposium on Virulence Mechanisms of Veterinary Bacterial Pathogens held in Ames in June 1987.

Journal

Veterinary microbiology [1395]

Other Journals

Journal of applied bacteriology (and *Letters in applied microbiology*)
Journal of bacteriology

BEHAVIOUR

Dictionaries

1270   Heymer, A. *Ethological dictionary. German–English–French*. New York: Garland Publishing, 1978. 238pp.

1271   Hurnik, J. F., Webster, A. B. and **Siegel, P. B.** *Dictionary of farm animal behaviour*. Raithby House, Guelph, Ontario, Canada: University of Guelph, Office of Educational Practice, 1985. 175pp.

Books

1272   Craig, J. V. *Domestic animal behavior: causes and implications for animal care and management.* Englewood Cliffs: Prentice-Hall, 1981. 364pp.
Deals with farm animals only.

1273   Dawkins, M. *Unravelling animal behaviour.* Harlow: Longman, 1986. 159pp.
Not a textbook but a companion work reviewing some of the more interesting and puzzling aspects of animal behaviour.

1274   Fraser, A. F. *From animal behaviour to animal bioethics.* St John's, Newfoundland: MUN Printing Service, 1987. 105pp.

1275   Fraser, A. F. *Farm animal behaviour: an introduction to behaviour in the common farm species.* 2nd ed. London: Baillière Tindall, 1980. 291pp.
A new edition under the editorship of A. F. Fraser and D. F. Broom is due in 1989.

1276   Hafez, E. S. E. (ed.) *The behaviour of domestic animals.* 3rd ed. London: Baillière Tindall, 1975. 532pp.
For many years the standard text and still invaluable for the reviews of the basic literature on animal behaviour. Includes chapters on dogs, cats, quail, chickens and ducks as well as farm animals.

1277   Hart, B. L. *The behavior of domestic animals.* New York: W. H. Freeman, 1985. 390pp.
Five chapters describe the behaviour of adult animals, including social, sexual, maternal and feeding behaviour and four further chapters discuss the determinants of behaviour, including the theoretical background.

1278   Houpt, K. A. and **Wolski, T. R.** *Domestic animal behavior for veterinarians and animal scientists.* Ames: Iowa State UP, 1982. 356pp.
A similar work to Hart's [1277] but with more illustrations and references to the literature. Appendices contain charts describing the behavioural development of the dog and cat.

1279   Jensen, P., Algers, B. and **Ekesbo, I.** *Methods of sampling and analysis of data in farm animal ethology.* Basel: Birkhäuser Verlag, 1986. 86pp. (Animal Management/Tierhaltung, vol. 17.)
A discussion of the methodology employed in recording and analysing behaviour.

1280   Kilgour, R. and **Dalton, C.** *Livestock behaviour: a practical guide.* London: Granada, 1983. 320pp.

A readable account of the behaviour of domestic animals. Written for those working in agriculture and livestock farming. Has an emphasis on animal welfare.

1281   Wood-Gush, D. G. M. *Elements of ethology: a textbook for agricultural and veterinary students.* London: Chapman & Hall, 1983. 240pp.

Journals

1282   *Animal behaviour.* 1953–. London: Baillière Tindall. Bimonthly.
Journal of the Association for the Study of Animal Behaviour.

1283   *Applied animal behaviour science.* 1974–. Amsterdam: Elsevier. Monthly.
Formerly (until 1985) *Applied animal ethology.*

Other Journals

Behaviour
Ethology (formerly *Zeitschrift für Tierpsychologie*)

DENTISTRY

Books

1284   Eisenmenger, E. and **Zetner, K.** *Veterinary dentistry.* Philadelphia: Lea & Febiger, 1985. 165pp.
Useful for the many colour illustrations. Translation of a German text originally published in 1982.

1285   Harvey, C. E. (ed.) *Veterinary dentistry.* Philadelphia: W. B. Saunders, 1985. 322pp.
Covers all the domestic species, laboratory animals and captive wild animals. A complete textbook of the anatomy, pathogenesis, diagnosis and management of oral diseases.

1286   Miles, A. E. W. and **Grigson, C.** *Colyer's Variations and diseases of the teeth of animals.* Cambridge: CUP. Forthcoming.

1287   Tholen, M. A. *Concepts in veterinary dentistry.* Edwardsville: Veterinary Medicine Publishing, 1983. 164pp.
Concentrates on the principles, techniques and instrumentation for dentistry in dogs. There is no index but the text is well laid out and illustrated.

EPIDEMIOLOGY AND PREVENTIVE MEDICINE

Books

1288   Berrier, H. H. *Animal sanitation and disease prevention.* 2nd ed. Dubuque: Kendall/Hunt, 1977. 226pp.

1289   British Veterinary Association. *Health management information pack.* London: the Association, 1984–5. Books and pamphlets in folder.
The pack is for veterinary surgeons to support their work in marketing health management/preventive medicine schemes. The two main volumes cover dairy, pig, beef and sheep fertility packages, and young animal (cattle, pigs and sheep) packages, respectively.

1290   Hanson, R. P. and **Hanson, M. G.** *Animal disease control: regional programs.* Ames: Iowa State UP, 1983. 331pp.
Covers the establishment and maintenance of systems for the tackling of animal diseases that require co-ordinated programmes for their control.

1291   Ingram, D. G., Mitchell, W. R. and **Martin, S. W.** *Animal disease monitoring.* Springfield: C. C. Thomas, 1975. 215pp.
Describes local, national and international recording of animal disease data.

1292   Leech, F. B. and **Sellers, K. C.** *Statistical epidemiology in veterinary science.* London: Charles Griffin, 1979. 158pp.
Guide to methods for planning the collection of survey data and for its handling and analysis.

1293   Martin, S. W., Meek, A. H. and **Willeberg, P.** *Veterinary epidemiology: principles and methods.* Ames: Iowa State UP, 1987. 343pp.
Outlines basic principles and discusses methods of studying disease in animal populations, including surveys and field trial design. Also contains a chapter on the economics of animal health and describes the purposes to which epidemiology may be applied.

1294   Radostits, O. M. and **Blood, D. C.** *Herd health: a textbook of health and production management of agricultural animals.* Philadelphia: W. B. Saunders, 1985. 456pp.
Textbook on the development of planned herd health and production programmes. Mostly concerned with dairy cattle, but also has sections on beef cattle, swine and sheep.

1295   Schnurrenberger, P. R., Sharman, R. S. and **Wise, G. H.** *Attacking animal diseases: concepts and strategies for control and eradication.* Ames: Iowa State UP, 1987. 200pp.

Describes the reasons for attempting to control animal diseases, discusses practical problems involved and outlines methods for improving disease control and eradication in the Western hemisphere.

1296 Schwabe, C. W. *Veterinary medicine and human health.* 3rd ed. Baltimore: Williams & Wilkins, 1984. 680pp.
Covers zoonoses and veterinary public health and the links and contributions veterinary medicine has and, will in future, make to human welfare. An important source of historical information on the development of veterinary medicine in these areas.

1297 Schwabe, C. W., Riemann, H. P. and **Franti, C. E.** *Epidemiology in veterinary practice.* Philadelphia: Lea & Febiger, 1977. 303pp.

1298 Thrusfield, M. V. *Veterinary epidemiology.* London: Butterworths, 1986. 280pp.
The only recent British text. Particularly strong in its treatment of quantitative aspects of the subject. Gives many references to the literature.

1299 Woods, G. T. (ed.) *Practices in veterinary public health and preventive medicine in the United States.* Ames: Iowa State UP, 1986. 347pp.
Outlines the background, execution, current status, and projected future of American initiatives to eradicate certain animal diseases that threaten public health.

Journals

1300 *Foreign animal disease report.* 1972–. Hyattsville: USDA–APHIS. Quarterly.
News items and reviews on diseases exotic to the United States focusing on their incidence and epidemiology.

1301 *Preventive veterinary medicine.* 1982–. Amsterdam: Elsevier. Quarterly.

HAEMATOLOGY, CYTOLOGY AND CLINICAL CHEMISTRY

(see also *Pathology)*

Review Series

1302 *Advances in clinical chemistry.* 1958–. Edited by H. E. Spiegel. San Diego: Academic Press. Irregular.

Data Collections

1303   Mitruka, B. M. and **Rawnsley, H. M.** *Clinical biochemical and hematological reference values in normal experimental animals*. New York: Masson Publishing, 1977. 272pp.
Clinical biochemical and haematological data are given for fourteen species and compared to values reported in humans. Introductory sections describe sample handling and the materials and methods used in such work.

1304   Rushton, B. *Veterinary laboratory data*. London: BVA Publications, 1981. 55pp.
Provides a series of tables giving representative results for many of the haematological, biological and other laboratory tests commonly performed on domestic animals.

Books

1305   Agar, N. S. and **Board, P. G.** (eds) *Red blood cells of domestic animals*. Amsterdam: Elsevier, 1983. 420pp.

1306   Archer, R. K. and **Jeffcott, L. B.** (eds) *Comparative clinical haematology*. Oxford: Blackwell, 1977. 737pp.
Has chapters devoted to each of the domestic animals, birds, exotic species and laboratory animals.

1307   Coles, E. H. *Veterinary clinical pathology*. 4th ed. Philadelphia: W. B. Saunders, 1986. 486pp.
A general textbook on the principles of clinical pathology. Includes sections on examinations for parasites, immunological techniques and avian clinical pathology. Another popular American text which describes the testing procedures used in domesticated animals is M. M. Benjamin's *Outline of veterinary clinical pathology* (3rd ed., Ames: Iowa State UP, 1978, 351pp.).

1308   Duncan, J. R. and **Prasse, K. W.** *Veterinary laboratory medicine: clinical pathology*. 2nd ed. Ames: Iowa State UP, 1986. 285pp.
Highly structured text, written in note form, and intended to show how abnormalities identified by laboratory procedures can be related to organ dysfunctions or lesions. Uses twenty-five case studies to indicate the points discussed in the text.

1309   Hawkey, C. M. and **Dennett, T. B.** *A colour atlas of comparative veterinary haematology*. London: Wolfe Publishing, 1989. 192pp.
Illustrates normal and abnormal blood cells from mammals, birds and reptiles. Blood parasites are covered in a section by M. A. Peirce.

1310   Kaneko, J. J. (ed.) *Clinical biochemistry of domestic animals*. 4th ed. San Diego: Academic Press, 1989. 932pp.
Classic work on the changes in the blood, other body fluids, organ function and other metabolic processes caused by disease.

1311   Kerr, M. G. *Veterinary laboratory medicine: clinical biochemistry and haematology*. Oxford: Blackwell, 1989. 270pp.
Comprehensive guide to establishing and running a practice laboratory with details of all the commonly required tests. Covers test interpretation and sampling techniques and discusses the use of external laboratories.

1312   Rowley, A. F. and **Ratcliffe, N. A.** *Vertebrate blood cells*. Cambridge: CUP, 1988. 444pp.
Comprises chapters on fish, amphibians, reptiles, birds, mammals and the comparative aspects of vertebrate and invertebrate blood cells. Primarily for researchers into comparative haematology.

1313 *Schalm's Veterinary haematology*. 4th ed. Edited by N. C. Jain. Philadelphia: Lea & Febiger, 1986. 1221pp.
Comprehensive work on the fundamentals of veterinary haematology and their application to the understanding of haematologic abnormalities. The haematology of common domestic, laboratory, zoo and wild animals is described in detail. The author has also written a series of works on the haematology of particular species. These have been published by Veterinary Practice Publishing as *Manual of . . . feline and canine hematology* (1980, 272pp.), *equine hematology* (1984, 80pp.) and *bovine hematology: anemias/leukocytes/testing* (1984, 82pp.).

Journals

1314 *Clinical chemistry: reference edition*. 1955–. 2029 K Street NW, Washington, DC 20006: American Association for Clinical Chemistry. Monthly.
Rarely includes papers on domestic animals. One issue each year is a reference edition with information on the Scientific Program of the Association's annual meeting.

1315 *Veterinary clinical pathology*. 1977–. Santa Barbara: Veterinary Practice Publishing. Quarterly.
Was *Bulletin of the American Society of Veterinary Clinical Pathologists*.

Other Journal

Journal of clinical pathology

HISTORY

Information Guides

1316   Corsi, P. and **Weindling, P.** *Information sources in the history of science and medicine.* London: Butterworths, 1983. 531pp. (Butterworths Guides to Information Sources.)

1317   *A world bibliography of bibliographies.* Compiled by T. Besterman. 4th ed. Lausanne: Societas Bibliographica, 1965–6. 5 vols. 8425 columns.
Has details of a number of bibliographies of early veterinary works in columns 6408–6414 of volume IV. Supplemented by *A world bibliography of bibliographies 1964–1974* (Compiled by A. F. Toomey, Totowa, New Jersey: Rowman and Littlefield, 1977, 2 vols).

Bibliographies

1318   *Bibliography of the history of medicine.* 1965–. Bethesda: National Library of Medicine. Annual with quinquennial cumulations.
Has a section on veterinary medicine.

1319   Morton, L. T. *A medical bibliography an annotated check-list of texts illustrating the history of medicine: Garrison and Morton.* 4th ed. Aldershot: Gower, 1983. 1000pp.

1320   Royal College of Veterinary Surgeons. *Catalogue of modern works 1900–1954, with a section showing periodicals and reports.* 2nd ed. London: RCVS, 1955. 98pp.
Supplements have been published for the years 1955–6 (16pp.) and 1957–8 (14pp.) There is an author catalogue and subject listing.

1321   Royal College of Veterinary Surgeons. *Catalogue of the historical collection: books published before 1850.* London: RCVS, 1953. 36pp. Plus supplement 1959, 6pp.
An author list with a list of periodicals appended.

1322   Royal Veterinary College Library. *A catalogue of the books, pamphlets and periodicals up to 1850: with an introduction by Professor L. P. Pugh.* Compiled by R. Catton. London: University of London, 1965. 48pp. (Supplement to *Veterinary record*, 1 May 1965.)

Books

1323   Gráy, E. A. *The trumpet of glory: the military career of John Shipp, first veterinary surgeon to join the British Army.* London: Robert Hale, 1985. 127pp.

1324   Katic, I. *World atlas of veterinary emblems.* Copenhagen: Veterinærhistorisk Forskning, 1987. 119pp.
Contains about four hundred logos from forty-eight countries. Supplements to the atlas will be issued.

1325   Ministry of Agriculture, Fisheries and Food. *Animal health: a centenary 1865–1965: a century of endeavour to control diseases of animals.* London: HMSO, 1965. 396pp.
An historical survey of government veterinary work in Great Britain.

1326   Pattison, I. *The British veterinary profession 1791–1948.* London: J. A. Allen, 1984. 207pp.

1327   Pattison, I. *John McFadyean: a great British veterinarian.* London: J. A. Allen, 1981. 240pp.

1328   Schwabe, C. W. *Cattle, priests, and progress in medicine.* Minneapolis: University of Minnesota Press, 1978. 277pp. (The Wesley W. Spink Lectures on Comparative Medicine, vol. 4.)

1329   Smith, F. *The early history of veterinary literature and its British development.* London: J. A. Allen, 1976. 4 vols.
The first three volumes are revisions of material originally published in the *Journal of comparative pharmacology and therapeutics* and the *Veterinary journal* (1912–30). The fourth volume covers the period 1823–80 and the manuscript was published after the author's death in 1929, edited by F. Bullock in 1933.

1330   Smithcors, J. F. *The veterinarian in America: 1625–1975.* Santa Barbara: American Veterinary Publications, 1975. 160pp.
Well illustrated history of the veterinary profession in the United States.

1331   Smithcors, J. F. *Evolution of the veterinary art: a narrative account to 1850.* Kansas City: Veterinary Medicine Publishing, 1957. 408pp.

1332   Smithcors, J. F. *The American veterinary profession: its background and development.* Ames: Iowa State UP, 1963. 704pp.

1333   Toynbee, J. M. C. *Animals in Roman life and art.* London: Thames & Hudson, 1973. 431pp.
Includes an appendix on Roman veterinary medicine (pp. 301–43) by R. F. Walker.

1334   '100 years of animal health: 1884–1984'. *Journal of the National Agricultural Library Associates* **11** (1987): (1/4) 230pp.

Journals

1335 *Historia medicinae veterinariae.* 1976–. Søndergade 39, DK-4130 Viby Sjælland, Denmark. Quarterly.

1336 *Medical history: devoted to the history and bibliography of medicine and the related sciences.* 1957–. 183 Euston Road, London NW1 2BP, England: Wellcome Institute for the History of Medicine Library. Quarterly.
The Institute also publish *Current work in the history of medicine: an international bibliography* (1954–, quarterly).

1337 *Veterinary history.* 1973–. London: Veterinary History Society. Two a year.
Formerly *Bulletin of the Veterinary History Society.*

Other Journals

Acta historiae medicinae, stomatologie, pharmaciae, veterinae
Bulletin of the history of medicine
Dansk veterinærhistorisk Årbog
Japanese journal of veterinary history

IMMUNOLOGY

Review Series

1338 *Immunological reviews.* 1969–. Copenhagen: Munksgaard. Bimonthly.

1339 *Progress in vaccinology.* 1987–. Edited by G. P. Talwar. Berlin: Springer-Verlag. Annual.

Other Review Series

Advances in immunology
The year in immunology

Books

1340 **Barta, O.** (ed.) *Laboratory techniques of veterinary clinical immunology.* Springfield: C. C. Thomas, 1984. 189pp.

1341 **Halliwell, R. E. W.** and **Gorman, N. T.** *Veterinary clinical immunology.* Philadelphia: W. B. Saunders, 1989. 548pp.
The first work to be devoted to the immunological aspects of disorders of animals. R. M. Lewis and C. A. Picut's *Veterinary clinical immunology: from*

classroom to clinic (Philadelphia: Lea & Febiger, 1989, 267pp.) is another recent work on the diagnosis and treatment of spontaneous immunologically mediated disease.

1342   Hay, J. B. (ed.) *Animal models of immunological processes*. London: Academic Press, 1982. 295pp.
Has reviews on the canine immune response, amphibian immunity and lympho-cyte migration patterns in sheep. The four other chapters concern aspects of the immunology of rodents and rabbits.

1343   Mayr, A., Eissner, G. and **Mayr-Bibrack, B.** *Handbuch der Schutzimp-fungen in der Tiermedizin*. Berlin: Paul Parey, 1984. 1006pp.
The only work devoted solely to immunization in domestic animals. The methods of immunization against fifty-nine diseases are described in addition to sections reviewing basic concepts in vaccination and immunology.

1344   Outteridge, P. M. *Veterinary immunology*. London: Academic Press, 1985. 280pp.
The principles of immunity are reviewed and there are chapters on immunity to parasites and pathogens. There is a glossary and an appendix gives immunological and serological techniques.

1345   Soulsby, E. J. L. (ed.) *Immune responses in parasitic infections: immunology, immunopathology and immunoprophylaxis*. Boca Raton: CRC Press, 1987. 4 vols. 336 + 220 + 349 + 344pp.
The volumes deal with **I**: *Nematodes*, **II**: *Trematodes and cestodes*, **III**: *Protozoa* and **IV**: *Protozoa, arthropods and invertebrates*.

1346   Tizard, I. *Veterinary immunology: an introduction*. 3rd ed. Philadelphia: W. B. Saunders, 1987. 401pp.
The fullest and most recent discussion of the topic. The book is divided into the following sections: the immune system, serology, protective immunity, hypersen-sitivity, inflammation and immunological diseases.

Conferences

1347   *Chemical regulation of immunity in veterinary medicine. Proceedings of a symposium held in Bethesda, Maryland, September 19–20, 1983*. Edited by M. Kende, J. Gainer and M. Chirigos. New York: Alan R. Liss, 1984. 599pp. (Progress in Clinical and Biological Research, vol. 161.)

1348   Morris, B. and **Miyasaka, M.** (eds) *Immunology of the sheep*. Basel: Editiones Roche, 1985. 520pp.
Contributions are grouped in the following sections: ontogeny and dif-ferentiation, primary lymphoid organs, lymphocyte migration and immune responses.

1349   Morrison, W. I. (ed.) *The ruminant immune system in health and disease.* Cambridge: CUP, 1986. 570pp.

1350   *Veterinary immunology. Proceedings of the 1st international veterinary immunology symposium. Held at the University of Guelph, Ontario, Canada, 1–4 July 1986.* Edited by B. N. Wilkie and P. E. Shewen. *Veterinary immunology and immunopathology* **17** (1987): (1–4) 518pp.

Journals

Comparative immunology, microbiology and infectious diseases [104]
Infection and immunity [1394]

1351   *Veterinary immunology and immunopathology.* 1979–. Amsterdam: Elsevier. Monthly.

Vaccine [134]

Other Journals

Developmental and comparative immunology
European journal of immunology
Immunology
Immunology today
Journal of immunological methods
Journal of immunology
Molecular immunology

LABORATORY MANUALS

1352   *Australian standard diagnostic techniques for animal diseases.* PO Box 89, East Melbourne, Victoria 3002, Australia: CSIRO, 1988–.
Each of the fifty-one booklets describes diagnostic tests and the interpretation of the results obtained from the tests for a particular disease/condition.

1353   Carter, G. R. *Veterinarian's guide to the laboratory diagnosis of disease.* Lenexa: Veterinary Medicine Publishing, 1986. 326pp.
Gives brief notes on over 200 diseases concentrating on the techniques used in laboratory diagnosis.

1354   Dobson, H. *A radioimmunoassay laboratory handbook: with special reference to hormones of reproduction.* Liverpool: LUP, 1984. 90pp.
Describes specific techniques and has tables giving the expected concentrations of hormones in the peripheral plasma of eight domesticated species.

1355   Hawken, M. L. (ed.) *Manual of laboratory techniques*. 2nd ed. Cheltenham: BSAVA, 1983. 108pp.
An introduction to the methods used in clinical pathology.

1356   *Manual of veterinary investigation laboratory techniques*. 3rd ed. London: HMSO, 1984. 2 vols. 219 + 196pp. (MAFF Reference Books 389 + 390.)
Volume 1 deals with safety precautions, media preparation, microscopy, bacteriology, mycology and virology; Volume 2 with biochemistry, haematology, histopathology and parasitology.

1357   *Manual of veterinary parasitological laboratory techniques*. 3rd ed. London: HMSO, 1986. 159pp. (MAFF Reference Book 418.)
Guide to techniques used in protozoology, helminthology and entomology, and to some serological tests used in diagnosis and research. Compiled by the staff of the Parasitology Department at the Central Veterinary Laboratories at Weybridge.

LEGISLATION AND REGULATORY MATTERS

1358   Animal Air Transportation Association. *Handbook*. Fort Washington, Maryland: the Association. Annual with quarterly supplements.
Provides summaries of laws, regulations and guidelines covering animal handling and shipping, including the IATA *Live animals regulations* and of veterinary procedures and animal health regulations.

1359   Blood, D. C. *Veterinary law: ethics, etiquette and convention*. 44 Waterloo Road, North Ryde, New South Wales 2113, Australia: Law Book Co., 1985. 368pp.
Although based on Australian law the book is of general interest since it provides an excellent account of the duties and responsibilities of the veterinary practitioner and of good professional practice.

1360   'Code of practice for storage and dispensing of medicines by veterinary surgeons'. *Veterinary record* **123** (1988): 47–8.
The code has been approved by the BVA and RCVS. It includes details of the statutory requirements.

1361   Cooper, M. E. *An introduction to animal law*. London: Academic Press, 1987. 213pp.
Written for those dealing with animals and relatively ignorant of the law and for those knowledgeable on legal topics but unfamiliar with veterinary matters. Has lists of legislation relating to the United Kingdom and Europe and of relevant international legislation.

1362   Dale, J. R. and **Appelbe, G. E.** *Pharmacy law and ethics*. 4th ed. London: Pharmaceutical Press, 1989. 586pp.

1363   Favre, D. S. and **Loring, M.** *Animal law*. Westport, Connecticut: Quorum Books, 1983. 253pp.

1364   *Guide to good pharmaceutical manufacturing practice 1983*. 3rd ed. Edited by J. R. Sharp. London: HMSO, 1983. 110pp.
Compiled by the Medicines Inspectorate of the DHSS and outlines recommended procedures for the manufacture of drugs.

1365   International Air Transportation Association. *Live animals regulations*. 15th ed. Publication Assistant, 2000 Peel Street, Montreal, Quebec H3A 2R4, Canada: the Association, 1986. Ringbound.
Gives information on the shipping and holding/carriage procedures and on sedation and euthanasia. Also includes national and international (CITES) regulations and requirements.

1366   *International zoo-sanitary code: rules recommended for trade in animals and animal products*. 5th ed. Paris: OIE, 1986. 509pp. (with annual updates)
A guide and reference document to assist international trade. Outlines measures to prevent the spread of disease and includes recommended norms for diagnostic procedures and biological products.

1367   *Legislation affecting the veterinary profession in the United Kingdom*. 5th ed. London: RCVS, 1987. 118pp.
Updated by amendment sheet incorporating changes in the legislation which have taken place in the previous twelve months and now relates to the law as it stood at 1 June 1988.

1368   Sandys-Winsch, G. *Animal law: a concise guide to the law relating to animals*. 2nd ed. London: Shaw & Sons, 1984. 260pp.
Covers UK legislation as stated on 1 October 1983. Contains lists of statutes, statutory instruments and cases discussed in the text.

1369   Soave, O. and **Crawford, L. M.** *Veterinary medicine and the law*. Baltimore: Williams & Wilkins, 1981. 146pp.

1370   Tannenbaum, J. *Veterinary ethics*. Baltimore: Williams & Wilkins. Forthcoming.

1371   Williams, D. R. *Animal feeding stuffs legislation in the UK: a concise guide*. London: Butterworths, 1987. 135pp.

A comprehensive work for those responsible for ensuring stuffs are manufactured, sold and distributed in accordance with statutory regulations.

Journals

1372   *FDA veterinarian.* 1986–. 5600 Fishers Lane, Rockville, Maryland 20857: FDA Veterinarian. Bimonthly.
Articles on regulatory issues, safety of animal drugs, news of interest to those involved in drug regulation. Includes lists of new FDA publications and of newly approved drugs in the United States.

1373   *Food and agricultural legislation.* 1952–. Rome: FAO. Twice per year.
Covers new and existing food and agriculture laws and legislation in FAO member countries.

1374   *Food chemical news.* 1959–. 1101 Pennsylvania Avenue, SE, Washington, DC 2000: Food Chemical News Inc. Weekly.
Concentrates on the US scene. Has news items on regulatory and related matters related to food, including additives, contaminants, labelling, feed and standards. The same publishers issue *Pesticide & toxic chemical news.*

1375   *MAIL: Medicines Act information letter.* 1980–. Market Towers, Nine Elms Lane, London SW8 5NQ, England: Department of Health. Quarterly.
News on the UK drug regulatory scene.

1376   *Regulatory affairs bulletin.* 1980–. Musselburgh EH21 7UB, Scotland: Inveresk Research International. Quarterly.
Covers national and international developments in the registration of veterinary drugs and other chemicals.

1377   *Veterinary drug registration newsletter.* 1987–. Paris: OIE. Two per year.
A forum for the exchange of news on regulatory matters. Sometimes includes lists of newly registered products and details of the registration procedures in selected countries. Published in Spanish, French and English.

1378   *WHO drug information.* 1987–. Geneva: WHO. Quarterly.
News and information, in particular on regulatory matters, about both medical and veterinary drugs. Includes details on new and proposed *International nonproprietary names.*

Other Journal

Food additives and contaminants

MICROBIOLOGY

Dictionary

1379   Singleton, P. and **Sainsbury, D.** *Dictionary of microbiology and molecular biology*. 2nd ed. Chichester: John Wiley, 1987. 1019pp.

Books

1380   Buxton, A. and **Fraser, G.** *Animal microbiology*. Oxford: Blackwell, 1977. 2 vols. 830pp.
The first volume deals with bacteriology and mycology, the second with rickettsias and viruses.

1381   Carter, G. R. *Essentials of veterinary bacteriology and mycology*. 3rd ed. Philadelphia: Lea & Febiger, 1986. 261pp.
A basic undergraduate textbook with lists of supplementary reading.

1382   Carter, G. R. (ed.) *Diagnostic procedures in veterinary bacteriology and mycology*. 4th ed. Springfield: C. C. Thomas, 1984. 515pp.
Has sections on methods of dealing with clinical specimens and chapters on each of the major groups of organisms of veterinary importance.

1383   Collins, C. H. *Laboratory-acquired infections*. 2nd ed. London: Butterworths, 1988. 295pp.
Useful reading for all working in microbiological laboratories.

1384   Collins, C. H. and **Grange, J. M.** (eds) *Isolation and identification of microorganisms of medical and veterinary importance*. London: Academic Press, 1985. 387pp. (Society for Applied Bacteriology Technical Series, no. 21.)
Each of the twenty-four contributions describes techniques applicable to a specific pathogen, group of pathogens or disease. Acts as an update of Cottral's manual and Carter's work.

1385   Cottral, G. E. (ed.) *Manual of standardized methods for veterinary microbiology*. Ithaca: Cornell UP, 1978. 731pp.

1386   Gyles, C. L. and **Thoen, C. O.** (eds) *Pathogenesis of bacterial infections in animals*. Ames: Iowa State UP, 1986. 227pp.
Describes the mechanisms of bacterial disease.

1387   *Hagan and Bruner's Microbiology and infectious diseases of domestic animals: with reference to etiology, epizootiology, pathogenesis, immunity, diagnosis and antimicrobial susceptibility*. 8th ed. By J. F. Timoney, J. H. Gillespie, F. W. Scott and J. E. Barlough. Ithaca: Cornell University Press, 1988. 951pp.

A standard textbook which describes each taxonomic group in detail, with sections devoted to each of the major diseases that they cause. There are also review chapters on general topics relevant to bacterial, fungal and viral diseases. Similar in scope to Buxton and Fraser's text.

1388 Olds, R. J. *A colour atlas of microbiology.* London: Wolfe Medical Publications, 1987. 288pp.
Uses almost 400 photographs to illustrate the common bacteria and fungi.

1389 *Topley and Wilson's Principles of bacteriology, virology and immunity.* 7th ed. General editors Sir G. Wilson, Sir A. Miles and M. T. Parker. London: Edward Arnold, 1983–4. 4 vols.
The basic reference text for microbiologists. Aspects of the immunology of infectious disease are covered in volume 1. The four volumes and their editors are:

1. *General microbiology and immunity.* Sir G. Wilson and H. M. Dick. 1983. 450pp.
2. *Systematic bacteriology.* M. T. Parker. 1983. 562pp.
3. *Bacterial diseases.* G. R. Smith. 1984. 610pp.
4. *Virology.* F. Brown and Sir G. Wilson. 1984. 584pp.

1390 Zak, O. and **Sande, M. A.** (eds) *Experimental models in antimicrobial chemotherapy.* London: Academic Press, 1986. 3 vols. 380 + 387 + 398pp.

Conferences

1391 *Advances in carriers and adjuvants for veterinary biologics.* Compiled by R. M. Nervig, P. M. Gough, M. L. Kaeberle and C. A. Whetstone. Ames: Iowa State UP, 1986. 202pp.
Proceedings of a symposium held in May 1984 discussing advances in carriers, adjuvants and delivery systems for vaccines.

1392 *Immunoassays for veterinary and food analysis – 1.* Edited by B. A. Morris, M. N. Clifford and R. Jackman. London: Elsevier Applied Science, 1988. 392pp.
Based on the proceedings of the second international symposium on advances in immunoassays for veterinary and food analysis held at Guildford, 15–17 July 1986.

Journals

1393 *Epidemiology and infection.* 1901–. Cambridge: CUP. Bimonthly.
Publishes original reports and reviews on all aspects of infection in man and animals. Until 1987 known as the *Journal of hygiene.*

1394   *Infection and immunity.* 1970–. 1913 I Street NW, Washington, DC 20006: American Society for Microbiology. Monthly.
Publishes research on infections caused by all kinds of pathogenic microbes and fungi, on related aspects of host resistance and susceptibility to infection and the immunology of infection.

1395   *Veterinary microbiology.* 1976–. Amsterdam: Elsevier. Monthly.

Other Journals

Antimicrobial agents and chemotherapy
Journal of antimicrobial chemotherapy
Journal of clinical microbiology
Journal of infection
Journal of general microbiology
Journal of infections diseases
Reviews of infectious diseases

MYCOLOGY AND MYCOTOXICOSES

Abstracting Service

1396   *Review of medical and veterinary mycology.* 1943–. Wallingford: CAB International. Quarterly.

Dictionary

1397   *Ainsworth and Bisby's Dictionary of the fungi.* 7th ed. Edited by D. L. Hawksworth, B. C. Sutton and G. C. Ainsworth. Farnham Royal: CAB, 1983. 445pp.
Lists generic names, defines mycological terms and gives brief accounts of most aspects of mycology.

History

1398   **Ainsworth, G. C.** *Introduction to the history of medical and veterinary mycology.* Cambridge: CUP, 1986. 228pp.

Books

1399   **Ainsworth, G. C.** and **Austwick, P. K. C.** *Fungal diseases of animals.* 2nd ed. Farnham Royal: CAB, 1973. 216pp. (Commonwealth Bureau of Animal Health Review Series, no. 6.)
Covers the literature to about mid–1971.

1400   Howard, D. H. (ed.) *Fungi pathogenic for humans and animals*. New York: Marcel Dekker, 1983–5. 3 vols. 672 + 576 + 381pp. (Mycology Series Volume 3.)
Part A deals with the basic biology of the fungi, the two volumes in Part B are concerned with pathogenicity and detection.

1401   Jungerman, P. F. and **Schwartzman, R. M.** *Veterinary medical mycology*. Philadelphia: Lea & Febiger, 1972. 200pp.

1402   Marasas, W. F. O. and **Nelson, P. E.** *Mycotoxicology: introduction to the mycology, plant pathology, chemistry, toxicology and pathology of naturally occurring mycotoxicoses in animals and man*. University Park, Pennsylvania: Pennsylvania State University Press, 1987. 102pp.
Deals with eleven mycotoxicoses considered to be of greatest economic importance. Designed for use as a teaching text and the forty-eight colour plates are also available as slide sets.

1403   Smith, J. E. and **Moss, M. O.** *Mycotoxins: formation, analysis and significance*. Chichester: John Wiley, 1985, 148pp.
An introductory work with a chapter reviewing the implications of mycotoxins in animal diseases.

1404   Wyllie, T. D. and **Morehouse, L. G.** (eds) *Mycotoxic fungi, mycotoxins, mycotoxicoses: an encyclopedic handbook*. New York: Marcel Dekker, 1977–8. 3 vols. 568 + 600 + 232pp.
Volume 1 is entitled *Mycotoxic fungi and chemistry of mycotoxins*, Volume 2 is *Mycotoxicoses of domestic and laboratory animals, poultry and aquatic invertebrates and vertebrates*, Volume 3 is *Mycotoxicoses of man and plants: mycotoxin control and regulatory aspects*.

Conference

1405   Lloyd, D. H. and **Sellers, K. C.** (eds) *Dermatophilus infection in animals and man*. London: Academic Press, 1976. 322pp.
Proceedings of a symposium held at the University of Ibadan, Nigeria, and sponsored by the Agricultural Research Council of Nigeria.

Journal

1406 *Journal of medical and veterinary mycology*. 1961–. PO Box 25, Abingdon, Oxfordshire OX14 3EU, England: Carfax Publishing. Bimonthly.
Sponsored by the International Society for Human and Animal Mycology. Until 1986 known as *Sabouradia: journal of medical and veterinary mycology*.

NEUROLOGY

Books

1407   de Lahunta, A. *Veterinary neuroanatomy and clinical neurology.* 2nd ed. Philadelphia: W. B. Saunders, 1983. 471pp.

1408   King, A. S. *Physiological and clinical anatomy of the domestic mammals. Volume 1. Central nervous system.* Oxford: Clarendon Press, 1987. 325pp.
Textbook with discussions based on a generalized mammal with occasional specific details of man and domestic animals. Forthcoming volumes will cover the head, thorax, abdomen and pelvis.

1409   Oliver, J. E. Jr, Hoerlein, B. F. and **Mayhew, I. G.** (eds) *Veterinary neurology.* Philadelphia: W. B. Saunders, 1987. 554pp.
Replaces B. F. Hoerlein's *Canine neurology* and now covers all domestic animals. Describes neurologic examination and diagnosis, then covers the various diseases of the nervous system and the medical and surgical therapy which is available.

1410   Oliver, J. E. Jr and **Lorenz, M. D.** *Handbook of veterinary neurologic diagnosis.* Philadelphia: W. B. Saunders, 1983. 371pp.

NUTRITION AND DIGESTION

Abstracting Services

1411   *Nutrition abstracts and reviews, Series B: livestock feeds and feeding.* 1931–. Wallingford: CAB International. Monthly.
There is a companion journal: *Nutrition abstracts and reviews. Series B: human and experimental.* The separate Series A and B journals began in 1977.

1412   *Food science and technology abstracts.* 1969–. Wallingford: CAB International. Monthly.

Review Series

1413   *Comparative Animal Nutrition.* 1976–. Edited by M. Rechigl. Basel: Karger.

    6 *Use of animal models for research in animal nutrition.* 1988. 190pp. (A. C. Benyon and C. E. Wert, editors)
    4 *Physiology of growth and nutrition.* 1981. 341pp.
    3 *Nitrogen, electrolytes, water and energy metabolism.* 1979. 260pp.
    2 *Nutrient elements and toxicants.* 1977. 205pp.
    1 *Carbohydrates, lipids and accessory growth factors.* 1976. 223pp.

1414   Haresign, W. and **Cole, D. J. A.** (eds) *Recent developments in ruminant nutrition.* London: Butterworths, 1981 and 1988. 2 vols. 367 + 352pp.
Reprints articles which have previously been published in *Recent advances in animal nutrition.* The same editors have produced *Recent developments in poultry nutrition* (London: Butterworths, 1989, 244pp.) and *Recent developments in pig nutrition* (1985, 321pp.).

1415   *Recent advances in animal nutrition.* 1977–. Edited by W. Haresign and D. J. A. Cole. London: Butterworths. Annual.
Each volume provides a collection of detailed reviews grouped around a number of areas of research and are the proceedings of the University of Nottingham Feed Manufacturers' Conferences.

Book Series

1416   National Research Council. *Nutrient Requirements of Domestic Animals.* Washington, DC: National Academy Press.
Each volume in the series comprises a comprehensive review of the nutritional requirements of the animal(s), the effects of deficiency states, and other nutritional disorders. The composition of specific feeds is presented in tables. The titles available are *Nutrient requirements of . . .:*

Cats. 2nd ed. 1986. 78pp
Dogs. 2nd ed. 1985. 79pp.
Horses. 4th ed. 1978. 33pp. (5th ed. due 1989)
Beef cattle. 6th ed. 1984. 90pp.
Dairy cattle. 6th ed. 1988. 168pp.
Goats: angora, dairy and meat goats in temperate and tropical countries. 1981.
   91pp.
Non-human primates. 1978. 84pp.
Laboratory animals: rat, mouse, gerbil, guinea pig, hamster, vole, fish. 3rd ed.
   1978. 96pp.
Coldwater fishes. 1981. 63pp.
Mink and foxes. 2nd ed. 1982. 72pp.
Warmwater fishes and shellfishes. 2nd ed. 1983. 102pp.
Poultry. 8th ed. 1984. 71pp.
Rabbits. 2nd ed. 1977. 30pp.
Sheep. 6th ed. 1985. 99pp.
Swine. 9th ed. 1988. 93pp

Books

1417   Anderson, N. V. (ed.) *Veterinary gastroenterology.* 2nd ed. Philadelphia: Lea & Febiger, 1980. 720pp.
A complete review of the physiology and functioning of the gastrointestinal tract in health and disease. Concentrates on clinical evaluation of patients, radiography and endoscopy, and discusses diseases in detail. A third edition is in preparation.

1418   Bondi, A. A. *Animal nutrition.* Chichester: John Wiley, 1987. 540pp.
A general textbook on the principles of nutrition, including metabolic and physiological aspects, dealing with both ruminant and monogastric animals including poultry.

1419   Christie, W. W. (ed.) *Lipid metabolism in ruminant animals.* Oxford: Pergamon, 1981. 452pp.

1420   Church, D. C. (ed.) *The ruminant animal: digestive physiology and nutrition.* Englewood Cliffs: Prentice-Hall, 1988. 564pp.
Chapters cover all the major aspects of nutrient consumption, metabolism and requirements and of digestive physiology. An updating of *Digestive physiology and nutrition of ruminants* (O & B Books, 1971–9, 3 vols).

1421   Church, D. C. (ed.) *Livestock feeds and feeding.* 2nd ed. Englewood Cliffs: Prentice-Hall, 1986. 549pp.

1422   Cullison, A. E. and **Lowrey, R. S.** *Feeds and feeding.* 4th ed. Englewood Cliffs: Prentice-Hall, 1987. 645pp.
Covers the nutrition and feeding of ruminants, swine and horses.

1423   Czerkawski, J. W. *An introduction to rumen studies.* Oxford: Pergamon, 1986. 236pp.
Integrates current knowledge on the functioning of the rumen with extensive discussions of the experimental techniques used in these studies.

1424   *Energy allowances and feeding systems for ruminants.* 2nd ed. London: HMSO, 1984. 85pp. (MAFF Reference Book 433.)

1425   Forbes, J. M. *The voluntary food intake of farm animals.* London: Butterworths, 1986. 206pp.
Review of the physiology of food intake control, of the factors affecting food intake and of the measurement, prediction and manipulation of voluntary intake.

1426   Hacker, J. B. and **Termouth, J. H.** (eds) *The nutrition of herbivores.* London: Academic Press, 1987. 552pp.

1427   Hobson, P. N. (ed.) *The rumen microbial system.* London: Elsevier Applied Science, 1988. 527pp.
Comprehensive guide to the rumen ecosystem describing the organisms found in the rumen and the physiology and functioning of that organ. R. E. Hungate's *The rumen and its microbes* (New York: Academic Press, 1966, 533pp.) is an earlier work on the same topic.

1428   McDonald, P., Edwards, R. A. and **Greenhalgh, J. F. D.** *Animal nutrition.* 4th ed. Harlow: Longman, 1988. 543pp.
Covers animal nutrition in both temperate and tropical zones. Describes the

chemical nature, digestion and metabolism of foods, covers their evaluation and the development of feeding standards and deals with the nutritive value of individual foods. Standard textbook for agricultural and veterinary students.

1429   McDowell, L. R. *Vitamins in animal nutrition: comparative aspects to human nutrition*. San Diego: Academic Press, 1989. 486pp. (Animal Feeding and Nutrition.)
Reviews the roles of vitamins and discuses deficiency diseases and supplementation in farm and laboratory animals and man.

1430   McDowell, L. R. (ed.) *Nutrition of grazing ruminants in warm climates*. Orlando: Academic Press, 1985. 443pp. (Animal Feeding and Nutrition.)
Describes the nutritional requirements of animals reared in the tropics and methods of dietary supplementation.

1431   Mertz, W. (ed.) *Trace elements in human and animal nutrition – fifth edition*. San Diego: Academic Press, 1986–7. 2 vols. 480 + 499pp.
Contains definitive reviews on each of the significant trace elements. Also has sections on methods of trace element research, quality assurance for trace element analysis and a chapter on soil–plant–animal and human inter-relationships in trace elements nutrition. Editions 1 to 4 were edited by E. J. Underwood.

1432   Ministry of Agriculture, Fisheries, and Food, Standing Committee on Tables of Feed Composition. *Feed composition: UK tables of feed composition and nutritive values for ruminants*. Marlow: Chalcombe Publications, 1985. 69pp.
Gives information, derived from *in vivo* evaluations, on the composition and nutritive value of 882 feeds.

1433   National Research Council, Subcommittee on Biological Energy. *Nutritional energetics of domestic animals and glossary of energy terms*. 2nd ed. Washington, DC: National Academy Press, 1981. 54pp.

1434   National Research Council, Subcommittee on Mineral Toxicity in Animals. *Mineral tolerance of domestic animals*. Washington, DC: National Academy of Sciences, 1980. 577pp.
The first chapter gives the suggested maximum tolerable levels for 35 minerals. Subsequent chapters review the literature on the adverse effects of these minerals in domestic animals. Other recent publications from the Council on nutritional topics include: *Vitamin tolerance of animals* (1987, 106pp.) and *Predicting feed intake of major food producing animals* (1987, 96pp.).

1435   *The nutrient requirements of ruminant livestock: technical review by an Agricultural Research Council Working Party*. Farnham Royal: CAB, 1980. 351pp.
Comprehensive reference work surveying and assessing the literature relevant to nutrient requirements. *The nutrient requirements of ruminant livestock: supplement no. 1* (1984, 45pp.) revises the work to provide the most recent guidance on the measurement of protein value in ruminants.

1436 Ørskov, R. *The feeding of ruminants: principles and practice.* Marlow: Chalcombe Publications, 1987. 92pp.
Introductory guide for farmers.

1437 Ørskov, E. R. *Protein nutrition in ruminants.* London: Academic Press, 1982. 160pp.

1438 Owen, J. *Complete diets for cattle and sheep.* Ipswich: Farming Press, 1979. 159pp.

1439 Perry, T. W. *Animal life-cycle feeding and nutrition.* New York: Academic Press, 1984. 319pp. (Animal Feeding and Nutrition.)
Reviews the nutrients, their evaluation, and feedstuffs, and gives recommendations for the feeding of animals. Uses the National Research Council's publications to devise the list of recommendations for cattle, pigs, goats, sheep, horses and poultry.

1440 Scott, M. L. *Nutrition of humans and selected animal species.* New York: John Wiley, 1986. 537pp.
Useful text on comparative nutrition.

1441 Rook, J. A. F. and **Thomas, P. C.** (eds) *Nutritional physiology of farm animals.* London: Longman, 1983. 704pp.
Considers the dynamic aspects of nutrient supply and intake in the regulation of metabolism and the relationship between diet and animal performance.

1442 Shirley, R. L. *Nitrogen and energy nutrition of ruminants.* Orlando: Academic Press, 1986. 358pp. (Animal Feeding and Nutrition.)
Detailed scientific review that emphasizes the activity of rumen microbes in nitrogen and energy nutrition.

1443 Underwood, E. J. *The mineral nutrition of livestock.* 2nd ed. Farnham Royal: CAB, 1981. 180pp.
A concise review of the requirements of livestock for minerals and of the detection and correction of dietary deficiencies of both the major mineral elements and of trace elements.

1444 Van Soest, P. J. *Nutritional ecology of the ruminant: ruminant metabolism, nutritional strategies, the cellulolytic fermentation and the chemistry of forages and plant fibers.* Ithaca: Comstock Publishing, 1982. 373pp.

1445 Wilson, P. N. and **Brigstocke, T. D. A.** *Improved feeding of cattle and sheep: a practical guide to modern concepts of ruminant nutrition.* London: Granada, 1981. 238pp.
Survey of the theory and practice of ruminant nutrition suitable for farmers, advisers and applied nutritionists.

1446   Wilson, P. N. and **Brigstocke, T. D. A.** *Improved feeding of pigs and poultry: a practical guide to modern concepts of pig and poultry nutrition.* London: Granada, 1985. 238pp.

1447   Wiseman, J. (editor and translator) *Feeding of non-ruminant livestock.* London: Butterworths, 1987. 214pp.
The majority of the text comprises dietary recommendations for the feeding of pigs, rabbits, broiler and laying hens, turkeys, guinea-fowl, ducks, geese, Japanese quail, pheasants and partridges. Translated from a French work written by the staff of the Institut National de la Recherche Agronomique.

Conferences

1448   Batt, R. M. and **Lawrence, T. L. J.** (eds) *Function and dysfunction of the small intestine. Proceedings of the second George Durrant Memorial Symposium.* Liverpool: LUP, 1984. 246pp.

1449   Dobson, A. and **Dobson, M. J.** (eds) *Aspects of digestive physiology in ruminants.* Ithaca: Cornell University Press, 1988. 311pp.

1450   Milligan, L. P., Grovum, W. L. and **Dobson, A.** (eds) *Control of digestion and metabolism in ruminants.* Englewood Cliffs: Prentice-Hall, 1986. 567pp.
Contains the proceedings of the sixth international symposium on ruminant physiology. The seventh symposium is to be held in Sendai, Japan during 1989 and the proceedings will be published (Secretariat: International Communications, Kasko Building, 2F, 2–14–9 Nihombashi, Chuo-ku, Tokyo 103, Japan).

1451   *Physiology of ruminant nutrition. Proceedings of the IV international symposium on physiology of ruminant nutrition, High Tatras, Czechoslovakia.* Edited by K. Boda. Kosice: Slovak Academy of Sciences, Institute of Animal Physiology, 1987. 551pp.

1452   *Proceedings 36th annual Pfizer research conference.* New York 10017: Pfizer Agricultural Division, 1988. 200pp.
Has reviews of developments in nutrition research during 1987 for ruminants, swine, dairy cattle and poultry and a review of bacterial antimicrobial resistance.

1453   *Trace elements in man and animals – TEMA 5. Proceedings of the fifth international symposium on trace elements in man and animals.* Edited by C. F. Mills, I. Bremner and J. K. Chesters. Farnham Royal: CAB, 1985. 977pp.
The first TEMA conference was held in 1969. Details of future meetings are available from the TEMA Symposium Secretary, Rowett Research Institute, Bucksburn, Aberdeen AB2 9SB, Scotland.

Journals

1454   *Animal feed science and technology.* 1976–. Amsterdam: Elsevier. Monthly.

1455   *Archives of animal nutrition (Archiv für Tierenährung).* 1950–. Berlin: Akademie Verlag. Monthly.

1456   *British journal of nutrition.* 1947–. Cambridge: CUP. Quarterly.

1457   *Feed compounder.* 1981–. Abney House, Baslow, Bakewell, Derbyshire DE4 1RZ, England: HGM Publications. Monthly.
This title and the next two journals publish reviews, brief technical articles and news on the feedstuffs industry.

1458   *Feed international.* 1980–. Mount Morris: Watt Publishing. Monthly.
Has an annual buyer's guide in the January issue.

1459   *Feedstuffs.* 1929–. Minnetonka: Miller Publishing. Weekly.
Publishes a reference issue each year which summarizes feed facts and figures and includes a buyer's guide.

Other Journals

Feed management
Journal of nutrition
Nutrition research
Proceedings of the Nutrition Society
Reproduction, nutrition, development

ONCOLOGY

Books

1460   Bostock, D. E. and **Owen, L. N.** *A colour atlas of neoplasia in the cat, dog and horse.* London: Wolfe Medical Publications, 1975. 144pp.
Illustrates the macroscopic and histological appearance of tumours and tumour-like conditions and discusses treatment and prognosis.

1461   Fiennes, R. N. T-W- *Infectious cancers of animals and man.* London: Academic Press, 1982. 166pp.
Has chapters on tumour systems in cats and cattle, neoplastic diseases of non-human primates and on the transmissible tumours of fowls.

1462   Gross, L. *Oncogenic viruses.* 3rd ed. Oxford: Pergamon, 1983. 2 vols. 1203pp.

1463   Moulton, J. E. (ed.) *Tumors in domestic animals.* 2nd ed. Berkeley: University of California Press, 1978. 465pp.
Deals with the tumours according to the tissues in which they are found. A new edition is in preparation.

1464   Priester, W. A. and **McKay, F. W.** *The occurrence of tumours in domestic animals.* Bethesda: National Cancer Institute, 1980. 210pp. (National Cancer Institute Monograph 54.)
Comprises statistical data on the tumours recorded in domestic animals in North America.

1465   Theilen, G. H. and **Madewell, B. R.** (eds) *Veterinary cancer medicine.* 2nd ed. Philadelphia: Lea & Febiger, 1987. 676pp.
Comprehensive work covering all aspects of veterinary oncology. Divided into three sections, the first on the principles of cancer management, the second on systemic cancer medicine and the third, consisting of a single chapter, on tumours in zoo animals and wildlife.

1466   Withrow, S. J. and **MacEwen, E. G.** (eds) *Clinical veterinary oncology.* Philadelphia: J. B. Lippincott. Forthcoming.

OPHTHALMOLOGY

History

1467   Magrane, W. G. *A history of veterinary ophthalmology.* 10661 Ellis Avenue, Suite A, Fountain Valley, California 92708: c/o American College of Veterinary Ophthalmologists, 1988. 76pp.

Books

1468   Barnett, K. C. *A colour atlas of veterinary ophthalmology.* London: Wolfe Medical Publications. Forthcoming.
Will concentrate on the dog and the horse.

1469   Bistner, S. I., Aguirre, G. and **Batik, G.** *Atlas of veterinary ophthalmic surgery.* Philadelphia: W. B. Saunders, 1977. 302pp.
Describes the techniques and equipment used but most of the book is an atlas of specific procedures with instructions and supporting text.

1470   Blogg, J. R. *The eye in veterinary practice.* Malvern, Australia: Chilcote
Publishing, 1987. 3 vols. 278 + 89 + 278pp.
Handbooks for the practitioner. Concisely written and with a large number of
diagrams, concentrating on diagnosis and treatment. The three volumes deal with
Extraocular diseases, Eye examination of the performance horse and *Eye injuries.* Available
in the UK from M. Blogg, 31 The White House, Vicarage Lane, London SW11
3LJ.

1471   Gelatt, K. N. (ed.) *Textbook of veterinary ophthalmology.* Philadelphia: Lea &
Febiger, 1981. 788pp.
There is an introductory section covering the basic sciences and clinical examination, a series of chapters on canine ophthalmology and a final section covering eye
diseases in other species. The most complete survey to appear thus far.

1472   Peiffer, R. L. Jr (ed.) *Comparative ophthalmic pathology.* Springfield: C. C.
Thomas, 1983. 359pp.

1473   Rubin, L. F. *Atlas of veterinary ophthalmoscopy.* Philadelphia: Lea & Febiger,
1974. 470pp.
Includes colour illustrations of most of the diseases affecting the fundus.

1474   Saunders, L. Z. and **Rubin, L. F.** *Ophthalmic pathology of animals: an atlas
and reference book.* Basel: Karger, 1975. 258pp.
A compendium of illustrations of diseases of the eye. There are brief clinical notes
accompanying the illustrations.

1475   Slatter, D. H. *Fundamentals of veterinary ophthalmology.* Philadelphia: W. B.
Saunders, 1981. 821pp.
An outline and introduction to clinical ophthalmology.

PARASITOLOGY

Abstracting Services

1476 *Helminthological abstracts. Series A: animal and human helminthology.* 1930–.
Wallingford: CAB International. Monthly.
Volumes 1–38 were published as *Helminthological abstracts* and included both
animal and plant helminthology. In 1970 this was divided into *Series A* and *Series B:
Plant nematology.*

1477 *Index-catalogue of medical and veterinary zoology.* 1932/52–. Prepared by the
USDA ARS's Animal Parasitology Institute. Washington, DC: US GPO. 18
vols plus supplements (1953–).

A bibliography of literature on the parasites of man and animals with strong coverage of literature on taxonomy. A description of the history and arrangement of the *Index-catalogue* is given in the *Journal of parasitology* (**55** (1969): 381–4). The basic catalogue was an author index in eighteen volumes. Incorporates and is a revision of the *Index-catalogue of medical and veterinary zoology-authors* published 1902–12 as Bureau of Animal Industry Bulletin 39. The supplements have most recently consisted of parasite subject catalogues divided by taxonomic group with author, host and subject heading and treatment indexes. Temporarily suspended publication with Supplement 24 (1982) (published by Oryx Press).

1478   *Review of applied entomology. Series B: medical and veterinary.* 1913–. Wallingford: CAB International. Monthly.

1479   *Tsetse and trypanosomiasis information quarterly.* 1978–. Central Avenue, Chatham Maritime, Chatham, Kent ME4 4TB, England: Overseas Development Natural Resources Institute. Quarterly.
Contains news items and abstracts of new literature.

Review Series

1480   *Advances in disease vector research.* Edited by K. F. Harris. 1983–. New York: Springer-Verlag. Occasional.
Most volumes contain three or four reviews on veterinary parasites or diseases and on aspects of their transmission. Originally entitled *Current topics in disease vector research*.

1481   *Advances in parasitology.* 1963–. London: Academic Press. Annual.

Bibliography

1482   **Hoogstraal, H.** *Bibliography of ticks and tickborne diseases from Homer (about 800 B.C.) to 31 December 1969.* Cairo: United States Naval Research Unit Number 3. 1970–82. 7 vols.
The first four volumes provide a list of the literature arranged according to author. Subsequent volumes update and revise the main work.

Identification Manuals

1483   *CIH keys to the nematode parasites of vertebrates.* Farnham Royal: CAB, 1974–83. 10 vols.
The first volume has a general introduction, glossary of terms and keys to subclasses, orders and superfamilies.

1484 Smith, K. G. V. (ed.) *Insects and other arthropods of medical importance.* London: British Museum (Natural History), 1973. 561pp.
A key for the identification of veterinary and medical pests. Includes brief discussions of their biology.

Books

1485 Alexander, J. O. *Arthropods and human skin.* Berlin: Springer-Verlag, 1984. 422pp.
Describes the eruptions caused by arthropods on human skin with background information on the pests themselves.

1486 *The anthelmintic index.* By J. H. Bard. Farnham Royal: CAB, 1972. 71pp. (Commonwealth Institute of Helminthology Technical Communication, no. 43.)
An index to the compounds noted in *Helminthological abstracts* (1966–72). Gives systematic chemical names and synonyms, and quotes the volume and abstract numbers in *Helminthological abstracts*.

1487 Campbell, W. C. and **Rew, R. S.** (eds.) *Chemotherapy of parasitic diseases.* New York: Plenum Press, 1986. 655pp.
Comprehensive text on antiparasitic agents. Covers the antiprotozoals, anthelmintics, insecticides and acaricides used against parasites of both man and animals. In most cases there are chapters on the chemistry of the drugs, the parasitic infections of man and one on those of domestic animals, a chapter on the biochemical action of the drugs and one on drug resistance. W. C. Campbell has also edited *Ivermectin and abamectin* (New York: Springer-Verlag, 1989, 363pp.).

1488 Cheng, T. C. *General parasitology.* 2nd ed. Orlando: Academic Press, 1986. 827pp.

1489 Drummond, R. O., George, J. E. and **Kunz, S. E.** *Control of arthropod pests of livestock: a review of technology.* Boca Raton: CRC Press, 1988. 245pp.
Comprises a review of the chemicals and application technology used to control insect and acarine pests.

1490 Dunn, A. M. *Veterinary helminthology.* 2nd ed. London: Heinemann, 1978. 323pp.
Overview of the taxonomy and biology of the parasites and of their effects in the host species.

1491 Georgi, J. R. *Parasitology for veterinarians.* 4th ed. Philadelphia: W. B. Saunders, 1985. 344pp.
Has three sections dealing with the biology of the parasites, control of parasitic diseases and diagnostic parasitology.

1492   Gibbons, L. M. *SEM guide to the morphology of nematode parasites of vertebrates.* Farnham Royal: CAB, 1986. 200pp.
Reproduces scanning electron micrographs of the major human and veterinary parasites. An aid to identification.

1493   Gibson, T. E. *Veterinary anthelmintic medication.* 3rd ed. Farnham Royal: CAB, 1975. 348pp. (Commonwealth Institute of Helminthology Technical Communication, no. 33.)
Has chapters on the treatment of parasitic infections in each major group of animals and a chapter on the methods of administration used.

1494   Graber, M. and **Perrotin, C.** *Helminthes et helminthoses des ruminants domestiques d'Afrique tropicale.* Maisons-Alfort: Éditions du Point Vétérinaire, 1983. 378pp.
Helminths, coccidia and microfilariae of cattle, goats and sheep are covered. There are almost 400 illustrations.

1495   *Grazing plans for the control of stomach and intestinal worms in sheep and in cattle.* Alnwick: MAFF, 1980. 17pp. (MAFF Booklet 2154.)

1496   Kettle, D. S. *Medical and veterinary entomology.* London: Croom Helm, 1984. 658pp.
Reviews the diseases transmitted as well as giving information on the insects and acarines themselves.

1497   Kim, K. C. and **Merritt, R. W.** (eds) *Black flies: ecology, population management and annotated world list.* University Park, Pennsylvania: Pennsylvania State University Press, 1988. 528pp.
The Simulidae are responsible for the transmission of onchocerciasis and avian malaria.

1498   Kim, K. C., Pratt, H. D. and **Stojanovich, C. J.** *The sucking lice of North America: an illustrated manual for identification.* University Park, Pennsylvania: Pennsylvania State University Press, 1986. 241pp.

1499   Laird, M. (ed.) *Blackflies: the future for biological methods in integrated control.* London: Academic Press, 1981. 399pp.

1500   Laird, M. and **Miles, J. W.** (eds) *Integrated mosquito control methodologies.* London: Academic Press, 1983–5. 358 + 464pp.
Volume 1 deals with conventional methods of control and volume 2 with biocontrol and the ecological and practical aspects of alternative methods of control.

1501   Lancaster, J. L. and **Meisch, M. V.** *Arthropods in livestock and poultry production*. Chichester: Ellis Horwood, 1985. 418pp. (Ellis Horwood Series in Entomology and Acarology.)
Review of the biology of all the important pests with data on the economic losses caused by them and on control techniques.

1502   Levine, N. D. *Nematode parasites of domestic animals and man*. 2nd ed. Minneapolis: Burgess Publishing, 1980. 477pp.
Primarily concerned with taxonomy rather than with the importance of the nematodes in disease or with their control.

1503   Marshall, A. G. *The ecology of ectoparasitic insects*. London: Academic Press, 1981. 459pp.

1504   Mehlhorn, H. (ed.) *Parasitology in focus: facts and trends*. Berlin: Springer-Verlag, 1988. 924pp.
A summary of the whole field of medical and veterinary parasitology outlining current knowledge and documenting recent progress.

1505   Mehlhorn, H., Duwel, D. and **Raether, W.** *Diagnose und Therapie der Parasiten von Haus-, Nutz- und Heimtieren*. Stuttgart: Gustav Fischer, 1986. 472pp.
Primarily intended as an identification manual to the parasites likely to be encountered by veterinarians. There are keys to the parasites and brief information on prophylaxis and therapy of infection. There are excellent colour and black and white illustrations.

1506   MSD AGVET. *Parasites of dogs*. Rahway, New Jersey: Merck & Co. 1988. 69pp.
Well illustrated description of arthropod and helminth parasites. Four other titles in the same series deal with the parasites of *Sheep* (1987), *Swine* (1986), *Cattle* (1985) and *Horses* (1985).

1507   Muirhead-Thomson, R. C. *Behaviour patterns of blood-sucking flies*. Oxford: Pergamon, 1982. 224pp.
Assesses the methods used and the results collected during field studies.

1508   Nunez, J. L. and **Moltedo, H. L.** *Sarna psoroptica en ovinos y bovinos*. Buenos Aires: Editorial Hemisferio Sur, 1985. 145pp.
Discussion of the biology and control of *Psoroptes* spp.

1509   Nunez, J. L., Munoz-Cobenas, M. E. and **Moltedo, H. L.** *Boophilus microplus: the common cattle tick*. Berlin: Springer-Verlag, 1985. 204pp.
Review of the biology and control of the cattle tick. The original Spanish edition was published in 1982 by Editorial Hemisferio Sur in Argentina and an updated edition was published in 1987.

1510   Nutting, W. B. (ed.) *Mammalian diseases and arachnids.* Boca Raton: CRC Press, 1984. 2 vols. 277 + 280pp.
The first volume deals with the biology of spiders, scorpions and ticks. The second with the diseases they cause and transmit including arachnid-related phobias.

1511   Pritchard, M. H. and **Kruse, G. O. W.** *The collection and preservation of animal parasites.* Lincoln: University of Nebraska Press, 1982. 141pp. (Harold W. Manter Laboratory Technical Bulletin, no. 1.)

1512   Reinecke, R. K. *Veterinary helminthology.* Durban, South Africa: Butterworths, 1983. 392pp.
A general survey covering the diagnosis of helminth infection, the individual parasites and the diseases they cause and the principles of chemotherapy and control.

1513   Rollinson, D. and **Simpson, A. J. G.** (eds) *The biology of schistosomes: from genes to latrines.* London: Academic Press, 1987. 472pp.
The chapters cover all aspects of schistosome biology including the epidemiology, treatment and control of schistosomiasis.

1514   Sauer, J. R. and **Hair, J. A.** (eds) *Morphology, physiology and behavioral biology of ticks.* Chichester: Ellis Horwood, 1986. 510pp. (Ellis Horwood Series in Acarology.)
Series of twenty-two reviews and original articles, most from the Seventeenth International Congress of Entomology (Hamburg 1984), on aspects of the biology of ticks. A companion volume is *Physiology of ticks* (edited by F. D. Obenchain and R. Galun, Oxford: Pergamon, 1982, 509pp.).

1515   Schmidt, G. D. *CRC handbook of tapeworm identification.* Boca Raton: CRC Press, 1986. 675pp.
Over 4,000 citations are listed in the bibliography. Mainly comprises an identification key but also has lists of hosts, geographical localities and synonyms and sections on methodology.

1516   Schofield, A. M. *A checklist of the helminth parasites of domestic animals in the United Kingdom.* Milton Keynes: Hoechst UK, 1983. 147pp.
Lists the parasites in taxonomic order and notes the hosts and site of infection. There are also lists of parasites according to hosts and an extensive bibliography.

1517   Service, M. W. *Mosquito ecology: field sampling methods.* London: Applied Science Publishers, 1976. 583pp.

1518   Singh, P. and **Moore, R. F.** (eds) *Handbook of insect rearing.* Amsterdam: Elsevier, 1985. 2 vols. 488 + 514pp.
Volume 1 has general chapters on insect rearing. Volume 2 gives specific techniques for many Diptera of veterinary importance.

1519   Sloss, M. W. and **Kemp, R. L.** *Veterinary clinical parasitology*. 5th ed. Ames: Iowa Street UP, 1978. 274pp.

Profusely illustrated work describing the diagnosis of various clinical and non-clinical parasitisms.

1520   Soulsby, E. J. L. *Helminths, arthropods and protozoa of domesticated animals*. 7th ed. London: Baillière Tindall, 1982. 809pp.

A standard textbook. Especially strong on its taxonomic data and useful for its extensive reference lists of key literature.

1521   Symons, L. E. A. *Pathophysiology of endoparasite infection: compared with ectoparasite infestation and microbial infection*. Sydney: Academic Press, 1989. 331pp.

'Endoparasites' includes both helminths and protozoa.

1522   Taylor, A. E. R. and **Baker, J. R.** (eds) *In vitro methods for parasite cultivation*. London: Academic Press, 1987. 465pp.

Gives detailed methods for the cultivation *in vitro* of protozoa and helminths, including a chapter on the preparation of helminth vaccines.

1523   Thienpont, D., Rochette, F. and **Vanparis, O. F. J.** *Diagnosing helminthiasis through coprological examination*. 2nd ed. Beerse, Belgium: Janssen Research Foundation, 1986. 205pp.

Illustrated procedural manual showing the characteristics of the most important worm eggs and larvae.

1524   Thompson, R. C. A. (ed.) *The biology of* Echinococcus *and hydatid disease*. London: Allen & Unwin, 1986. 290pp.

1525   Thompson, R. C. A. and **Allsop, C. E.** *Hydatidosis: veterinary perspectives and annotated bibliography*. Wallingford: CAB International, 1988. 246pp.

A seventeen page review is supplemented by an annotated bibliography of 591 items on echinococcosis/hydatidosis published between 1979 and 1986. There are author and subject indexes.

1526   *Ticks and tick-borne disease control: a practical field manual. Volume 1: tick control. Volume II: tick-borne disease control*. Rome: FAO, 1984. 2 vols. 621pp.

Guide for those involved in control operations.

1527   Urquhart, G. M., Armour, J., Duncan, J. L., Dunn, A. M. and **Jennings, F. W.** *Veterinary parasitology*. London: Longman, 1987. 286pp.

The text, which is extremely well illustrated, discusses each taxonomic group (usually at generic level) in three sections devoted to veterinary helminthology, entomology and protozoology. Five final chapters provide a broader perspective by reviewing topics of general interest: epidemiology, immunity, anthelmintics, ectoparasiticides and laboratory diagnosis. Other than in the final review chapter there are no references in the text.

1528   Vanden Bossche, H., Thienpont, D. and **Janssens, P. G.** (eds) *Chemotherapy of gastrointestinal helminths.* Berlin: Springer-Verlag, 1985. 719pp. (Handbook of Experimental Pharmacology, vol. 77.)
There are chapters on epidemiology and pharmacology in general and chapters review the therapeutic efficacy, pharmacology, pharmacokinetics, toxicology and mode of action of anthelmintics used in man, ruminants, equines, pigs, carnivores and birds.

1529   Verderame, M. (ed.) *CRC Handbook of chemotherapeutic agents.* Boca Raton: CRC Press, 1986. 2 vols. 276 + 354pp.
Volume 1 covers sulpha drugs, beta-lactams, non-lactam antibiotics, antimyco-bacterials and antifungals. Volume 2 covers synthetic antibacterials, antimalarials and other antiprotozoals, anthelmintics, antineoplastic agents and antiviral chemotherapy. Other handbooks in the CRC Series in Medicinal Chemistry are: *CNS agents and local anesthetics, Autonomic drugs and autocoids, Anti-inflammatory and cardiovascular agents* and *Hormones, vitamins, and radiopaques.*

1530   Williams, R. E., Hall, R. D., Broce, A. B. and **Scholl, P. J.** *Livestock entomology.* New York: John Wiley, 1985. 335pp.
An overview for non-entomologists of the important arthropod pests of livestock covering their biology, effects on animals and control.

1531   Woolley, T. A. *Acarology: mites and human welfare.* New York: John Wiley, 1988. 484pp.
A general text on the biology, morphology and systematics of the Acari.

1532   Youdeowei, A. and **Service, M. W.** (eds) *Pest and vector management in the tropics: with particular reference to insects, ticks, mites and snails.* London: Longman, 1983. 399pp.

Conferences

1533   *ACAROLOGY VI.* Edited by D. A. Griffiths and C. E. Bowman. Chichester: Ellis Horwood, 1984. 2 vols. 1296pp.
Proceedings of the Sixth International Congress of Acarology.

1534   Anderson, N. and **Waller, P. J.** *Resistance in nematodes to anthelmintic drugs.* Glebe: CSIRO Australia and Australian Wool Corporation, 1985. 189pp. (Australian Wool Corporation Technical Publication.)
Has reviews on all aspects of the problem of anthelmintic resistance.

1535   Crompton, D. W. T., Nesheim, M. C. and **Pawlowski, Z. S.** (eds)
Ascariasis and its public health significance. London: Taylor & Francis, 1985.
289pp.

1536   *Integrated tse-tse fly control: methods and strategies.* Edited by R. Cavalloro.
Rotterdam: A. A. Balkema, 1987. 203pp.
Papers describe the current and future programmes for tse-tse fly control of
national and international organizations, cover biological and biotechnological
control methods and review the safety and efficacy of chemical control.

1537   Ticks and tick-borne diseases: proceedings of an international workshop
on the ecology of ticks and epidemiology of tick-borne diseases, held at Nyanga,
Zimbabwe, 17–21 February 1986. Edited by R. W. Sutherst. *Australian Centre
for International Agricultural Research proceedings* **17** (1987): 159pp.
A theme for many of the contributions is the use of computer modelling in the
solution of tick-related problems. Available from Inkata Press, 13/170 Forster
Road, Mt Waverly, Victoria 3149, Australia.

Journals

1538   *Experimental and applied acarology.* 1985–. Amsterdam: Elsevier. Quarterly.

1539   *Experimental parasitology.* 1951/2–. Duluth: Academic Press. Bimonthly.

1540   *International journal for parasitology.* 1971–. Oxford: Pergamon. Bimonthly.
The journal of the Australian Society for Parasitology. As well as about fifteen
scientific papers each issue has a 'Parasitological calendar' and an address list of
'Parasitological societies of the World'. The Proceedings of the Sixth International Congress of Parasitology were published in **17** (1987): (1) and (2).

1541   *Journal of helminthology.* 1923–. London: Bureau of Hygiene and Tropical
Diseases. Quarterly.

1542   *Journal of parasitology.* 1915–. 1041 New Hampshire Street, Lawrence,
Kansas 66044: American Society of Parasitologists. Bimonthly.

1543   *Journal of veterinary parasitology.* 1987–. c/o K. D. Prasad, College of
Veterinary Sciences, Birsa Agricultural University, Ranchi 834 007, India:
Indian Association for the Advancement of Parasitology. Quarterly.

1544   *Medical and veterinary entomology.* 1987–. Oxford: Blackwell. Quarterly.

1545   *Parasitology.* 1908–. Cambridge: CUP. Bimonthly. 2 vols a year.
The first volume each year has a supplement containing the proceedings of sympo-
sia of the British Society of Parasitology. Most issues have a review article in the
'Trends and perspectives' series.

1546   *Parasitology research.* 1928–. Berlin: Springer-Verlag. Bimonthly. Founded as *Zeitschrift für Parasitenkunde.*

1547   *Parasitology today.* 1985–. 68 Hills Road, Cambridge CB2 1LA: Elsevier Publications Cambridge. Monthly.
A blend of news, reviews and topical information.

1548   *Veterinary parasitology.* 1975–. Amsterdam: Elsevier. Sixteen issues per year.

Other Journals

Annales de parasitologie humaine et comparée
Annals of tropical medicine and parasitology
Bulletin of entomological research
Helminthologia
Journal of the American Mosquito Control Association
Journal of economic entomology
Journal of medical entomology
Molecular and biochemical parasitology
Nematologica
Parasite immunology
Parasitology research
Pesticide science
Proceedings of the Helminthological Society of Washington

PATHOLOGY

(see also *Haematology and Clinical Chemistry*)

Multivolume Works

1549   *Handbuch der speziellen pathologischen Anatomie der Haustiere.* 3rd ed. Edited by J. Dobberstein, G. Pallaske and H. Stünzi. Berlin: Paul Parey. 1968–85.
The first edition was begun by E. Joest in 1919. In the third edition contributions by English-speaking authors are in English and all the captions to the illustrations are bilingual. The volumes/editors are:

I   *Musculoskeletal system.* J. Dobberstein. 1969. 557pp.
II   *Circulatory and haematopoietic system.* H. Stünzi. 1970. 820pp.
III   *Endocrine glands, nervous systems, sense organs.* J. Dobberstein and H. Stünzi. 1968. 680pp.
IV   *Genital system, skin, skeleton.* H. Stünzi. 1985. 649pp.
V   *Alimentary system, part I.* G. Pallaske. 1970. 543pp.
VI   *Alimentary system, part II.* J. Dobberstein. 1967. 704pp.
VII   *Respiratory system.* G. Pallaske and H. Stünzi. 1971. 556pp.

Books

1550   Cheville, N. F. *Introduction to veterinary pathology.* Ames: Iowa State UP, 1988. 537pp.
The most recent general work.

1551   Cheville, N. F. *Cell pathology.* 2nd ed. Ames: Iowa State UP, 1983. 681pp.
Deals with pathological changes caused by disease in domestic animals. A comprehensive textbook on histopathology.

1552   Jones, T. C. and **Hunt, R. D.** *Veterinary pathology.* 5th ed. Philadelphia: Lea & Febiger, 1983. 1792pp.
The most detailed of the single volume texts.

1553   Jubb, K. V. F., Kennedy, P. C. and **Palmer, N.** *Pathology of domestic animals.* 3rd ed. Orlando: Academic Press, 1985. 3 vols. 574 + 582 + 527pp.
The basic reference text in veterinary pathology. The contents of the volumes are as follows: Volume 1 – bones and joints, muscles and tendons, nervous system, eye and ear, skin and appendages; Volume 2 – alimentary system, liver and biliary system, pancreas, peritoneum, retroperitoneum and mesentery, urinary system and respiratory system; Volume 3 – cardiovascular system, haematopoietic system, endocrine glands, female genital system (including the mammary gland) and the male genital system.

1554   Mims, C. A. *The pathogenesis of infectious disease.* 3rd ed. London: Academic Press, 1987. 342pp.
Discusses the principles by which organisms cause disease and the relationships between the disease agent and host.

1555   Mouwen, J. M. V. M. and **de Groot, E. C. B. M.** (eds) *A colour atlas of veterinary pathology.* London: Wolfe Medical Publications, 1983. 160pp.
Uses 516 photographs to illustrate macro- and microscopic morphological changes occurring in animals.

1556   Robinson, W. F. and **Huxtable, C. R. R.** (eds) *Clinicopathologic principles for veterinary medicine.* Cambridge: CUP, 1988. 440pp.
Relates the effects of disease at tissue level to the clinical signs seen by practising veterinary surgeons.

1557   Strafuss, A. C. *Necropsy: procedures and basic diagnostic methods for practicing veterinarians.* Springfield: C. C. Thomas, 1988. 244pp.
Complete review of post-mortem techniques. The appendices describe staining techniques and other necropsy-related procedures.

1558   Thomson, R. G. (ed.) *Special veterinary pathology*. Toronto: B. C. Decker, 1988. 661pp.
Each of the fifteen chapters deals with a body system. In each case the pathology of each of the specific diseases and lesions are described. Tropical diseases are included. There are many illustrations and comprehensive reference lists.

1559   Thomson, R. G. *General veterinary pathology*. 2nd ed. Philadelphia: W. B. Saunders, 1984. 463pp.
A general survey of pathology which relates the pathological processes to the clinical problems likely to be encountered in practice. The main sections of the work are: degeneration and necrosis, circulatory disturbances, inflammation and repair, disturbances of growth, neoplasia, and host-parasite relationships.

Journals

1560   *Comparative pathology bulletin*. 1969–. Washington, DC: Registry of Comparative Pathology. Quarterly.
Each issue has three or four brief review articles plus news items.

1561   *Veterinary pathology*. 1964–. Allen Press, 1041 New Hampshire Street, Lawrence, Kansas 66044: American College of Veterinary Pathologists. Bimonthly.
Publishes articles on both natural and experimental disease in animals. Cumulative indexes have been produced for **1–15** (1964–78) and **16–20** (1978–83). Originally (until 1971) entitled *Pathologia veterinaria*.

PHYSIOLOGY AND METABOLISM

Books

1562   *Duke's Physiology of the domestic animals*. 10th ed. Edited by M. J. Swenson. Ithaca: Cornell UP, 1984. 922pp.
Comprehensive textbook on physiology for undergraduates. Has brief discussions of comparative aspects of physiology where appropriate.

1563   Eckert, R., Randall, R. and **Augustine, G.** *Animal physiology: mechanisms and adaptations*. New York: W. H. Freeman, 1988. 683pp.
General textbook on animal physiology.

1564   Hanrahan, J. P. (ed.) *Beta-agonists and their effects on animal growth and carcass quality*. London: Elsevier Applied Science, 1987. 201pp.

1565   Heady, E. O. and **Bhide, S.** *Livestock response functions*. Ames: Iowa State UP, 1984. 331pp.
Presents statistical data relating to the response of cattle, pigs and poultry to differing feeding and husbandry conditions.

1566   Larson, B. L. (ed.) *Lactation*. Ames: Iowa State UP, 1985. 276pp.
Complete review of the physiology and biochemistry of milk production. Includes sections on milk production and on mastitis. *Physiology of lactation* (by T. B. Mepham, Milton Keynes: Open University Press, 1987, 207pp.) is another recent multidisciplinary work on the topic.

1567   Lawrence, T. L. J. (ed.) *Growth in animals*. London: Butterworths, 1980. 308pp. (Studies in the Agricultural and Food Sciences.)
A series of reviews on aspects of the nature and control of animal growth including methods used to improve growth.

1568   Lawrence, T. L. J. and **Fowler, V. R.** *Growth of farm animals*. London: Butterworths, 1988. 272pp.
Covers cell and tissue growth and the processes controlling growth. Methods of modifying and improving growth are also discussed. *Biotechnology in growth regulation* (edited by R. B. Heep, C. G. Prosser and G. E. Lamming, London: Butterworths, 1989, 286pp.) is a more recent work. It is the proceedings of an international symposium held in 1988 and concentrates on growth hormone and growth factors, especially the contributions made in biotechnology and genetic engineering in this field.

1569   Lister, D. (ed.) *In vivo measurement of body composition in meat animals*. London: Elsevier Applied Science, 1984. 241pp.

1570   Norris, D. O. *Vertebrate endocrinology*. 2nd ed. Philadelphia: Lea & Febiger, 1985. 505pp.

1571   Payne, J. M. *Metabolic diseases in farm animals*. London: Heinemann, 1977. 206pp.

1572   Payne, J. M. and **Payne, S.** *The metabolic profile test*. Oxford: OUP, 1987. 179pp.
Mainly concerned with the use of the test in dairy cows. The test relies on the use of autoanalyser equipment to indicate the metabolic and nutritional status of animals via blood analysis.

1573   Phillis, J. W. (ed.) *Veterinary physiology*. Bristol: Wright/Scientechnica, 1976. 882pp.
Textbook on the fundamental principles of physiology especially as they relate to the health of domestic animals.

1574   Yousef, M. K. (ed.) *Stress physiology in livestock*. Boca Raton: CRC Press, 1985. 3 vols. 217 + 261 + 159pp.
Volume 1 covers the basic principles of the effects of thermal stress and discusses the regulation of body temperature in farm animals. Volumes 2 and 3 deal with the effects of heat and cold on ungulates and poultry respectively.

Journal

1575   Domestic animal endocrinology. 1984–. Department of Physiology and Pharmacology, College of Veterinary Medicine, Auburn University, Alabama 36849: DOMENDO, Inc. Quarterly.

Other Journal

Journal of veterinary physiology and allied sciences

PRACTICE MANAGEMENT

Books

1576   Erlewein, D. L. and **Kuhns, L.** *Instructions for veterinary clients*. Goleta: American Veterinary Publications, 1988. 341pp. in ring binder.
Provides model information in a form suitable for clients on 335 subjects. Designed to be photocopied and given to clients.

1577   Fry, P. D. (ed.) *A manual of practice improvement*. 2nd ed. Cheltenham: BSAVA, 1982. 144pp.
Covers the design of premises, and their effective use. Gives guidelines on specific methods of improving the practice's effectiveness and on introducing modern techniques.

1578   Knapp, E. J. *The floor plan book of veterinary hospital design*. Lenexa: Veterinary Medicine Publishing, 1986. 198pp.

1579   McCurnin, D. M. (ed.) *Veterinary practice management*. Philadelphia: J. B. Lippincott, 1988. 401pp.
A multi-authored American text covering the acquisition, disposal, management and development of veterinary practices.

1580   *Successful financial management for the veterinary practice*. Denver: AAHA, 1987. 115pp.

Audiovisual Materials

1581 *Audiotape programs*. Goleta: American Veterinary Publications.
Twelve titles on aspects of practice management and marketing.

Newsletters and Journals

1582 *The Dooley letter*. 1986–. Goleta: American Veterinary Publications.
Monthly.

1583 *DVM management consultants' report*. 1970–. Goleta: American Veterinary
Publications. Monthly.
These two titles give tips and suggestions to allow practice managers, staff veterinarians, technicians and reception staff to improve the efficiency of both
themselves and the practice.

1584 *DVM: the newsmagazine of veterinary medicine*. 1970–. 7500 Old Oak
Boulevard, Cleveland, Ohio 44130: Edgell Communications. Monthly.

1585 *Marketing & practice strategies*. 1988–. Schaumberg: AVMA. Quarterly.
Two versions are produced, one for large animal practitioners and one for companion animal practitioners.

1586 *Practice marketing and management: veterinary edition*. 1983–. 67 Peachtree Park
Drive, NE, Atlanta, Georgia 30309: American Health Consultants. Monthly.

1587 *Veterinary economics: the veterinarian's business magazine*. 1960–. Lenexa:
Veterinary Medicine Publishing. Monthly.
This and the next title are issued free to practising veterinarians in the United
States.

1588 *Veterinary forum*. 1982–. 1610 A Frederica Road, St Simons Island, Georgia
31522: Forum Publications. Monthly.

1589 *Veterinary practice management*. 1985–. Epsom: A. E. Morgan. Two or three
a year.
Issued as a supplement to *Veterinary practice*.

PROTOZOOLOGY

Abstracting Service

1590 *Protozoological abstracts*. 1977–. Wallingford: CAB International. Monthly.
Both medical and veterinary protozoology are covered.

Multivolume Works

1591   Kreier, J. P. (ed.) *Parasitic protozoa.* New York: Academic Press, 1977–8. 4 vols.
Flagellates of fish are dealt with in volume 1, other flagellates, amoebae and ciliates in volume 2, coccidia and plasmodia in volume 3 and *Babesia, Theileria, Anaplasma, Ehrlichia* and microsporidia in volume 4.

1592   Levandowsky, M., Hutner, S. H. and **Provasoli, L.** (eds) *Biochemistry and physiology of protozoa.* 2nd ed. New York: Academic Press, 1979–81. 4 vols.

Books

1593   Anderson, O. R. *Comparative protozoology: ecology, physiology, life history.* Berlin: Springer-Verlag, 1988. 482pp.

1594   Canning, E. U., Lom, J. and **Dykova, I.** *The microsporidia of vertebrates.* London: Academic Press, 1986. 304pp.
Has sections on the microsporidia of fish, amphibians and reptiles, and birds and mammals, plus a chapter on techniques.

1595   Dubey, J. P. and **Beattie, C. P.** *Toxoplasmosis of animals and man.* Boca Raton: CRC Press, 1988. 220pp.

1596   Dubey, J. P., Speer, C. A. and **Fayer, R.** *Sarcocystosis of animals and man.* Boca Raton: CRC Press. Forthcoming.

1597   Jordan, A. M. *Trypanosomiasis control and African rural development.* London: Longman, 1986. 357pp.
Written from an entomological viewpoint but providing a reflective survey of the disease, its control and the impact effective control would make on animal production in Africa.

1598   Kreier, J. P. and **Baker, J. R.** *Parasitic protozoa.* London: Allen & Unwin, 1987. 241pp.
Brief review of medical and veterinary species.

1599   Levine, N. D. *Veterinary protozoology.* Ames: Iowa State UP, 1985. 414pp.
A comprehensive survey. Has thirteen chapters devoted to the taxonomic groups of major importance. The genera and species are described fully with information on their hosts, prevalence, pathogenesis, diagnosis, control and treatment. There is a chapter on the laboratory diagnosis of protozoan infections.

1600   Levine, N. D. and **Ivens, V.** *The coccidian parasites (Protozoa, Apicomplexa) of Artiodactyla.* Urbana: University of Illinois Press, 1986. 265pp. (Illinois Biological Monographs 55.)
Latest in a series of works dealing with the Coccidia of animals (*Rodents*, 1965; *Ruminants*, 1970; *Carnivores*, 1981).

1601   Long, P. L. (ed.) *The biology of the Coccidia.* London: Edward Arnold, 1982. 502pp.
Comprehensive monograph of the biology of the Coccidia including chapters on chemotherapy, resistance and control. Concentrates on the Coccidia of poultry.

1602   Molyneux, D. H. and **Ashford, R. W.** *The biology of* Trypanosoma *and* Leishmania, *parasites of man and domestic animals.* London: Taylor & Francis, 1983. 294pp.

1603   Peters, W. and **Killick-Kendrick, R.** (eds) *The leishmaniases in biology and medicine.* London: Academic Press, 1987. 2 vols. 550 + 390pp.
The first volume deals with biology and epidemiology, the second with clinical aspects and control.

1604   Ristic, M. (ed.) *Babesiosis of domestic animals and man.* Boca Raton: CRC Press, 1988. 255pp.

1605   Scholtyseck, E. *Fine structure of parasitic protzoa: an atlas of micrographs and diagrams.* Berlin: Springer-Verlag, 1979. 206pp.

1606   Stephen, L. E. *Trypanosomiasis: a veterinary perspective.* Oxford: Pergamon, 1986. 551pp.
A detailed reference work of use to research workers and those engaged in the control of trypanosomiasis.

Journals

Journal of protozoology
Protistologica

PUBLIC HEALTH (INCLUDING ZOONOSES) AND HYGIENE

Abstracting Service

1607   *Abstracts on hygiene and communicable diseases.* 1926–. Keppel Street, London WC1E 7HT, England: Bureau of Hygiene and Tropical Diseases. Monthly.

A continuation (from 1981) of *Abstracts on hygiene*. Publishes 4,500 abstracts per year on aspects of health and disease worldwide. Covers food hygiene and zoonotic diseases. The Bureau also compile the *Tropical diseases bulletin*. These data are available online as the PUBLIC HEALTH AND TROPICAL MEDICINE database.

Multivolume Works

1608 *CRC Handbook Series in Zoonoses*. Editor-in-chief J. H. Steele. Boca Raton: CRC Press, 1979–.
The volumes published are:

Section A: *Bacterial, rickettsial and mycotic diseases*. 1979/80, 2 vols. 643 + 568pp.
Section B: *Viral zoonoses*. 1981. 2 vols. 510 + 488pp.
Section C: *Parasitic zoonoses*. 1981. 3 vols. 361 + 360 + 337pp.
Section D: *Antibiotics, sulphonamides and public health*. 1984. 397pp.

Books

1609 **Acha, P. N.** and **Szyfres, B.** *Zoonoses and communicable diseases common to man and animals*. 2nd ed. Washington, DC: Pan American Health Organization, 1987. 963pp. (Scientific Publication, no. 503.)
Has brief but detailed reviews of nearly all known zoonotic infections. It covers 176 diseases, each being identified according to the WHO's International Classification of Diseases. Available in English and Spanish.

1610 **Bell, J. C., Palmer, S. R.** and **Payne, J. M.** *The zoonoses: infections transmitted from animals to man*. London: Edward Arnold, 1988. 241pp.
Concise pocketbook guide to 121 zoonoses which are listed alphabetically.

1611 **Brack, M.** *Agents transmissible from simians to man*. Berlin: Springer-Verlag, 1987. 454pp.

1612 **Bremner, A. S.** *Poultry meat hygiene and inspection*. London: Baillière Tindall, 1977. 186pp.

1613 **Cunningham, F. E.** and **Cox, N. A.** (eds) *The microbiology of poultry meat products*. Orlando: Academic Press, 1987. 359pp.

1614 **Doyle, M. P.** (ed.) *Foodborne bacterial pathogens*. New York: Marcel Dekker. Forthcoming. (Food Science and Technology Series, vol. 31.)

1615 **Gil, J. I.** *A colour atlas of meat inspection*. London: Wolfe Medical Publications. Forthcoming.
Will cover cows, sheep, pigs and horses.

1616   Gracey, J. F. *Meat hygiene.* 8th ed. London: Baillière Tindall, 1986.
   517pp.
The standard text. Surveys all the factors affecting the quality and safety of meat.
Covers the whole process of the meat trade to the final cutting and preserving of
prepared meat.

1617   Hagstad, H. V. and **Hubbert, W. T.** *Food quality control: foods of animal
   origin.* 2nd ed. Ames: Iowa State UP, 1986. 148pp.
Describes the potential hazards and critical control points in the food production
chain. Includes information on the food processing techniques and inspection
regulations of the USDA.

1618   Hubbert, W. T., McCulloch, W. F. and **Schnurrenberger, P. R.** (eds)
   Diseases transmitted from animals to man. 6th ed. Springfield: C. C. Thomas, 1975.
   1206pp.
Detailed reference work covering all the principal diseases.

1619   Mitchell, J. R. *Guide to meat inspection in the tropics.* 2nd ed. Farnham
   Royal: CAB, 1980. 95pp.

1620   Wiggins, G. S. and **Wilson, A.** *A color atlas of meat and poultry inspection.*
   London: Wolfe Medical Publications, 1976. Unpaginated.

1621   Wilson, A. *Practical meat inspection.* 4th ed. Oxford: Blackwell, 1985.
   289pp.
Based on lecture notes on meat inspection. An introductory text on poultry and
meat inspection. Most of the book consists of reviews of the various body systems
of food animals.

1622   Wilson, N. R. P. *The meat hygienist's pocket book.* Barnet, Hertfordshire:
   Association of Meat Inspectors, 1980. 124pp.
Describes the slaughtering process, has notes on the lesions of diseases likely to be
encountered, and recommendations for condemnation.

Conference

1623   Freed, D. L. J. (ed.) *Health hazards of milk.* London: Baillière Tindall,
   1984. 281pp.

Journals

1624   *Animal & human health.* 1988–. 15 West 44th Street, New York 10036:
   AgResources. Quarterly.
Publishes review and general articles on zoonoses, consumer and environmental
protection and veterinary preventive medicine.

Other Journals

Dairy, food and environmental sanitation
Journal of food protection
The meat hygienist
Meat science

RADIOLOGY

Radiography is an important diagnostic tool and there are a number of specialized texts on aspects of its use with both large and small animals. Because of the subject matter these are usually exceptionally well illustrated.

Standards

1625 *Guidelines for radiology service in veterinary medicine.* Compiled by D. L. Barber and R. E. Lewis. Schaumberg: AVMA, 1982. 25pp.
Compiled on behalf of the American College of Veterinary Radiology Committee to Formulate Standards for Radiology in Veterinary Medicine.

1626   National Radiological Protection Board and **Health and Safety Executive.** *Guidance notes for the protection of persons against ionising radiations arising from veterinary use.* London: HMSO, 1988. 20pp.
These notes replace the booklet *Radiation safety in veterinary practice* (1970, amendments 1974). They are a guide to the implementation of procedures to cover the statutory requirements for the protection of persons exposed to radiation in veterinary practice.

Nomenclature Guide

1627   Smallwood, J. E., Shively, M. J., Rendano, V. T. and **Habel, R. E.** 'A standardized nomenclature for radiographic projections used in veterinary medicine'. *Veterinary radiology* **26** (1985): 2–9.

Books

1628   Douglas, S. W., Herrtage, M. E. and **Williamson, H. D.** *Principles of veterinary radiography.* 4th ed. London: Baillière Tindall, 1987. 371pp.
A respected work providing theoretical and practical guidance for students and practitioners. The bulk of the work is an atlas for the radiographic positioning of animals with detailed notes and illustrations describing appropriate techniques and the results obtained. A unique feature is the provision of space for the user to develop their own technique charts and notes for each anatomical region.

1629   Morgan, J. P. *Radiography in veterinary orthopedics*. Philadelphia: Lea & Febiger, 1972. 406pp.

1630   Morgan, J. P. and **Silverman, S.** *Techniques of veterinary radiography*. 4th ed. Ames: Iowa State UP, 1984. 334pp. (Venture Series in Veterinary Medicine.)
A textbook and reference work which includes discussions of many special radiographic procedures.

1631   Suter, P. F. and **Gomez, J. A.** *Diseases of the thorax: radiographic diagnosis*. Ames: Iowa State UP, 1981. 78pp. (Venture Series in Veterinary Medicine.)
An edited version of lecture notes on the radiology of the thorax (especially of dogs and cats). There are illustrations and tables listing differential diagnoses but no reproductions of radiographs.

1632   Thrall, D. E. (ed.) *Textbook of veterinary diagnostic radiology*. Philadelphia: W. B. Saunders, 1986. 563pp.
Concerned only with horses and companion animals, including aviary birds. Each chapter describes the normal signs and radiographic findings, then discusses the abnormalities.

1633   Ticer, J. W. (ed.) *Radiographic technique in veterinary practice*. 2nd ed. Philadelphia: W. B. Saunders, 1984. 511pp.
A comprehensive work for the practitioner covering the radiography of both small and large animals and the manner in which X-ray departments should be designed and run.

Journal

1634 *Veterinary radiology*. 1959–. Hagerstown: J. B. Lippincott. Bimonthly.
Official journal of the American College of Veterinary Radiology and the International Veterinary Radiology Association. Until 1980 known as *Journal of the American Veterinary Radiology Society*.

REPRODUCTION AND GENETICS

(see also *Animal Husbandry and Production*)

Indexing Service

1635 *Bibliography of reproduction*. 1963–. 141 Newmarket Road, Cambridge CB5 8HA, England: Reproduction Research Information Service. Monthly.
Items appear in one or more of forty-seven broad subject sections. There are author and animal indexes in each issue and six-monthly keyword indexes.

Abstracting Service

1636 *Animal breeding abstracts.* 1933–. Wallingford: CAB International. Monthly.

Review Series

1637 *Oxford reviews of reproductive biology.* 1979–. Edited by J. R. Clarke. Oxford: OUP. Annual.

Multivolume Works

1638 Austin, C. R. and **Short, R. V.** (eds) *Reproduction in mammals.* 2nd ed. Cambridge: CUP, 1982–6. 5 vols.
Provides a synthesis of knowledge on mammalian reproduction. The volumes are:
1. *Germ cells and fertilization.* 1982. 177pp.
2. *Embryonic and fetal development.* 1982. 190pp.
3. *Hormonal control of reproduction.* 1984. 244pp.
4. *Reproductive fitness.* 1985. 241pp.
5. *Manipulating reproduction.* 1986. 235pp.

There are two other volumes from the first edition:
6. *The evolution of reproduction.* 1976. 189pp.
7. *Mechanisms of hormone action.* 1979. 239pp.

1639 *Marshall's Physiology of reproduction.* 4th ed. Edinburgh: Churchill Livingstone. 1984–. 6 vols planned.
Thus far only *Volume 1: Reproductive cycles of vertebrates* (edited by G. E. Lamming, 1984, 842pp.) has appeared. Will cover reproduction in all vertebrates not just mammals.

1640 *The physiology of reproduction.* Editors-in-chief E. Knobil and J. D. Neill. New York: Raven Press, 1988. 2 vols. 2413pp.

Books

1641 Arthur, G. H., Noakes, D. E. and **Pearson, H.** *Veterinary reproduction and obstetrics (theriogenology).* 6th ed. London: Baillière Tindall, 1989. 641pp.
The standard British text. Covers all aspects of reproductive function and dysfunction in animals.

1642 Cunningham, E. P. (ed.) *Modern techniques in animal breeding.* London: Butterworths, 1988. 288pp.
Reviews the latest work in the field under the following headings: breeding value estimation theory, gene flow theory, crossbreeding theory, and genetic aspects.

1643   *Current therapy in theriogenology 2: Diagnosis, treatment and prevention of reproductive disorders in small and large animals.* Edited by D. A. Morrow. Philadelphia: W. B. Saunders, 1986. 1143pp.
A unique and comprehensive multiauthored work which uses a problem-oriented approach to provide a concise source of current information for veterinarians supported by selected references to the literature. Nineteen tables in an appendix provide much comparative numerical data.

1644   Dalton, D. C. *An introduction to practical animal breeding.* 2nd ed. London: Granada, 1985. 192pp.
Guide to the scientific principles of animal breeding.

1645   Evans, G. and **Maxwell, W. M. C.** *Salamon's Artificial insemination of sheep and goats.* Sydney: Butterworths, 1987. 194pp.
A complete handbook and manual for those wishing to develop artificial insemination programmes.

1646   Foley, C. W., Lasley, J. F. and **Osweiler, G. D.** *Abnormalities of companion animals: analysis of heritability.* Ames: Iowa State UP, 1979. 270pp.
Describes inherited conditions and defects in cats, dogs and horses with selected references to the source literature.

1647   Gordon, I. *Controlled breeding in farm animals.* Oxford: Pergamon, 1983. 436pp.
Has sections on the control and manipulation of reproduction in cattle, sheep, pigs and horses.

1648   Hafez, E. S. E. (ed.) *Reproduction in farm animals.* 5th ed. Philadelphia: Lea & Febiger, 1987. 649pp.
The classic text dealing with reproductive physiology and its application to farm animals. Has a section on methods used for improving reproductive efficiency. Appendices provide much useful information.

1649   Herman, H. A. and **Madden, F. W.** *The artificial insemination and embryo transfer of dairy and beef cattle (including techniques for goats, sheep, horses, and swine): a handbook and laboratory manual for students, herd operators, and workers in the AI field.* 7th ed. Danville: Interstate Printers and Publishers, 1987. 279pp.

1650   Hunter, R. H. F. *Physiology and technology of reproduction in female domestic animals.* London: Academic Press, 1980. 393pp.
Concentrates on aspects of reproduction amenable to manipulation. The same author has also written a popular introduction: *Reproduction of farm animals* (London: Longman, 1982, 149pp. Longman Handbooks in Agriculture).

1651   Laing, J. A., Morgan, W. J. B. and **Wagner, W. C.** (eds) *Fertility and infertility in veterinary practice*. 4th ed. London: Baillière Tindall, 1988. 280pp.
Within each chapter the different species are dealt with in turn. The text reviews normal reproductive function and then deals with the infectious and non-infectious causes of infertility.

1652   McDonald, L. E. and **Pineda, M. H.** (eds) *Veterinary endocrinology and reproduction*. 4th ed. Philadelphia: Lea & Febiger, 1989. 571pp.
A standard text on reproductive endocrinology.

1653   Mason, I. L. (ed.) *Evolution of domesticated animals*. London: Longman, 1984. 452pp.
Describes the wild ancestor, date and place of domestication and history of breeding of sixty-nine species groups.

1654   Nicholas, F. W. *Veterinary genetics*. Oxford: OUP, 1987. 580pp.
The first section covers basic genetics and recombinant DNA, the second discusses genetics in relation to animal disease, the third is a more conventional discussion of genetics and animal breeding.

1655   Roberts, S. J. *Veterinary obstetrics and genital diseases (theriogenology)*. 3rd ed. North Pomfret, Vermont: David & Charles Inc., 1986. 981pp.
Comprehensive text on veterinary obstetrics, genital diseases and animal reproduction.

1656   Szabo, K. T. *Congenital malformations in laboratory and farm animals*. New York: Academic Press. Forthcoming.

1657   Van Vleck, L. D., Pollak, E. J. and **Oltenacu, E. A. B.** *Genetics for the animal sciences*. New York: W. H. Freeman, 1987. 391pp.
Covers the principles of animal genetics and their application to practical breeding problems. A similar text is J. F. Lasley's *Genetics of livestock improvement* (4th ed., Englewood Cliffs: Prentice-Hall, 1987, 466pp.).

Conference

1658   *11th International congress on animal reproduction and artificial insemination, Dublin, Ireland 1988. Belfield Campus, University College Dublin. Congress proceedings.* Dublin: Organizing Committee, 1988. 5 vols.
Abstracts of the presentations are given in volume 1, the Brief Communications are in volumes 2–4, volume 5 contains the Plenary and Symposia papers. The congresses are held every four years.

1659 Smith, C., King, J. W. B. and **McKay, J. C.** (eds) *Exploiting new technologies in animal breeding: genetic developments*. Oxford: OUP, 1986. 202pp.

Journals

1660 *Animal genetics*. 1970–. Oxford: Blackwell. Quarterly.

1661 *Animal reproduction science*. 1978–. Amsterdam: Elsevier. Monthly.

1662 *Journal of reproduction and fertility*. 1960–. 22 Newmarket Road, Cambridge CB5 8DT, England: The Journals of Reproduction and Fertility. Bimonthly. Official journal of the Society for the Study of Fertility. The *Journal of reproduction and fertility abstract series* (1988–) contains the abstracts of the SSF's meetings and conferences. The *Supplements* are also distinct from the journal. They contain the proceedings of many important conferences, the most recent being:

35 Equine reproduction IV. 1987. 761pp.
34 Reproduction in domestic animals. 1987. 291pp.
33 Control of pig reproduction II. 1985. 266pp.

1663 *Theriogenology*. 1974–. 80 Montvale Avenue, Stoneham, Massachusetts 02180: Butterworths. Monthly.

Other Journals

Archiv für Tierzucht/Archives of animal breeding
Biology of reproduction (plus supplements)
International journal of fertility
Reproduction, nutrition, development
Genetics, selection, evolution
Journal of animal breeding and genetics. Zeitschrift für Tierzuchtung und Zuchtungsbiologie
Zuchthygiene

SURGERY

Books

1664 Dougherty, R. W. *Experimental surgery in farm animals*. Ames: Iowa State UP, 1981. 146pp.
Describes a variety of experimental procedures and techniques. Stresses the correct selection of animals for experimental surgery, gives guidelines for care during the pre- and post-operative periods and describes humane methods of restraint and anaesthesia.

1665 Hickman, J. and **Walker, R. G.** *An atlas of veterinary surgery.* 2nd ed. Bristol: Wright, 1980. 244pp.
Uses line drawings and diagrams to illustrate the standard surgical procedures employed in veterinary operative surgery. A new edition is in preparation.

1666 Hurov, L. *Handbook of veterinary surgical instruments and glossary of surgical terms.* Philadelphia: W. B. Saunders, 1978. 214pp.
Illustrates all the common equipment and gives lists of instrument sets for special purposes. The second part is a glossary of definitions and descriptions of surgical conditions.

1667 Hofmeyr, C. F. B. *Ruminant urogenital surgery.* Ames: Iowa State UP, 1987, 174pp.
Several surgical alternatives are described for each of the conditions discussed. Deals with the urinary systems, male and female genital tracts and mammary glands.

1668 Knecht, C. D., Allen, A. R., Williams, D. J. and **Johnson, J. H.** *Fundamental techniques in veterinary surgery.* 3rd ed. Philadelphia: W. B. Saunders, 1987. 349pp.
Covers all the basic surgical techniques including operating room conduct and pre-operative care, suture materials and technique, and bandaging and splinting. Also describes a range of surgical procedures for small animals.

1669 *Methods of Animal Experimentation.* 1965–. Edited by W. I. Gay. Orlando: Academic Press. Occasional.
The most recent volume (**VII** 1986) deals with *Research surgery and the care of the research animal:* Part A. *Patient care, vascular access and telemetry* (272pp.), Part B. *Surgical approaches to the organ systems* (269pp.).

1670 Sumner-Smith, G. (ed.) *Bone in clinical orthopaedics: a study in comparative osteology.* Philadelphia: W. B. Saunders, 1982. 435pp.

1671 Swindle, M. M. and **Adams, R. J.** (eds) *Experimental surgery and physiology: induced animal models of human disease.* Baltimore: Williams & Wilkins, 1988. 350pp.
Concentrates on surgically induced models. Neoplasia, infectious diseases and spontaneous or genetic models are excluded.

1672 Zaslow, I. M. (ed.) *Veterinary trauma and critical care.* Philadelphia: Lea & Febiger, 1984. 584pp.
Comprehensive review of the evaluation, management and monitoring of patients needing intensive care. Special procedures such as hyperalimentation, tracheostomy and endoscopy are discussed in detail.

Journals

1673 *Veterinary and comparative orthopaedics and traumatology.* 1988–. Stuttgart:
F. K. Schattauer. Quarterly.
Includes a 'literature survey' – classified list of new literature in surgery, bio-
mechanics and related topics.

1674 *Veterinary surgery.* 1971–. Hagerstown: J. B. Lippincott. Bimonthly.
Offical journal of the American College of Veterinary Surgeons and the American
College of Veterinary Anesthesiologists. It has a special section on veterinary
anaesthesiology. Formerly entitled *Archives of the American College of Veterinary
Surgeons.*

THERAPEUTICS, PHARMACOLOGY AND PHARMACEUTICS

The drug and trade directories [214–273] are also sources of information about
veterinary drugs and their use.

Review Series

1675 *The antimicrobial agents annual.* 1986–. Edited by P. K. Peterson and J.
Verhoef. Amsterdam: Elsevier. Annual.

Other Review Series

Advances in drug research
Advances in pharmacology and chemotherapy
Advances in pharmaceutical sciences
Annual reports in medicinal chemistry
Progress in drug metabolism
Progress in drug research
Progress in medicinal chemistry

Book Series

1676 **Post-Graduate Committee in Veterinary Science, University of
Sydney.** 1983–. *The T. G. Hungerford Vade Mecum Series for Domestic Animals.*
Sydney: the Committee.
Each volume in Series A describes the control and therapy of the common diseases
of a species. Lists of drugs and dosages are included. *Series A Diseases of . . .*

11. Deer. 1988. 112pp. A. W. English
 7. Dogs. 1986. 256pp. C. W. Prescott

6. Pigs. 1985. 46pp. R. J. Love
5. Goats. 1984. 62pp. P. A. Howe
4. Cattle. 1984. 140pp. D. I. Bryden
3. Cats. 1984. 154pp. G. T. Wilkinson
2. Birds. 1983. 145pp. R. A. Perry
1. Horses. 1983. 125pp. R. J. Rose

Each volume in Series B is concerned with differential diagnosis. *Series B The diagnosis of the diseases of* . . .

9. Goats. 1987. 89pp. S. A. Baxendell
8. Pigs. 1986. 184pp. J. R. Buddle

The first title in Series C is:

10. Ferrets: a compendium. 1988. 53pp. J. H. Lewington.

Books

1677   Alexander, F. (ed.) *An introduction to veterinary pharmacology*. 4th ed. London: Longman, 1985. 429pp.
Concise account of the pharmacological properties of the principal veterinary drugs.

1678 *Animal drug analytical manual*. Edited by J. R. Markus and J. Sherma. 1111 North 19th St., Suite 210-P, Arlington, Virginia 22209: Association of Official Analytical Chemists, 1985. 352pp. Looseleaf.
Gives methods for determining drugs in feeds and drug residues in food animals. The following compounds are covered: carbadox, diethylstilbestrol, lasalocid, melengestrol acetate, morantel tartrate and sulfamethazine. Methods for other drugs are being prepared. Analytical methods for other compounds of veterinary interest are contained in the *Official methods of analysis of the AOAC* (14th ed., 1984 with annual supplements, 15th ed. due 1989).

1679   Baggott, J. D. *Principles of drug distribution in domestic animals: the basis of veterinary clinical pharmacology*. Philadelphia: W. B. Saunders, 1977. 238pp.

1680   Blodinger, J. (ed.) *Formulation of veterinary dosage forms*. New York: M. Dekker, 1983. 316pp. (Drugs and the Pharmaceutical Sciences, vol. 17.)

1681   Booth, N. H. and **McDonald, L. E.** (eds) *Veterinary pharmacology and therapeutics*. 6th ed. Ames: Iowa State UP, 1988. 1227pp.
Complete review of the pharmacologic, therapeutic and toxicologic action of drugs and chemicals. Organized according to the pharmacological activity of the compounds.

1682   Brander, G. C. *Chemicals for animal health control.* London: Taylor & Francis, 1986. 170pp.
A general survey of the chemicals currently in use with chapters on formulation and delivery methods and on legislation.

1683   Brander, G. C., Pugh, D. M. and **Bywater, R. J.** *Veterinary pharmacology and therapeutics.* 4th ed. London: Baillière Tindall, 1982. 582pp.
Most detailed of the single volume British texts.

1684   *The Bristol veterinary handbook of antimicrobial therapy.* 2nd ed. Edited by D. E. Johnston. Lawrenceville: Veterinary Learning Systems, 1987. 296pp.
A guide to the principles and practice of antimicrobial use in a quick reference format.

1685   *Goodman and Gilman's The pharmacological basis of therapeutics.* 7th ed. Edited by A. G. Gilman, L. S. Goodman, T. W. Rall and F. Murad. New York: Macmillan, 1985. 1839pp.
Describes the pharmacology of all the main classes of drugs.

1686   Klide, A. M. and **Kung, S. H.** (eds) *Veterinary acupuncture.* Pittsburgh: University of Pennsylvania Press, 1977. 297pp.
Monograph on the theory and practice of acupuncture describing techniques and equipment, animal acupuncture points and the physiology of acupuncture, and acupuncture therapy and analgesia. Equine acupuncture is described in E. Westermayer's *The treatment of horses by acupuncture* (Holsworthy: Health Science Press, 1979, 40pp.). An extensive bibliography on canine acupuncture appears in S. White's 'Some aspects of canine acupuncture' *Veterinary annual* **28th issue** (1988): 214–22.

1687   Linton, A. H., Hugo, W. B. and **Russell, A. D.** (eds) *Disinfection in veterinary and farm animal practice.* Oxford: Blackwell, 1987. 179pp.
Describes physical and chemical methods of disinfection and sterilization and the evaluation of disinfectants and disinfection processes. Has chapters on the legal control of veterinary disinfectants and on practical aspects of disinfection and infection control. A source of more detailed information on the activity of specific agents is *Disinfection, sterilization and preservation* (3rd ed., edited by S. S. Block, Philadelphia: Lea & Febiger, 1983, 1053pp.).

1688   Macleod, G. *A veterinary materia medica and clinical repertory with a materia medica of the nosodes.* Saffron Walden: C. W. Daniel, 1983. 193pp.
Guide to materials used in homeopathic veterinary medicine. Other books on veterinary homeopathy are noted in an article by C. E. I. Day (*The Henston veterinary vade mecum (small animals) 1987–88*, 1987, pp. 277–82). J. de Bairacli Levy's two works *The complete herbal handbook for farm and stable* (2nd ed., London: Faber, 1984, 383pp.) and . . . *for the dog and cat* (5th ed., 1985, 287pp.) are well

known and there is an English translation of the 1981 edition of H. G. Wolff's *Unsere Hunde: Gesund durch Homöopathie* (5th ed., Regensburg, Federal Republic of Germany: Johannes Sonntag, 1984, 269pp.) as *Homeopathic medicine for dogs: a handbook for vets and pet owners* (Wellingborough: Thorsons, 1984, 160pp.). Wolff has also written a book on cats, *Unsere Katze: . . .* (2nd ed., 1984, 159pp.).

1689   *Martindale: the extra pharmacopoeia.* 29th ed. Edited by J. E. F. Reynolds. London: Pharmaceutical Press, 1988. 1926pp.
Has monographs on all the common drugs and therapeutic agents. Side-effects, toxicity, uses and formulations (including international trade names) are included. Available online as MARTINDALE ONLINE.

1690   Michell, A. R., Bywater, R. J., Clarke, K. W., Hall, L. W. and **Waterman, A. E.** *Veterinary fluid therapy.* Oxford: Blackwell, 1988. 272pp.
Discusses the regulation of the body fluids, the disturbances which may occur and how these may be assessed. Therapeutic methods and procedures are then discussed in detail.

1691   Prescott, J. F. and **Baggot, J. D.** *Antimicrobial therapy in veterinary medicine.* Boston: Blackwell Scientific Publications, 1988. 367pp.
Describes the principles of drug selection and use, reviews data on the important compounds and types of drugs, and gives guidelines on drug dosages.

1692   Rabinovich, M. I. *Medicinal plants in veterinary practice* (in Russian). Moscow: Agropromizdat, 1987. 288pp.
Describes 204 plants which have uses in veterinary medicine.

1693   *Remington's Pharmaceutical sciences.* Edited by A. R. Gennaro. Easton, Pennsylvania: Mack Publishing, 1985. 1980pp.
Textbook and reference work for pharmacists and others dealing with the formulation and use of pharmaceutical and medicinal agents.

1694   Rico, A. G. (ed.) *Drug residues in animals.* London: Academic Press, 1986. 233pp. (Veterinary Science and Comparative Medicine.)
Eight reviews on various aspects of drug metabolism and residues.

1695   Upson, D. W. *Handbook of clinical veterinary pharmacology.* 3rd ed. 201 Cedar Drive, Manhattan, Kansas 66502: Ian Upson Enterprises, 1988. 729pp.

Conference

1696   *Antimicrobials and agriculture: the proceedings of the 4th international symposium on antibiotics in agriculture: benefits and malefits.* Edited by M. Woodbine. London: Butterworths, 1984. 583pp. (Studies in the Agricultural and Food Sciences.)
The majority of the forty-three contributions relate to the use of drugs in animals.

Journals

1697 *Biologische Tiermedizin.* 1984–. D-7570 Baden-Baden, Federal Republic of
Germany: Aurelia Verlag. Quarterly.

1698 *Journal of microencapsulation.* 1984–. 4 John Street, London WC1N 2ET:
Taylor & Francis. Quarterly.
Includes a 'Patent briefing' and 'Literature alerts' section in each issue. The
Controlled Release Society's *Journal of controlled release* is also of interest to those
working in the field of drug delivery.

1699 *Journal of veterinary pharmacology and therapeutics.* 1978–. Oxford: Blackwell.
Quarterly.

1700 *The pharmaceutical journal.* 1841–. London: Royal Pharmaceutical Society
of Great Britain. Weekly.
Contains news on aspects of pharmacy and technical articles and reviews on
pharmaceutical topics. *Medicines and ethics: a guide for pharmacists* (1988. no. 1,
58pp.) is an occasional supplement which provides a summary of the law on the
sale or supply of medicines and lists approved human and animal medicines.
Amendments are noted in *The pharmaceutical journal.*

Other Journals

Advanced drug delivery reviews
Chemotherapy
International journal of veterinary homeopathy
Journal of medicinal chemistry
Journal of parenteral science and technology
Journal of pharmaceutical sciences
Journal of pharmacy and pharmacology
Pharmaceutical technology
Pharmacology & therapeutics
Xenobiotica

TOXICOLOGY

Bibliographies

1701 **Hails, M. R.** and **Crane, T. D.** (Compilers) *Plant poisoning in animals: a
bibliography from the world literature, 1960–1979.* Farnham Royal: CAB, 1983.
153pp.
Supplemented by *Plant poisoning in animals: a bibliography from the world literature,*

no. 2. 1980–1982. (M. R. Hails, Farnham Royal: CAB, 1986, 93pp.) The entries are arranged taxonomically by plant family. There are indexes to authors, plant species, animals poisoned and a geographical index. The second volume has indexes on signs and pathology.

Compilations of Data

1702 *Clinical toxicology of commercial products.* 5th ed. Edited by R. E. Gosselin, R. P. Smith and H. C. Hodge. Baltimore: Williams & Wilkins, 1984. 2002pp.
Gives information on the composition and physiological effects of household products with recommendations for treatment and supportive care in cases of poisoning.

1703 *Dangerous properties of industrial materials.* 7th ed. N. I. Sax and R. J. Lewis Sr. New York: Van Nostrand Reinhold, 1989. 3 vols.
An index to more than 20,000 chemicals giving information on toxicity and hazards. Most of the toxicity data is taken from the RTECS (*Registry of toxic effects of chemical substances*) database.

Books

1704 *Analytical toxicology methods manual.* Edited by H. M. Stahr. Ames: Iowa State UP, 1977. 315pp.
Gives methods for the analysis and detection of toxicants, including metals, pesticides, feed additives and other substances. A *Supplement to 'Analytical toxicology methods manual' and cumulative index*, edited by H. M. Stahr and W. G. Hyde, was issued in 1981.

1705 *Casarett and Doull's Toxicology: the basic science of poisons.* 3rd ed. Edited by C. D. Klaassen, M. O. Amdur and J. Doull. New York: Macmillan, 1986. 974pp.
The best survey of the whole of modern toxicology.

1706 **Cheeke, P. R.** and **Shull, L. R.** *Natural toxicants in feeds and poisonous plants.* Westport: AVI, 1985. 492pp.
Has chapters on each of the major classes of naturally occurring toxicants and general chapters on their metabolism, biological effects and effects on livestock production and animal health. Each chapter has extensive reference lists.

1707 **Clarke, E. G. C.** *Poisoning in veterinary practice.* London: Association of the British Pharmaceutical Industry, 1975. 34pp.
Gives advice on the diagnosis and treatment of poisoning by the most common toxic agents. There are brief notes on the more important of these and a table of the symptoms caused by the common poisons.

1708   Cooper, M. R. and **Johnson, A. W.** *Poisonous plants in Britain and their effects on animals and man.* London: HMSO, 1984. 305pp. (MAFF Reference Book 161.)
The plants are arranged in alphabetical order of plant families, each is described, the poisonous principle(s) indicated and the poisoning they cause in animals and man discussed. The more important plants are illustrated in colour plates or line drawings. Thirty fungi are also described. There is a detailed bibliography. A popular version has been published as *Poisonous plants and fungi: an illustrated guide* (London: HMSO, 1988, 134pp.).

1709   Frohne, D. and **Pfänder, H. J.** translated by **N. G. Bisset.** *A colour atlas of poisonous plants.* London: Wolfe Publishing, 1984. 291pp.
Describes 140 flowering plant species. The toxic components are listed and treatment is discussed.

1710   Humphreys, D. J. *Veterinary toxicology.* 3rd ed. London: Baillière Tindall, 1988. 356pp.
The best single source of information. Current knowledge on each toxic agent is reviewed in brief articles, each having many references to the original literature.

1711   Kellerman, T. S., Coetzer, J. A. W. and **Naude, T. W.** *Plant poisonings and mycotoxicoses of livestock in Southern Africa.* Cape Town: Oxford University Press, 1988. 243pp.
Plant poisonings are a serious cause of loss of livestock in the area. This book covers all the 600 indigenous poisonous plants and illustrates each in colour.

1712   Osweiler, G. D., Carson, T. L., Buck, W. B. and **Van Gelder, G. A.** *Clinical and diagnostic veterinary toxicology.* 3rd edition. Dubuque: Kendall/Hunt, 1985. 494pp.
Reviews data on the major toxicants with much information presented in tabular form.

1713   Radeleff, R. D. *Veterinary toxicology.* 2nd ed. Philadelphia: Lea & Febiger, 1970. 352pp.
Useful for its reviews of the early literature on pesticide toxicity.

1714   Smith, G. J. *Pesticide use and toxicology in relation to wildlife: organophosphorus and carbamate compounds.* Matomic Building, Room 148, Washington, DC 20240: US Department of the Interior, Fish and Wildlife Service, 1987. 171pp. (Resource Publication 170.)
Gives basic data on the chemicals and details of toxicoses in mammals and birds. Covers the US scene. Summarizes the literature up to 1986.

Journals

1715 *Food and chemical toxicology.* 1963–. Oxford: Pergamon. Monthly.
Formerly *Food and cosmetics toxicology.* Published for the British Industrial Biological
Research Association.

1716 *Veterinary and human toxicology.* 1958–. Comparative Toxicology Laboratories, Kansas State University, Manhattan, Kansas 66506. Bimonthly.
Sponsored by the American Academy of Veterinary and Comparative Toxicology
and the American Board of Veterinary Toxicology. Contains news items, original
reports and comprehensive review articles. Formerly known as *Veterinary toxicology.*

Other Journals

Fundamental and applied toxicology
Regulatory toxicology and pharmacology
Toxicology and applied pharmacology
Toxicology in vitro

TROPICAL VETERINARY MEDICINE

Handbooks

1717 *Agricultural compendium for rural development in the tropics and subtropics.* 2nd ed.
Edited by ILACO BV. Amsterdam: Elsevier, 1985. 738pp.
A handbook on quantitative methods for assessing and improving agricultural
production. Covers topics such as climate, geodesy, water control, soil and land
classification etc., and has a chapter on managing animal production including
recommendations on health control.

1718 *Handbook on animal diseases in the tropics.* 3rd ed. Revised and edited by Sir A.
Robertson. London: BVA, 1976. 304pp.
The standard work giving a concise summary of all the important infections and
other conditions causing ill health in tropical and subtropical areas.

1719 *Handbook of tropical veterinary laboratory diagnosis.* Easter Bush: Centre for
Tropical Veterinary Medicine, 1980–. 5 booklets. 19 + 35 + 33 + 31pp.
Prepared under the editorship of Sir A. Robertson. Section 1 discusses the
laboratory and its equipment, Section 2 techniques and procedures, Section 3
protozoal and rickettsial diseases and the identification of ticks and tsetse flies,
Section 4 viral diseases and Section 5 (forthcoming) bacterial diseases. Another
recent work is *Manual of tropical veterinary parasitology* (IEMVT/CTA, Wallingford:
CAB International, 1989, 473pp.).

Books

1720   Auriol, P., Pagot, J. and **Tacher, G.** *L'élevage en pays tropicaux.* Paris: Éditions G-P. Maisonneuve & Larose, 1985. 526pp. (Techniques Agricoles et Productions Tropicales, vol. 34.)
A general work on animal production in the tropics.

1721   Crowder, L. V. and **Chheda, H. R.** *Tropical grass husbandry.* London: Longman, 1982. 562pp.

1722   Haan, C. de and **Nissen, N. J.** *Animal health services in sub-Saharan Africa.* Washington, DC: World Bank, 1985. 83pp. (World Bank Technical Paper 44.)
Describes the organization, functioning and financing of current veterinary services and discusses alternative approaches.

1723   Hall, H. T. B. *Diseases and parasites of livestock in the tropics.* 2nd ed. London: Longman, 1986. 328pp. (Intermediate Tropical Agriculture Series.)
A readable, well illustrated handbook for veterinary ancillary staff, agriculturalists, students and others with an interest in animal health and husbandry.

1724   Heath, E. and **Olusanya, S.** (eds) *Anatomy and physiology of tropical livestock.* London: Longman, 1985. 138pp. (Intermediate Tropical Agriculture Series.)

1725   *Livestock manual for the tropics.* Newport East, PO Box 36, Kingston, Jamaica, West Indies: Jamaica Livestock Association Limited, 1983. 406pp.
A comprehensive and practical manual for farmers with particular relevance to the Caribbean.

1726   Losos, G. J. *Infectious tropical diseases of domestic animals.* Harlow: Longman, 1986. 938pp.
A remarkable work comprising twenty-five chapters each reviewing in depth current knowledge and the literature on a particular disease. The subjects have been reviewed up to 1982–3. There is no index but the chapters are well structured.

1727   *Traditional (indigenous) systems of veterinary medicine for small farmers.* Bangkok, Thailand: FAO Regional Office, 1980–.
Thus far reports have been issued for India (RAPA 80), Nepal (RAPA 81), Thailand (RAPA 82) and Pakistan (RAPA 86/3).

1728   Webster, C. C. and **Wilson, P. N.** *Agriculture in the tropics.* 2nd ed. London: Longman, 1980. 640pp. (Tropical Agriculture Series.)

1729   Williamson, G. and **Payne, W. J. A.** *An introduction to animal husbandry in the tropics.* 3rd ed. London: Longman, 1978. 755pp.

Conferences

1730   Della-Porta, A. J. (ed.) *Veterinary viral diseases: their significance in South-East Asia and the Western Pacific. Proceedings of an international seminar, held at the Australian National Animal Health Laboratory, CSIRO, Australia, 27–30 August 1984.* Sydney: Academic Press, 1985. 616pp.
Of the eighty-two papers, fifteen deal with FMD and ten with herpesviruses.

1731   *Livestock production and diseases in the tropics.* Edited by M. R. Jainudeen, M. Mahyuddin and J. E. Huhn. Serdang: Universiti Pertanian Malaysia, 1986. 352pp.
The proceedings of the scientific sessions of the Fifth International Conference of Institutions of Tropical Veterinary Medicine. Mainly consists of studies performed in Asia but also includes valuable papers on the provision of veterinary services in Africa.

Journals

1732   *Bulletin of animal health and production in Africa.* 1953–. Nairobi: Interafrican Bureau for Animal Resources. Quarterly.
Includes maps of the geographical distribution of animal diseases in Africa. Formerly known as the *Bulletin of epizootic diseases of Africa.*

1733   *Revue d'élevage et de médecine vétérinaire des pays tropicaux.* 1947–. Maisons-Alfort: IEMVT. Three a year.
About a dozen papers per issue on aspects of veterinary parasitology and disease.

1734   *Tropical animal health and production.* 1969–. Harlow: Longman. Quarterly.
Journal of the Centre for Tropical Veterinary Medicine, University of Edinburgh.

1735   *Tropical veterinarian.* 1983–. Ibadan, Nigeria: University of Ibadan, Faculty of Veterinary Medicine. Quarterly.

1736   *World review of animal production.* 1965–. Via di Tor Vergata 85/87, 00133 Rome: International Publishing Enterprises. Quarterly.

Other Journals

Acta tropica
Agriculture international
Annals of tropical medicine and parasitology
Tropical animal production
Tropische Landwirtschaft und Veterinärmedizin: Beiträge

VIROLOGY

Information Guide

1737 Nicholas, R. and **Nicholas, D.** *Virology, an information profile.* London: Mansell, 1983. 236pp.

Abstracting Service

1738 *Foot and mouth disease bulletin.* 1962–. Foot and Mouth Disease Vaccine Laboratory, Pirbright, Surrey: Coopers Animal Health. Quarterly.

Book Series

1739 *Advances in Medical & Veterinary Virology, Immunology and Epidemiology.* Edited by T. Mathew. New Delhi: Thajema.
   1 1987 *Cultivation and immunological studies on pox group of viruses with special reference to buffalo pox virus.* T. Mathew. 174pp.

1740 Appel, M. J. (ed.) *Virus infections of carnivores.* Amsterdam: Elsevier, 1987. 500pp. (Virus Infections of Vertebrates, vol. 1.)
Has sections on virus infections of dogs, cats, mink and ferrets, non-domestic carnivores and pinnipeds. Volumes **2** *Virus infections of porcines* by M. B. Pensaert and **3** *Virus infections of bovines* are in preparation. Other volumes in the series will deal with virus infections of rodents and lagomorphs, equines, avian species and fish.

1741 *Developments in Veterinary Virology.* 1985–. Boston: Kluwer Academic Publishers.
Most volumes are concerned with a single disease. The titles and editors of the volumes published thus far are:

   9 *Herpesvirus diseases of cattle, pigs and horses.* G. Wittmann. 1989, 345pp.
   8 *Rabies.* J. B. Campbell and K. M. Charlton. 1988, 431pp.
   7 *Newcastle disease.* D. J. Alexander. 1988, 378pp.
   6 *Virus diseases in laboratory and captive animals.* G. Darai. 1988, 568pp.
   5 *Classical swine fever and related viral infections.* B. Liess. 1988, 298pp.
   4 *Avian leukosis.* G. F. de Boer. 1987, 292pp.
   3 *African swine fever.* Y. Becker. 1987, 157pp.
   2 *Enzootic bovine leukosis and bovine leukemia virus.* A. Burny and M. Mammerickx. 1987, 283pp.
   1 *Marek's disease: scientific basis and methods of control.* L. N. Payne. 1985, 359pp.

Kluwer also publish two other book series in virology: *Developments in molecular virology* (1981–) and *Developments in medical virology* (1985–).

1742 *Perspectives in Medical Virology.* Series editor A. J. Zuckerman. 1985–. Amsterdam: Elsevier. Annual.

3 *Animal virus structure.* M. V. Nermut and A. C. Steven (eds). 466pp.
2 *Arenaviruses.* C. R. Howard. 254pp.
1 *Conquest of viral diseases.* J. Oxford and B. Oberg. 708pp.

Other Book Series

Advances in virus research
Monographs in virology
Progress in medical virology
Virology monographs

Books

1743 Gibbs, E. P. J. (ed.) *Virus diseases of food animals: a world geography of epidemiology and control.* London: Academic Press, 1981. 2 vols. 786pp.
Volume 1 (*International perspectives*) gives a global view of the surveillance and control of virus diseases in different regions of the world and has chapters reviewing the virus diseases of each group of food animals. Volume 2 (*Disease monographs*) has chapters on eighteen individual diseases.

1744 Fenner, F., Bachmann, P. A., Gibbs, E. P. J., Murphy, F. A., Studdert, M. J. and **White, D. O.** *Veterinary virology.* Orlando: Academic Press, 1987. 660pp.
The first half of the book reviews the basic principles of animal virology; the second has chapters on each of the major families of viruses affecting domestic animals. There are tables listing the virus infections and a glossary of terms. A concise reference work for veterinarians and all dealing with viruses affecting domestic animals.

1745 Fenner, F. and **Gibbs, A.** (eds) *Portraits of viruses: a history of virology.* Basel: Karger, 1988. 344pp.
Has chapters on FMD virus, picornaviruses and herpesviruses.

1746 *Foot and mouth disease: ageing of lesions.* London: HMSO, 1986. 54pp. (MAFF Reference Book 400.)
Colour plates depict the lesions.

1747 Mahy, B. W. J. (ed.) *Virology: a practical approach.* Oxford: IRL Press, 1985. 264pp.
Has practical recipes and protocols for handling most animal viruses of current interest.

1748   Mims, C. A. and **White, D. O.** *Viral pathogenesis and immunology*. Oxford: Blackwell, 1984. 398pp.

1749   Odend'hal, S. *The geographical distribution of animal viral diseases*. New York: Academic Press, 1983. 493pp.
Presents maps illustrating the known distribution of 110 virus diseases with brief notes on the viruses themselves supported by key references to the literature. The sources of the information are given in an appendix.

1750   Olson, R. G., Krakowka, S. and **Blakeslee, J. R. Jr.** *Comparative pathobiology of viral disease*. Boca Raton: CRC Press, 1985. 2 vols.
Has chapters on a variety of infections in domestic animals.

1751   Porterfield, J. S. *Andrewes' Viruses of vertebrates*. 5th ed. London: Baillière Tindall. Forthcoming.
Most recent edition of a definitive reference work on the taxonomy and morphology of viruses affecting vertebrates.

1752   Russell, P. H. and **Edington, N.** *Veterinary viruses*. 19A Chalcot Square, London NW1 8JY, England: the Authors, 1985. 266pp.
Concise introduction to veterinary virology.

1753   Versteeg, J. *A colour atlas of virology*. London: Wolfe Medical Publications, 1985. 240pp.
Six hundred and sixteen photographs are used to describe the techniques used in diagnostic and research virology. A set of slides is also available.

Journal

Veterinary microbiology [1395]

Other Journals

Articles on animal viruses appear in a wide range of general virology and microbiology journals. The most important virology titles are:

Antiviral research
Archives of virology
Intervirology
Journal of general virology
Journal of medical virology
Journal of virological methods
Journal of virology
Virology
Virus research

WELFARE

Directory

1754 *Directory of animal rights/animal welfare organizations.* Waltham, Massachusetts: National Association for BioMedical Research. Occasional.

Review Series

1755 *Advances in animal welfare science.* 1985–. Edited by M. W. Fox and L. D. Mickley. Dordrecht: Martinus Nijhoff.
Volumes have appeared for 1984, 1985 and 1986/7. Each has papers on a variety of issues in the scientific and ethical aspects of animal welfare.

Books and Pamphlets

1756 *Code of practice for the housing and care of animals used in scientific procedures.* London: HMSO, 1989. 33pp.
Issued under the Animals (Scientific Procedures) Act 1986.

1757 *Codes of recommendations for the welfare of livestock.* Alnwick: MAFF. Occasional. (MAFF Leaflets Series.)
Prepared by the Farm Animal Welfare Council. Each leaflet gives specifications for the management, housing and welfare of a group of animals. The titles available are: *Rabbits* (1987, L938), *Sheep* (1987, L705), *Ducks* (1987, L937), *Domestic fowls* (1987, L703), *Turkeys* (1987, L704), *Cattle* (1986, L701) and *Pigs* (1983, L702). New codes for goats and farmed deer and a revised code for sheep are in preparation.

1758 'Colloquium on recognition and alleviation of animal pain and distress'. *Journal of the American Veterinary Medical Association* **191** (1987): 1184–298.

1759 **Connell, J.** *International transport of farm animals intended for slaughter.* Luxembourg: Commission of the European Communities, 1984. 67pp.
Review of the literature on the transport of farm animals with an indication of future research needs. Has a bibliography of 174 items.

1760 **Dawkins, M. S.** *Animal suffering: the science of animal welfare.* London: Chapman & Hall, 1980. 149pp.
Introduction to the nature and recognition of animal suffering.

1761 **Folsch, D. W.** and **Nabholz, A.** *Ethical, ethological and legal aspects of intensive farm animal management.* Basel: Birkhauser, 1987. 158pp. (Animal Management/Tierhaltung, vol. 18.)

1762   Fox, M. W. *Laboratory animal husbandry: ethology, welfare and experimental variables*. Albany: State University of New York Press, 1986. 267pp.
Describes the conditions under which laboratory animals should be reared and used and discusses the ethical issues involved in experimental work using animals.

1763   Fox, M. W. *Farm animals: husbandry, behavior and veterinary practice*. Baltimore: University Park Press, 1984. 285pp.
A critical survey of production systems and a review of the issues they raise in animal welfare.

1764   *Guidelines on the use of living animals in scientific investigations*. Institute of Biology, 20 Queensberry Place, London SW7 2DZ, England: The Biological Council, 1987. 24pp.
Prepared by the Animal Research and Welfare Panel of the Council. Provides an indication of the aspects of animal welfare to be considered when planning experimental investigations and acts as a brief guide to the Animals (Scientific Procedures) Act 1986. Has a good reading list.

1765   Management and welfare of farm animals: the UFAW handbook. 3rd ed. London: Baillière Tindall, 1988. 260pp.
Has an introductory chapter on the concept of animal welfare and chapters on each of the major species of farm animals. The welfare implications of modern husbandry techniques are discussed. An excellent introduction to those concerned with improving the efficiency and standards of farm animal production.

1766   Office of Technology Assessment, Congress of the United States. *Alternatives to animal use in research, testing and education*. New York: Dekker, 1988. 441pp.
A survey of the technologies available for reducing the use of animals and of the ethical considerations behind this objective. It also contains chapters on the federal, state, institutional and self-regulation of animal use in the USA and on the regulation of animal use in selected countries.

1767   Paton, W. *Man and mouse: animals in medical research*. Oxford: OUP, 1984. 174pp.
Puts forward the arguments for the responsible use of animals in experiments.

1768   Regan, T. *The case for animal rights*. Berkeley: University of California Press, 1983. 425pp.
The author has written a number of texts in the field including *Animal rights and human obligations* (2nd ed., Englewood Cliffs: Prentice-Hall, forthcoming), *Animal sacrifices: religious perspectives on the use of animals in science* (Philadelphia: Temple University Press, 1986, 270pp.) and *The struggle for animal rights* (Clarks Summit, Pennsylvania: International Society for Animal Rights, 1987, 197pp.).

1769 *Report on the welfare of . . .* London: HMSO. Occasional.
Prepared by the Farm Animal Welfare Council. The most recent are: *farmed deer* (1985, available from MAFF: Alnwick), *livestock when slaughtered by religious methods* (1985, MAFF Reference Book 262), *livestock (red meat animals) at the time of slaughter* (1984, MAFF Reference Book 248), *livestock at markets* (1986, MAFF Reference Book 265) and *poultry at the time of slaughter* (1982, UR59 available from MAFF: Alnwick). The FAWC has also issued an *Assessment of egg production systems* (1985).

1770 Rowan, A. N. *Of mice, models and men: a critical evaluation of animal research.* Albany: State University of New York Press, 1984. 323pp.
Readable review of the historical, social and scientific aspects of the use of animals in research.

1771 Russell, W. M. S. and **Burch, R. L.** *The principles of humane experimental technique.* London: Methuen, 1959. 252pp.

1772 Sainsbury, D. *Farm animal welfare: cattle, pigs and poultry.* London: Collins, 1986. 175pp.
A balanced review of the criteria to be considered in ensuring the welfare of farm animals.

Conferences

1773 Dodds, W. J. and **Orlans, F. B.** (eds) *Scientific perspectives on animal welfare.* London: Academic Press, 1982. 131pp.
Proceedings of a conference held in 1981 and organized by the Scientists' Center for Animal Welfare. Most of the papers relate to the situation in the United States.

1774 Kitchell, R. L. and **Erickson, H. H.** (eds) *Animal pain: perception and alleviation.* Bethesda: American Physiological Society, 1983. 221pp.

1775 Moberg, G. P. (ed.) *Animal stress.* Bethesda: American Physiological Society, 1985. 324pp.
The papers describe the determination of animal well-being, the nature and effects of stress in animals and the welfare of laboratory animals.

MISCELLANEOUS SUBJECTS

1776 Baker, J. and **Brothwell, D.** *Animal diseases in archaeology.* London: Academic Press, 1980. 235pp. (Studies in Archaeological Science.)

1777 Gill, J. L. *Design and analysis of experiments in the animal and medical sciences.* Ames: Iowa State UP, 1978. 3 vols. 410 + 302 + 174pp.
The third volume contains appendices and tables for use with the first two volumes.

1778   Hall, L. W. (ed.) *Veterinary nephrology*. London: Heinemann, 1983. 256pp. Deals with the anatomy, physiology and pathology of the mammalian and avian kidney and covers renal disease and therapy.

1779   Harrison, R. M. and **Wildt, D. E.** *Animal laparoscopy*. Baltimore: Williams & Wilkins, 1980. 256pp.
Comprehensive monograph with chapters on the use of laparoscopy in all the common species.

1780   Klemm, W. R. *Applied electronics for veterinary medicine and animal physiology*. Springfield: C. C. Thomas, 1976. 470pp.

1781   *Safety precautions for use in veterinary laboratories*. Weybridge: MAFF, 1978. 59pp. + index.
General guide to safe practice in veterinary laboratories.

1782   Sard, D. M. *Dealing with data: the practical use of numerical information*. London: BVA, 1981. 47pp.
Practical approach to statistics as applied to veterinary medicine. A collection of fifteen articles orginally published in *Veterinary record*. MAFF have also prepared a set of five videos (also a training booklet) covering safety in the laboratory: *Be aware! An introduction to laboratory safety* (Room 404, Government Buildings, Garrison Lane, Chessington, Surrey KT9 2LW, England: MAFF Publicity, 1989).

PART III

Directory of Organizations

Directory of Organizations

SELECTED LIST OF VETERINARY LIBRARIES

International

1783   British Library Document Supply Centre, Boston Spa, Wetherby, West Yorkshire LS23 7BQ, England. Tel. (0937) 843434. Telex: 557381

1784   Food and Agriculture Organization of the United Nations, David Lubin Memorial Library, Via delle Terme di Caracalla, 00100 Rome, Italy. Tel. 57971 (ext. 3703). Telex: 610181 FAO I

1785   Inter-American Institute for Cooperation on Agriculture, Biblioteca Conmemorativa Orton, Apartado Postal 55, 2200 Coronado, San José, Costa Rica. Tel. 290222. Telex: 2144 IICA. Fax: 294741

1786   Centro Internacional de Agricultura Tropical, Library and Documentation Unit, Apartado Áereo 6713, Cali, Colombia. Tel. 675050. Telex: 05769 CIAT CO

1787   International Laboratory for Research on Animal Diseases (ILRAD), Training and Information Services, PO Box 30709, Nairobi, Kenya. Tel. 592311. Telex: 963–22040 ILRAD. Fax: 593499

1788   International Livestock Centre for Africa (ILCA), Library, Information Section, PO Box 5689, Addis Ababa, Ethiopia. Tel. 183215. Telex: 21207 ILCA ET. Fax: 188191

Australia

1789 The Library, McMaster Laboratory, Private Mail Bag No. 1, Glebe, New South Wales 2037. Tel. (02) 660 4411. Telex: 21376. (Houses both the AVA Library (Max Henry Memorial Library) and the CSIRO's Division of Animal Health Collection)

1790 Badham Library, University of Sydney, Sydney, New South Wales 2006. Tel. (02) 692 2728. Telex: FISHLIB 20056

1791 Central Library, University of Queensland, St Lucia, Queensland 4067

1792 Main Library, James Cook University of North Queensland, James Cook University, Queensland 4811. Tel. (077) 81 4472. Telex: AA47009. Fax: (077) 79 6371. (Emphasis on tropical veterinary science)

1793 Central Library, Department of Primary Industries, GPO Box 46, Brisbane, Queensland 4001. (Emphasis on grazing animals)

1794 Baillieu Library, University of Melbourne, Parkville, Victoria 3052

Austria

1795 Veterinärmedizinische Universität Wien, Universitätsbibliothek, Linke Bahngasse 11, A-1030 Vienna. Tel. (0222) 735581

Belgium

1796 Institut National de Recherches Vétérinaires, Bibliothèque, Groeselenberg 99, B-1180 Brussels. Tel (02) 375 44 55

1797 Bibliothèque, Faculté de Médecine Vétérinaire de l'Université de Liège, Rue des Vétérinaires 45, 1070 Brussels. Tel. (02) 522 73 05. Telex: 41397 UNIV LG B

Brazil

1798 Biblioteca da Escola de Veterinária da Universidade Federal de Minas Gerais, Pampulha, Belo Horizonte, Minas Gerais, CEP 31271. Tel. 031–441-8077 R.1150

1799 Biblioteca, Universidade de São Paulo USP, Faculdade de Medicina Veterinária e Zootecnia, Universidade de São Paulo, Cidade Universitária, Butanta, CEP 05508, São Paulo. Tel. 011-210-2122 R.461

Bulgaria

1800 Higher Institute of Animal Husbandry and Veterinary Medicine, D Blagoev str 62, 6000 Stara Zagora. Telex: 88 465

Canada

1801   Robertson Library, Atlantic Veterinary College, University of Prince Edward Island, Charlottetown, Prince Edward Island C1A 4P3. Tel. (902) 566 0460

1802   Bibliothèque de Médecine Vétérinaire, Université de Montréal, C.P. 5000, St. Hyacinthe, Quebec J2S 7C6. Tel. (514) 773 8521. Telex: FMVSTHY 05830505

Denmark

1803   The Royal Veterinary and Agricultural University, Danish Veterinary and Agricultural Library, Bülowsvej 13, DK-1870 Frederiksberg C. Tel. (01) 35 17 88. Telex: 15061 DVJBIB DK

Finland

1804   College of Veterinary Medicine Library, Hämeentie 57, SF-00550 Helsinki 55. Tel. (0) 393 101. Telex: 123203 ELKK SF

France

1805   Bibliothèque, École Nationale Vétérinaire d'Alfort, 7 Rue du Général de Gaulle, Maisons Alfort 94704. Tel. (1) 43 96 71 00. Telex: 213863F ECAL-FOR. Fax: (1) 43 96 71 25

1806   Institut d'Élevage et de Médecine Vétérinaire des Pays Tropicaux (IEMVT), Bibliothèque, 10 Rue Pierre-Curie, 94704 Maisons Alfort. Tel (1) 43 68 88 73

1807   Laboratoire Central de Recherches Vétérinaires, 22 Rue Pierre-Curie, BP-67, 94703 Maisons Alfort

Federal Republic of Germany

1808   Veterinärmedizinische Bibliothek (Freie Universität Berlin), Koserstrasse 20, D-1000 Berlin 33. Tel. (030) 838 3512

1809   Tierärztliche Hochschule Hannover, Bibliothek, Bischofsholer Damm 15, D-3000 Hanover. Tel (0511) 856 464. Telex: 922034 TIHO D

Hungary

1810   Veterinary University of Budapest, Landler Jenő utca 2, 1078 Budapest, Tel. (01) 222 660. Telex: 224439 AAOE H

Ireland

1811   Veterinary Medicine Library, University College Dublin, Veterinary College, Ballsbridge, Dublin 4. Tel. (01) 687988

Italy

1812 Biblioteca della Facolta di Medicina Veterinaria, Universitaria Degli Studi di Milano, Via Celoria 10, 20133 Milan. Tel. (02) 884 6248

Japan

1813 Library, College of Agriculture and Veterinary Medicine, Nihon University, Fugisawa-shi, Kanagawa-Ken 252

Kenya

1814 Kenya Agricultural Research Institute, POB 30148, Nairobi

1815 Library, Ministry of Livestock Development, Veterinary Services Division, PO Kabete

Mexico

1816 Biblioteca de la Facultad de Medicina Veterinaria y Zootecnia, Universidad Autónoma de México, Ciuadad Universitaria, 04510 México DF. Tel. 5 50 52 15 (ext. 4992)

Morocco

1817 Institut Agronomique et Vétérinaire Hassan 2, Bibliothèque, B.P. 6202, Rabat. Tel. 743-51/52. Telex: AGKOVET 318737° M

Netherlands

1818 Central Veterinary Institute, Postbus 65, 8200 AB Lelystad. Tel. (03200) 73911. Telex: 40227

1819 Bibliothek, Faculteit der Diergeneeskunde, Rijksuniversiteit te Utrecht, Yalelaan 1, 3508 TD Utrecht. Tel. (30) 531118/532116

New Zealand

1820 Massey University Library, Massey University, Palmerston North. Tel. (063) 69–099

1821 Agricultural Library Information Centre, Ministry of Agriculture and Fisheries, Private Bag, Upper Hutt. Tel. (04) 286–089

Nigeria

1822 Library and Documentation Division, National Veterinary Research Institute, Vom near Jos, Plateau State

Norway

1823 Norges Veterinærhogskoles Bibliotek, Postboks 8146 DEP, N-0033 Oslo 1. Tel. (02) 693690

Poland

1824 Central Agricultural Library, PO Box 360, 00–950 Warsaw. Tel. 26 60 41. Telex: 816481 CBROL PL

1825 Veterinary Research Institute, Library, 24–100 Pulawy. Tel. 30 51. Telex: 642401 IWET PL

Portugal

1826 Escola Superior de Medicina Veterinaria, Biblioteca, Rua Gomes Freire, 1199 Lisboa Codex. Tel. (019) 562596/7

South Africa

1827 Veterinary Research Institute, Library, PO, Onderstepoort, 0110. Tel. (012) 554141. Telex: 3-22088 SA

Spain

1828 Biblioteca, Facultad de Veterinaria, Universidad Complutense de Madrid, Calle Noviciado 3, 28015 Madrid

Sweden

1829 Statens Veterinarmedicinska Anstalts, Bibliotek, Norra Ultuna 2, S-750 07 Uppsala. Tel. (018) 15 58 20

1830 Sveriges Lantbruksuniversitets, Bibliotek – Ultunabiblioteket, S-750 07 Uppsala. Telex: 76062 ULTBIBL S

Union of Soviet Socialist Republics

1831 Central Scientific Agricultural Library of the All-Union Lenin Academy of Agricultural Sciences, 107804 Moscow, B-139, Orlicov per. 3, Korpus V. Tel. 204 48 19

1832 Moscow Veterinary Academy, Zuz'minskaya ZH-349, Moscow

United Kingdom

1833 British Library Science Reference and Information Service (Aldwych), 9 Kean Street, London WC2B 4AT. Tel. 01-323 7288 (life science enquiries). Telex: 22717

1834 British Library Science Reference and Information Service (Holborn), 25 Southampton Buildings, London WC2A 1AW. Tel. 01-323 7494 (general enquiries), 01-323 7919 (patents), 01-323 7454 (business enquiries). Telex: 266959

1835   Central Veterinary Laboratory (MAFF) Library, New Haw, Weybridge, Surrey KT15 3NB. Tel. (09323) 41111. Telex: 262318 VETWEY. Fax. (09323) 47046

1836   Royal College of Veterinary Surgeons' Wellcome Library, 32 Belgrave Square, London SW1X 8QP. Tel. 01-235 6568

1837   The Royal Veterinary College (University of London), The Library, Royal College Street, London NW1 0TU. Tel. 01-387 2898 (ext. 331). (Pre-clinical and historical materials)

1838   The Royal Veterinary College (University of London), The Library, Hawkshead House, Hawkshead Lane, North Mymms, Hatfield, Hertfordshire AL9 7TA. Tel. (0707) 55486 (ext. 312). (Core veterinary collection)

United States of America

1839   Cornell University – Flower Veterinary Library, New York State College of Veterinary Medicine, Schurman Hall, Ithaca, New York 14853. Tel. (607) 253 3000

1840   Louisiana State University, School of Veterinary Medicine Library, Baton Rouge, Louisiana 70803. Tel. (504) 346 3172

1841   National Agricultural Library, US Department of Agriculture, Beltsville, Maryland 20705. Tel. (301) 344 3778. Telex: 710 828 0506

1842   National Library of Medicine, Bethesda, Maryland 20894. Tel. (301) 496 6097

1843   US Department of Agriculture, National Animal Disease Center, Library, Dayton Road, PO Box 70, Ames, Iowa 50010. Tel. (515) 239 8201

1844   US Department of Agriculture, Plum Island Animal Disease Center, Library, PO Box 848, Greenport L. I., New York 11944. Tel. (516) 323 2500. Fax: (516) 323 2500 (ext. 295)

NATIONAL VETERINARY ASSOCIATIONS

An asterisk indicates that the country is a member of the World Veterinary Association [2328] and identifies the member organization. A dagger (†) indicates that the country is a member of the Commonwealth Veterinary Association [2148].

†*Antigua

1845 *Antigua Veterinary Association, c/o Veterinary & Livestock Division, c/o Ministry of Agriculture, Lands, Fishing and Housing, PO Box 1282, St. John's, Antigua, West Indies. Tel. 21081

*Argentina

1846 Academia Nacional de Agronomía y Veterinaria, Avenida Alvear 1711, 1014 Buenos Aires. Tel. (1) 44–4168

1847 Consejo Professional de Medicos Veterinarios, Pasana 467–1, 1017 Buenos Aires. Tel. (1) 40 7392

1848 Federación Veterinaria Argentina, *see* Sociedad de Medicina Veterinaria

1849 *Sociedad de Medicina Veterinaria, Calle Chile 1856, 1227 Buenos Aires. Tel. (1) 38–7415, (1) 37–8760

†*Australia

1850 *Australian Veterinary Association, 134–136 Hampden Road, Artarmon, New South Wales 2064. Tel. (02) 411 2733. Fax: (02) 411 5089

*Austria

1851 Berufsverband freiberuflich tätiger Tierärzte Österreichs, Aignerstrasse 26, A-8952 Irdning. Tel. (03682) 2937

1852 *Bundeskammer der Tierärzte Österreichs, Biberstrasse 22, A-1010 Vienna. Tel. (0222) 5121766, (0222) 5131265

1853 *Österreichische Gesellschaft der Tierärzte, c/o Veterinärmedizinische Universität Wien, Linke Bahngasse 11, A-1030 Vienna. Tel. (0222) 735581 (ext. 504)

†The Bahamas

1854 Veterinary Medical Association of the Bahamas, PO Box N-9547, Nassau. Tel. 809 32 58416

†Bangladesh

1855 Bangladesh Veterinary Association, Directorate of Livestock Services, 48 Kazi Allaudin Road, Dhaka 1000

†Barbados

1856 Barbados Veterinary Association, RSPCA, Cheltenham Lodge, Fontabelle, St. Michael, Bridgetown, Barbados, West Indies

*Belgium

1857   Ordre des Médecins Vétérinaires, Rue des Vétérinaires 45, 1070 Brussels. Tel (02) 521 03 14

1858   Orde der Dierenartsen, Nederlandstalige Gewestelijke Raad, Casinoplein 24, Gent. Tel. (091) 23 37 65

1859   *Union Syndicale Vétérinaire Belge, Avenue Fonsny 41, 1060 Brussels. Tel. (02) 538 17 54

†Belize

1860   Belize Veterinary Association, c/o Ministry of Natural Resources, Belmopan, Cayo

Bolivia

1861   Asociación Nacional de Clínicas y Farmacias, same address as next entry

1862   Asociación Nacional de Veterinarios, Avda. Irala No. 303, Santa Cruz. Tel. 2941

1863   Dr C. Justiniano Melgar, Director General de Ganadería, Ministerio de Asuntos Campesinos y Agropecuarios, Avenida Camacho 1471, La Paz

†Botswana

1864   Botswana Veterinary Association, c/o Private Bag 0032, Gaborone

*Brazil

1865   Conselho Federal de Medicina Veterinaria, SCS-Ed. Ceará-14° andar, 70303 Brasilia-D.F. Tel. (061) 226 7708. Telex: 0612281 CFMV BR

1866   Federação Nacional dos Medicos Veterinarios, Rua Anita Garibaldi, 19–503, 88010 Florianopolis, S. C.

1867   *Sociedade Brasileira de Medicina Veterinaria, SRTQ 702, Bloco E, Lote I e II, Sala 220, Palácio do Rádio II, 70303 Brasilia-D. F.

†British Virgin Islands

1868   Dr J. Mathew, Department of Agriculture, Tortola

*Bulgaria

1869   Bulgarian Scientific Veterinary Association, 73 Lenin Boulevard, Sofia. Tel. Sofia 7223

1870   *Prof. Vulo Dikov, General Secretary, The Veterinary Administration of the Ministry of Agriculture, Sofia. Telex: 23242 NPOVD BG

†*Canada

1871   *Canadian Veterinary Medical Association, 339 Booth Street, Ottawa, Ontario K1R 7K1. Tel. (613) 236 1162. Fax: (613) 236 9681

†Cayman Islands

1872   Cayman Islands Veterinary Association, c/o Department of Agriculture, PO Box 459 (GT), Grand Cayman

Central African Republic

1873   Director General for Animal Husbandry and Animal Industries, Ministry of Rural Development, PO Box 707, Bangui

Chile

1874   Colegio Médico Veterinario de Chile, Estado no. 337, Oficina 729, Casilla 13384 – Correo 21, Santiago

1875   Comité Chileno Veterinario de Zootecnia, Casilla 16202, Correo 9, Santiago

1876   Sociedad de Medicina Veterinaria de Chile, Estado no. 337, Oficina 729, Casilla 13384 – Correo 21, Santiago. Tel. 397866

People's Republic of China

1877   Chinese Animal Husbandry and Veterinary Society, c/o China Association for Science and Technology, Sanlihe, Beijing. Tel. 89–6963. Telex: 20035

Colombia

1878   Asociación Colombiana de Médicos Veterinarios y de Zootecnistes ''Acovez'', Calle 13 10–14 of, 405 Bogotá

*Congo People's Republic

1879   *Centre de Recherche Vétérinaire et Zootechnique, B. P. 235, Brazzaville. Tel. 81 03 51

*Costa Rica

1880   *Colegio de Médicos Veterinarios de Costa Rica, Apartado 4134, San José. Tel. (506) 234664

*Cuba

1881   *Consejo Científico Veterinario de Cuba, Paseo 604, e/25 y 27 Vedado, La Habana 4. Tel. 30–8064 and 30–8076. Telex: 051 1333

†*Cyprus

1882   *Pancyprian Veterinary Association, PO Box 5284, Nicosia

1883   Pancyprian Veterinary Practitioners Association, PO Box 6269, Limassol

***Czechoslovakia**

1884   Československa Společnost pro Vědy Zemědělské, Lesnické, Veterinární a Potravinářské, 160 21 Prague 6-Suchdol VSZ. Tel. 32 36 40

1885   *State Veterinary Administration (Státní veterinární sprava CSR), Ministry of Agriculture and Food, Těšnov 17, 117 05 Prague 1. Tel. 282111

***Denmark**

1886   *Den Danske Dyrlaegeforening (Danish Veterinary Association), Rosenlunds Allé 8, 2720 Vanløse. Tel. 01 71 0888. Fax. 01 71 0322

Dominica

1887   Dominica Veterinary Association, c/o Division of Agriculture, Botanic Gardens, Roseau, Dominica, West Indies

Dominican Republic

1888   Asociación Dominicana de Médicos Veterinarios, Apartado Postal 196, Ciudad Ganadera, Recinto Feria Ganadera, Santo Domingo

Ecuador

1889   Federación de Médicos Veterinarios del Ecuador, Garcia Moreno 1517 y Esmeraldas, 4 Piso Casilla N 4083, Quito

***Egypt**

1890   *The Egyptian Veterinary Medical Association, 8 Sharia 26 July Street, App. 52, PO Box 2366, Cairo. Telex: 20664 VOSAG UN

El Salvador

1891   Asociación de Médicos Veterinarios de El Salvador, Apartado Postal 1079, San Salvador

***Ethiopia**

1892   *Ethiopian Veterinary Medical Association, PO Box 2462, Addis Ababa

†Fiji Islands (CwVA membership via Australia)

1893   Fiji Veterinary Association, c/o Ministry of Primary Industries, PO Box 358, Rodwell Road, Suva

*Finland

1894 Finnish Veterinary Association of Specialized Practitioners, c/o Dr Heikki Saarinen, Peltola, 16300 Orimattila. Tel. (918) 74830

1895 *Suomen Eläinlääkäriliitto (Finnish Veterinary Association), Akavatalo, Rautatieläisenkatu 6, SF-00520 Helsinki 52. Tel. (0) 150 2382

*France

1896 Académie Vétérinaire de France, 60 Boulevard de Latour-Maubourg, 75007 Paris. Tel. (01) 47 05 59 72

1897 *Comité Français de l'Association Mondiale Vétérinaire, École National Vétérinaire d'Alfort, 7 Avenue Général de Gaulle, 94704 Maisons Alfort. Tel. (01) 48 93 71 31

1898 L'Ordre National des Vétérinaires Français, 10 Place Léon Blum, 75011 Paris. Tel. (01) 43 79 11 52

1899 Syndicat Genérále de la Médecine Vétérinaire, Le Bourg-Sainte-Catherine, 69440 Mornant. Tel. (7) 88 185 44

1900 Société Nationale des Groupements Techniques Vétérinaires, *see* [1898]

1901 Syndicat National des Vétérinaires Français, *see* [1898]

†The Gambia

1902 The Gambia Veterinary Medical Association, c/o International Trypanotolerance Centre, Private Mail Bag 14, Banjul

*Federal Republic of Germany

1903 Bundesverband praktischer Tierärzte eV, Hamburger Allee 12, 6000 Frankfurt am Main 90. Tel. (069) 70 30 03

1904 *Deutsche Tierärzteschaft eV Geschaftsstelle, Steubenstrasse 34, Postfach 2144, 6200 Wiesbaden 1. Tel. (06121) 37 31 16

1905 Deutsche Veterinärmedizinische Gesellschaft, Veterinärstrasse 13, 8000 Munich 22. Tel. (0641) 24466

1906 Verband der Tierheilpraktiker Deutschlands, c/o Dr E. Veil, Friedenstrasse 13, 7060 Schorndorf

†Ghana

1907 Ghana Veterinary Medical Association, PO Box 143, Legon

*Greece

1908   *Chambre Géotechnique de Grèce, 64 rue Venizelou, Thessaloniki. Tel. (31) 278817

1909   Elliniki Ktiniatriki Etairia (Hellenic Veterinary Medical Society), PO Box 3546, 102 10 Athens. Tel. (01) 524 46 53, 883 64 20

†Grenada

1910   Grenada Veterinary Association, c/o Ministry of Agriculture, St. Georges, Grenada, West Indies

Guatemala

1911   Colegio de Médicos Veterinarios y Zootecnistas de Guatemala, Avenida Elena 14–45, Zona 1 Guatemala

†Guyana

1912   Guyana Veterinary Association, PO Box 10851, Georgetown. Tel. 066-2657/02-64639

Honduras

1913   Colegio de Médicos Veterinarios de Honduras, Clínica Veterinaria Matamoros, Av. Juan Lindo No. 107, Col. Palmira, Tegucigalpa, D. C.

*Hong Kong

1914   *Hong Kong Veterinary Association, c/o President – Mr D. K. Manson, Equine Hospital, Shatin Racecourse, New Territories. Tel. (0) 6956608. Telex: 65581 RHKJC HX

*Hungary

1915   *MAE Allatorvosok Társasaga (Veterinary Association of the Hungarian Society of Agricultural Sciences), H-1055 Budapest, Kossuth Lajos ter 6–8. Tel. (1) 533333

*Iceland

1916   *The Icelandic Veterinary Association (Dýralæknafélag Íslands), Lágmúla 7, 108 Reykjavik

†*India

1917   *Indian Veterinary Association, No. 123, 7th Main Road, IV Block West, Jayanagar, Bangalore 560 011, Karanataka. Tel. (0812) 641200

Indonesia

1918   Indonesian Veterinary Association (Perhimpunan Dokter Hewan Indonesia), 16 Jalan Salemba Raya, Jakarta Pusat 10430. Tel. 331180. Telex: 48125 DJPJKTIA

***Iran**

1919 *Iranian Veterinary Association, Tohid Square, Parcham Avenue No. 89, PO Box 14335–383, Postal Code No. 14, Tehran. Tel. (21) 932744

Iraq

1920 Iraqi Veterinary Medical Association, Medical Union Building, Al-Mari Street, Al-Mansur, Baghdad

***Ireland**

1921 Irish Veterinary Association, 53 Lansdowne Road, Ballsbridge, Dublin 4. Tel. (01) 685263

1922 Irish Veterinary Union, 32 Kenilworth Square, Dublin 6

1923 *Veterinary Council, 53 Lansdowne Road, Ballsbridge, Dublin 4. Tel. (01) 688402

***Israel**

1924 *Israel Veterinary Medical Association, Secretary's Office, PO Box 1871, Tel Aviv. Tel. (03) 521 251

1925 Israel Veterinary Scientific Council, PO Box 9610, Haifa. Tel. (04) 0521251

***Italy**

1926 *Federazione Nazionale degli Ordini dei Veterinari Italiani, Via del Tritone 125, 00186 Rome. Tel. (06) 48 59 23, (06) 46 11 90

1927 Sindicato Nationale Veterinari Liberi Professionisti, Via Turali 19, 54031 Avenza Carrara

1928 Società Italiana delle Scienze Veterinarie, Via Antonio Bianchi 1, 25100 Brescia. Tel. (030) 525 16

†*Jamaica

1929 *The Jamaica Veterinary Association, Secretary's Office, PO Box 309, Kingston 6, Jamaica, West Indies. Tel. 9276475–6, 92777711

***Japan**

1930 *Japan Veterinary Medical Association, Room 2357 West, 1–1–1 Minami Aoyama, Minato-ku, Tokyo 107. Tel. (03) 475 1601. Telex: 34799 ITCINBTH J

1931 Nihon Ju-i Gakkai (Japanese Society of Veterinary Science), Rakuno-Kaikan Bldg, 37–20 Yoyogi-1, Shibuya-Ku, Tokyo 151. Tel. (03) 379 0636

*Jordan

1932 *Jordanian Veterinary Medical Association, PO Box 7224, Amman. Tel. (6) 44502

†*Kenya

1933 *The Kenya Veterinary Association, PO Box 29089, Kabete. Tel. 59223

1934 Veterinary Surgeons Board, Veterinary Research Laboratory, PO Kabete

*Korea

1935 *Korean Veterinary Medical Association, 104–41 Daehyeon-dong, Suadeun-gu, Seoul 120. Tel. (2) 392 2526

Lebanon

1936 Lebanese Veterinary Association, Ministry of Agriculture, Beirut

†Lesotho

1937 Lesotho Veterinary Association, PO Box 24, Maseru

*Luxembourg

1938 *Syndicat des Vétérinaires du Grande-Duché de Luxembourg, Rue de Luxembourg 15, 3392 Roedgen. Tel. 378977

†*Malawi

1939 *The Malawi Veterinary Association, Ministry of Agriculture, Department of Veterinary Services, Headquarters, PO Box 30372, Lilongwe 3

†Malaysia

1940 Association of Veterinary Surgeons Malaysia, d/a Jabatan Perkhidmatan Haiwan Selangor, Off Jalan Barat, 46630 Petaling Jaya

1941 Malaysian Veterinary Association, c/o Balai Ikhtisas Malaysia, Bim Building, 51B, Jalan SS 21/56B, Damansara Utama, 47400 Petaling Jaya
These organizations are to merge to form the Veterinary Association of Malaysia.

Malta

1942 The Malta Veterinary Association, 8 St. Vincent Street, Sliema

†Mauritius

1943 Mauritius Veterinary Association, c/o Division of Veterinary Services, Reduit

*Mexico

1944 *Confederación Unidad Nacional Veterinaria, Rodriguez Saro N° 100–502, 03100 México D. F. Tel. (5) 5347428

†Montserrat

1945 Montserrat Veterinary Association, Ministry of Agriculture, Trade, Lands & Housing, Plymouth (PO Box 275), Montserrat, West Indies

*Morocco

1946 *Association Nationale des Vétérinaires du Maroc, BP 572 Rabat, Chellah

*Mozambique

1947 *Universidade Eduardo Mondlane, Faculdade de Veterinaria, PO Box 4527, Maputo

*Namibia

1948 *South West Africa Veterinary Association, P. B. 296, Windhoek 900. Tel. (61) 37720

*Nepal

1949 *Nepal Veterinary Association, PO Box 3130, Tripureswar, Kathmandu. Tel. 2-15316

*Netherlands

1950 *The Royal Netherlands Veterinary Association, Julianalaan 10, Postbus 14031, 3508 SB Utrecht. Tel. (30) 510111

†*New Zealand

1951 *New Zealand Veterinary Association, PO Box 524, Wellington. Tel. (04) 843 632

1952 Veterinary Surgeons Board, c/o Ministry of Agriculture and Fisheries, Box 2526, Wellington. Tel. (04) 739 410. Telex: 31532 NZ. Fax. (04) 729 071

1953 Veterinary Surgeons Council, PO Box 417, Wellington. Tel. (04) 718 300

Nicaragua

1954 Asociación de Medicos Veterinarios de Nicaragua, Apartado Postal No. RP-70, Managua

†*Nigeria

1955 *Nigeria Veterinary Medical Association, c/o Dr Chidi O. Ogboso (National Secretary), Harmony Project Limited, PO Box 4911, Lagos

1956 Veterinary Council of Nigeria, P.O. 38, Vom, Plateau-Jos

*Norway

1957 *Den Norske Veterinaerforening, Sognsveien 4, N-0451 Oslo. Tel. (02) 46 05 13

*Oman

1958   *Director, Animal Resources, Ministry of Agriculture and Fisheries, PO Box 467, Muscat

Pakistan

1959   Pakistan Veterinary Medical Association, PO Box 10622, P.E.C.H.S. Shahrah-e-Faisal, Karachi 29

*Panama

1960   *Asociación Panameña de Médicos Veterinarios, Apartado 6–2198, El Dorado

†*Papua New Guinea

1961   *Papua New Guinea Veterinary Association, PO Box 6372, Boroko. Tel. 21 7005/21 7405

1962   Veterinary Surgeons Board, Department of Primary Industry, Livestock Division, PO Box 2141, Boroko, N.C.D. Tel. 217005. Telex: NE 23076. Fax. 211337

Paraguay

1963   Paraguay Veterinary Association, c/o Dr Baumgarten, Facultad de Veterinaria, Ciudad Universitaria, San Lorenzo, Casilla de Correo 1061, Asuncion. Tel. (595–21) 500930

*Peru

1964   *Asociación de Médicos Veterinarios del Perú, Pedro Irigoyen Diez Canseco 208, Urb. Santa Rità, Surco, Lima. Tel. 45 64 29. Telex: C. P. 25424–25–257

Philippines

1965   Philippine Veterinary Medical Association, c/o College of Veterinary Medicine, University of the Philippines, Diliman, Quezon City 3004. Tel. 995436

*Poland

1966   *Polskie Towarzystwo Nauk Weterynaryjnych, ul. Grochowska 272, 03-849 Warsaw. Tel. (2) 10 33 97

1967   Zrzeszenie Dekarzy i Techników Weterynarii, ul. Przyjaciol 1, PO Box 118, 00-950 Warsaw

*Portugal

1968   Sindicato Nacional des Médicos Veterinários, Rua D. Dinis 2, 1°D, Lisbon 2. Tel. (1) 68 05 25

1969   *Sociedade Portuguesa de Ciências Veterinárias, Rua D. Dinis 2-A, 1200 Lisbon. Tel. (1) 68 01 88

Qatar

1970   Veterinary Association, PO Box 3107

Romania

1971   Academia de Științe Agricole și Silvice, Bucharest, Bd. Mărăști 61. Tel. 18 06 99

1972   Romanian Veterinary Medicine Association, Bul. Respublici Nr. 24, COD 70033, Bucharest

†St Kitts/Nevis

1973   St Kitts/Nevis Veterinary Association, c/o Ministry of Agriculture, PO Box 39, Basseterre, St Kitts/Nevis, West Indies

†St Lucia

1974   Chief Veterinary Officer, Dr Keith Scotland, c/o Ministry of Agriculture, Lands, Fisheries and Co-operatives, Castries, St Lucia, West Indies

†St Vincent

1975   St Vincent Veterinary Association, c/o Ministry of Agriculture, Kingstown, St Vincent, West Indies

†Western Samoa

1976   Western Samoa Veterinary Association, c/o PO Box L1874, Apia

San Salvador

1977   Asociación de Médicos Veterinarios del Salvador, Avenida los Girasoles No. 165, Colonia Miramonte Poniente No. 2, San Salvador CA

*Senegal

1978   *Association Nationale des Vétérinaires Sénégalais, c/o Dr P. I. Thiongane, Inst. Sénégalais de Recherches Agricoles, 3 Rue de Thiong prolongée angle Valmy, B. P. 3120, Dakar

*Seychelles

1979   *Veterinary Division, Ministry of National Development, PO Box 199, Victoria, Mahe. Tel. Mahe 222190

†Sierra Leone

1980   Sierra Leone Veterinary Medical Association, c/o Veterinary Services Division, Ministry of Agriculture and Natural Resources and Forestry, Youyi Buildings, Brookfields, PO Box 1127, Freetown

†*Singapore

1981 *Singapore Veterinary Association, c/o City Veterinary Centre, 40 Kampong Java Road, Singapore 0922. Tel. 2511203, 2515687

†Solomon Islands

1982 Chief Veterinary Officer, c/o Ministry of Agriculture and Lands, PO Box G.13, Honiara

*South Africa

1983 *South African Veterinary Association, PO Box 25033, Monument Park, Pretoria 0105. Tel. (012) 346–1150/1

1984 South African Veterinary Council, PO Box 933, Pretoria 0001. Tel. (012) 28–7 348. Telex: 32–0245. Fax. (012) 325 5980

South West Africa

1985 South West African Veterinary Council, Department of Agriculture and Nature Conservation, Private Bag 13184, Windhoek. Tel. (061) 3029111. Telex: 908–3109. Fax. (061) 224566

*Spain

1986 Asociación del Cuerpo Nacional Veterinario, Calle Carranza 3–6°, 28004 Madrid. Tel. (91) 446 57 25

1987 Asociación Nacional de Veterinarios Titulares, Calle Plaza España, Edificio Espana, Planta 21, 28008 Madrid. Tel. (91) 247 97 17

1988 *Consejo General de Colegios Veterinarios de España, Calle Villanueva, 11–5ª Planta, 28001 Madrid. Tel. (91) 276 73 30

1989 Sociedad Veterinaria de Zootecnia de España, Calle Isabel La Católica 12–4° izda, 28013 Madrid. Tel (91) 247 18 38

†Sri Lanka

1990 The Sri Lanka Veterinary Association, c/o President – Dr M Kopalasum-tharum, Ministry of Rural Industrial Development, 45 St Michael's Road, Colombo 3

Sudan

1991 Sudan Veterinary Association, PO Box 2382, Khartoum

†Swaziland

1992 Swaziland Veterinary Association, Box 30, Manzini. Tel. 52204

*Sweden

1993   *Sveriges Veterinärförbund, Kungsholms Hamnplan 7, S-112 20 Stockholm. Tel. (08) 54 24 80

*Switzerland

1994   *Gesellschaft Schweizerischer Tierärzte/Société des Vétérinaires Suisses, Postfach 1518, 3001 Bern. Tel. (031) 24 55 00

Syria

1995   Syrian Medical Veterinary Association, Aleppo University, Aleppo

*Taiwan

1996   *The Chinese Society of Veterinary Science, 142 Chou-San Road, Taipei. Tel. (02) 3510231 (ext. 2753)

1997   Taiwan Association of Veterinary Medicine and Animal Husbandry, 250 Kao-Kuang Road, Taichung

1998   Taiwan Veterinary Association, RM 1, 8/F, 70 Chem-An West Road, Taipei. Tel. (02) 5224958, (02) 5624333

†*Tanzania

1999   *Tanzania Veterinary Association, PO Box 40452, Dar es Salaam. Tel. 63191

2000   Registrar, Veterinary of Tanzania, Dr V. B. Merdard, c/o Livestock Development Division, Ministry of Agriculture, PO Box 9152, Dar es Salaam

Thailand

2001   The Royal Veterinary Medical Association, 69/26 Athens Theater, Phya Thai Road, Bangkok 10400. Tel. 2528773

†Tonga

2002   Tonga Veterinary Association, c/o Regional Livestock Development Project, PO Box 14, Nuku'olofa

†*Trinidad and Tobago

2003   *Trinidad and Tobago Branch – Caribbean Veterinary Association, c/o Ministry of Agriculture, St Clair, Port-of-Spain, Trinidad and Tobago, West Indies. Tel. (809) 662–5678/62–22072/662–7113

*Tunisia

2004   *Conseil National de l'Ordre des Vétérinaires Tunisiens, 18 Rue de Russie, Tunis

*Turkey

2005   Türk Veteriner Hekimleri Derneği (Turkish Veterinary Medical Union), Sağlik Sokak, No. 21, Yenişehir, Ankara. Tel. (4) 1316274

2006   *Veteriner Isleri genel Mudurlugugida, Tarim ve Hayvancilik Bakanligi, Ankara

†*Uganda

2007   *Uganda Veterinary Association, Secretariat, PO Box 16338, Kampala

2008   Uganda Veterinary Board, Department of Veterinary Services and Animal Industry, PO Box 7141, Kampala

*Union of Soviet Socialist Republics

2009   All-Union V. I. Lenin Academy of Agricultural Sciences (Veterinary Department), 107078 Moscow, Bolshoi Kharitonevsky per. 21

2010   *Dr A. D. Tretyakov, Chief – Main Veterinary Department, State Agro-industrial Committee of the USSR, Moscow 107139, Orlikov per. 1/11. Tel. 2035917. Telex: 411258 ZERNO SU

†*United Kingdom

2011   *British Veterinary Association, 7 Mansfield Street, London W1M 0AT, England. Tel. 01–636 6541, 01–636 6544. Fax. 01–436 2970

2012   Royal College of Veterinary Surgeons, 32 Belgrave Square, London SW1X 8QP, England. Tel. 01–235 4971/2. Telegrams: CENTAURUM LONDON SW1

*United States of America

2013   *American Veterinary Medical Association, 930 North Meacham Road, Schaumberg, Illinois 60196. Tel. (312) 885 8070

*Uruguay

2014   Camara Uruguaya de Especialidades Medicinales, Plaza Cagancha 1342, Piso 2°, Esc 9, Montevideo. Tel. (2) 916816/985156

2015   *Sociedad de Medicina Veterinaria del Uruguay, Casa del Veterinario, Cerro Largo 1895, Montevideo. Tel. (2) 46174

Venezuela

2016   Federación de Colegios de Medicos Veterinarios de Venezuela, Avenida Matatlan, entre calles Caroni y Chama No. 29–18, Colinas de Bello Monte, Caracas

Yugoslavia

2017 Drustvo Veterinara SR Srbije, Bulevar JNA 18, 11000 Belgrade. Tel. (011) 684 597

2018 The Union of Veterinary Associations of SFR Yugoslavia, Sloserovestube 7, 41000 Zagreb

*Zaire

2019 *Association des Médecins Vétérinaires du Zaïre, B.P. 7298, Lubumbashi

†Zambia

2020 Zambia Veterinary Association, c/o Old Turf Showgrounds, Great East Road, Lusaka

†*Zimbabwe

2021 *Zimbabwe Veterinary Association, PO Box 8387, Causeway, Harare

2022 The Registrar, Council of Veterinary Surgeons, 4 Hill Road, Greendale, Harare. Tel. Harare 46254

VETERINARY ASSOCIATIONS AND SOCIETIES

2023 Academy of Veterinary Allergy, Department of Veterinary Clinical Medicine, University of Illinois, 1008 West Hazelwood Drive, Urbana, Illinois 61801, USA
Tel. (217) 333 2000
Contact point: President – Prof. Erwin Small
Publications: The veterinary allergist (quarterly); *Membership list* (occasional)

2024 Academy of Veterinary Cardiology, 25 Lumber Road, Roslyn, New York 11576, USA
Tel. (800) 652 2700, (516) 484 2700
Contact point: Executive Secretary – Dr Larry Patrick Tilley
Publications: Newsletter (quarterly); *Cardiac disease in the dog and cat: a diagnostic handbook*; *Membership directory* (biennial)

2025 Agricultural and Food Research Council, Central Office, Wiltshire Court, Farnsby Street, Swindon SN1 5AT, England
Tel. (0793) 514242. Fax. (0793) 481251
Contact point: Press Office
Publications: Annual report; *Index of agricultural and food research*; seminar reports, policy documents and occasional publications

2026   Agricultural Chemical and Animal Remedies Manufacturers' Association of New Zealand, 8th Floor, Cumberland House, 235–237 Willis Street, PO Box 27–283, Wellington 1, New Zealand
Tel. (04) 851 962. Fax. (04) 828 200
Contact point: Executive Director – C. Ian Blincoe
Publications: *NZ farm progress*; newsletters; membership list; *Safety with pesticides* (booklet); industry salary and benefits survey; production survey (based on quarterly invoice value); promotional materials

2027   Agricultural and Veterinary Chemicals Association of Australia, Private Bag 968, North Sydney, New South Wales 2059, Australia
Tel. (02) 963 7690. Telex: PROMED 177214. Fax. (02) 929 0213
Contact point: Executive Director – G. J. A. Digby
Publications: *Directory* (of members); *News in brief* (bimonthly); *Farm chemicals today* (occasional)

2028   American Academy of Veterinary and Comparative Toxicology, College of Veterinary Medicine, Drawer V, Mississippi State University, Mississippi 39762, USA
Contact point: Secretary-Treasurer – Dr C. Pat McCoy
Publications: *Veterinary and human toxicology*; Directory (annual, as a supplement to the journal)

2029   American Academy of Veterinary Dermatology, Box J126 JHMHC, College of Veterinary Medicine, University of Florida, Gainesville, Florida 32610, USA
Tel. (904) 392 3261
Contact point: President – Dr Gail Ann Kunkle
Publications: *Derm dialogue* (quarterly); *Newsletter* (biannual); *Membership directory* (annual)

2030   American Academy of Veterinary Nutrition, 452 Old Orchard Circle, Millersville, Maryland 21108, USA
Tel. (301) 981 3342
Contact point: Secretary/Treasurer – Dr Joseph E. Milligan
Publications: *Membership directory* (annual); *Newsletter* (biannual)

2031   American Academy of Veterinary Pharmacology and Therapeutics, Fort Dodge Laboratories, 800 5th Street NW, PO Box 518, Fort Dodge, Iowa 50501, USA
Tel. (515) 955 4600
Contact point: Secretary/Treasurer – Dr Daniel A. Gingerich
Publications: *Newsletter* (three a year); *Journal of veterinary pharmacology and therapeutics*

2032 American Academy of Veterinary Preventive Medicine, 1023 15th Street NW, Suite 300, Washington, DC 20005, USA
Contact point: Secretary – Dr E. L. Menning
Publications: Continuing education seminars with published proceedings

2033 American Animal Hospital Association, PO Box 150899, Denver, Colorado 80215, USA
Tel. (800) 252 2242, (303) 279 2500
Contact point: Director of Communication and Information – Marilyn L. Bergquist
Publications: Journal of the American Animal Hospital Association; Proceedings of the annual meetings (March or April) have been published since 1934 (55th, 1988); Atlases and manuals for ophthalmology, cytology, dermatology and cardiology; *Veterinary practice building: design starter kit* plus other materials on financial and practice management and staff training; *Directory of membership; Trends* (bimonthly magazine on practice management)

2034 American Association for Accreditation of Laboratory Animal Care, 9650 Rockville Pike, Bethesda, Maryland 20814, USA
Tel. (301) 571 1850
Contact point: Executive Director – Dr Albert E. New
Publications: AAALAC activities report (includes list of accredited units); *Brochure* (describes the organization of the association)
Corporation formed by thirty-one sponsoring member societies. Assesses standards for the maintenance and use of animals in institutions and grants accreditation to facilities meeting these standards of care.

2035 American Association of Animal Welfare Veterinarians, 502 North Eye Street, Tacoma, Washington 98403, USA
Tel. (206) 475 6750
Contact point: Secretary – Dr Bernard R. Pinckney

2036 American Association of Avian Pathologists, New Bolton Center, University of Pennsylvania, Kennett Square, Pennsylvania 19348, USA
Tel. (215) 444 5800 (ext. 257)
Contact point: Secretary-Treasurer – Dr Robert J. Eckroade
Publications: Avian diseases; Slide study sets (sixteen available, each comprises descriptive manuscript on the disease and about twenty colour slides); *Isolation and identification of avian pathogens* (2nd ed., 1980, 155pp.); *Avian disease manual* (2nd ed., 1983, 209pp.); *Avian histopathology* (1987, 93pp.); *A manual of methods for the laboratory diagnosis of avian chlamydiosis* (1987); *Proceedings: international symposium on Salmonella* (1984, 396pp.); *Proceedings: international symposium on Marek's disease* (1984)

2037   American Association of Bovine Practitioners, Box 2319, West Lafayette, Indiana 47906, USA

Tel. (317) 494 8560 (office), (317) 463 6063 (home)

Contact point: Executive Secretary – Dr Harold E. Amstutz

Publications: Newsletter (monthly); *AABP directory*; *Annual meeting program* (three months prior to meeting); *The bovine practitioner* (one month prior to meeting); *Proceedings of annual meeting* (four months after meeting) – 21st annual meeting 1988

2038   American Association of Equine Practitioners, 410 West Vine Street, Lexington, Kentucky 40507, USA

Tel. (606) 233 0147

Contact point: Executive Director – Michael J. Nolan

Publications: Proceedings of the annual convention (34th 1988) – includes cumulative subject and author indexes to papers published in all the proceedings; *Membership directory* (annual); *AAEP report* (bimonthly); abstracts (book of abstracts of articles on equine medicine published during the previous year); *AAEP Hospital planning manual*; *Official guide for determining the age of horses*; *Compendium of equine immunizing agents*; *Guide for veterinary service and judging of equestrian events*; *Index of equine medical research*; *International conference for equine sports medicine, August 11–13, 1986, San Diego* (1986, 124 + 35pp.)

2039   American Association of Feline Practitioners, Forest Hills Cat Hospital, 6902 Austin Street, Forest Hills, New York 11775, USA

Tel. (314) 846 6505

Contact point: Secretary-Treasurer – Jay Luger

Publication: Journal (biannual)

2040   American Association of Industrial Veterinarians, Box 1447, Sioux Falls, South Dakota 57117, USA

Tel. (605) 276 5741

Contact point: Dr Curtis Shafer

Publications: AAIV highlights (three a year); *Directory* (annual)

2041   American Association for Laboratory Animal Science, 70 Timber Creek Drive, Suite 5, Cordova, Tennessee 38018, USA

Tel. (901) 754 8620

Contact point: Executive Director – Donald W. Keene

Publications: Laboratory animal science; *AALAS bulletin*; *Membership directory*; *Effective animal care and use committees* (1987, 178pp.); *Manual for laboratory animal technicians* (1984, 248pp.); *Manual for assistant laboratory animal technicians* (1984, 454pp.); Other educational materials

2042   American Association of Small Ruminant Practitioners, 248 NW Garden Valley Road, Roseburg, Oregon 97470, USA

Tel. (503) 672 2829 (home), (502) 673 4403 (office)
Contact point: Executive Director – Dr Don E. Bailey
Publications: *Wool and wattles* (quarterly newsletter); Proceedings of the regional meetings and annual symposia

2043   American Association of Swine Practitioners, 5921 Fleur Drive, Des Moines, Iowa 50321, USA
Tel. (515) 285 7808
Contact point: Executive Secretary – Dr Tomas A. Neuzil
Publications: *Newsletter* (occasional); *Directory* (annual); Proceedings of the annual meetings

2044   American Association of Veterinary Anatomists, Department of Anatomy and Histology, College of Veterinary Medicine, Auburn University, Auburn, Alabama 36849, USA
Tel. (205) 826 4000
Contact point: President – James Ed Smallwood
Publications: *AAVA directory* (biennial); *Newsletter* (biannual)

2045   American Association of Veterinary Clinicians, 1024 Dublin Road, Columbus, Ohio 43215, USA
Tel. (614) 488 0617
Contact point: Secretary-Treasurer – Dr P. Mickell Davis
Publication: Directory of information on internship and residency programmes

2046   American Association of Veterinary Immunologists, USDA-ARS Animal Parasite Research Laboratory, PO Box 952, Auburn, Alabama 36830, USA
Contact point: Secretary-Treasurer – Dr P. H. Klesius
Publication: *Directory*

2047   American Association of Veterinary Laboratory Diagnosticians, PO Box 6023, Columbia, Missouri 65205, USA
Tel. (314) 882 6811
Contact point: Secretary-Treasurer – Dr Harvey S. Gosser
Publications: Proceedings of the annual meetings (31st 1988) now published in the *Journal of veterinary diagnostic investigation* (1988–, quarterly); international symposia (with the World Association of Veterinary Laboratory Diagnosticians); *Newsletter* (biannual)

2048   American Association of Veterinary Parasitologists, The Upjohn Company, Department 9690–190–41, Kalamazoo, Michigan 49001, USA
Tel. (616) 385 6523
Contact point: Executive Secretary-Treasurer – Dr S. D. 'Bud' Folz
Publications: *AAVP newsletter*; Proceedings of the annual meeting (33rd 1988); *Directory*

2049   American Association of Wildlife Veterinarians, Wyoming State Veterinary Laboratory, Department of Veterinary Science, 1190 Jackson Street, Laramie, Wyoming 82070, USA
Contact point: President – Dr Elisabeth S. Williams
Publications: Newsletter (quarterly); Membership directory

2050   American Association of Zoo Veterinarians, 34th Street and Girard Avenue, Philadelphia, Pennsylvania 19104, USA
Tel. (215) 243 1100
Contact point: Executive Director – Dr Wilbur B. Amand
Publications: Proceedings of the annual scientific conference; Directory of membership (annual); *Newsletter* (quarterly); *Journal of zoo animal medicine*

2051   American Board of Veterinary Practitioners, 9240 Highway 51 North, Southaven, Mississippi 38671, USA
Tel. (601) 393 4280 (office), (601) 342 0303 (home)
Contact point: Executive Secretary – Dr Bill R. Utroska
Publications: Brochure; *Diplomate directory* (biennial); *Newsletter* (quarterly); Newspage in the *Compendium on continuing education for the practicing veterinarian*

2052   American Board of Veterinary Toxicology, Texas Veterinary Medical Diagnostic Laboratory, 6610 Amarillo Boulevard West, Amarillo, Texas 79106, USA
Tel. (806) 353 7478
Contact point: Secretary-Treasurer – Dr John Haliburton
Publications: Directory of diplomates; Veterinary and human toxicology

2053   American College of Laboratory Animal Medicine, The Milton S. Hershey Medical Center, Pennsylvania State University, PO Box 850, Hershey, Pennsylvania 17033, USA
Tel. (717) 531 8462
Contact point: Secretary-Treasurer – Dr C. Max Lang
Publications: Newsletter (quarterly); *Membership directory*; sponsors a series of monographs on laboratory animal medicine (published by Academic Press)

2054   American College of Theriogenologists, 261 Large Animal Clinic, University of Illinois, 1008 West Hazelwood, Urbana, Illinois 61801, USA
Tel. (217) 333 2000
Contact point: Secretary – Dr Ted Lock
Publication: Directory (annual)

2055   American College of Veterinary Anesthesiologists, Department of Urban Practice, College of Veterinary Medicine, University of Tennessee, PO Box 1071, Knoxville, Tennessee 37901, USA
Tel. (615) 546 9240
Contact point: Executive Secretary-Treasurer – Dr Robert R. Paddleford
Publication: Veterinary surgery

2056   American College of Veterinary Dentistry, Animal Medical Center, 510 E. 62nd Street, New York 10021, USA
Tel. (212) 838 8100
Contact point: Dr Sandy Manfra Marretta
See also [2079]

2057   American College of Veterinary Dermatology, 595 Columbian Street, South Weymouth, Massachusetts 02190, USA
Tel. (617) 337 6622. Fax. (617) 329 7188
Contact point: Secretary – Dr Richard K. Anderson

2058   American College of Veterinary Internal Medicine, Suite C-1A, 620 N. Main Street, Blacksburg, Virginia 24060, USA
Tel. (703) 951 8543 or (800) 245 9081
Contact point: Secretary – Inge E. Pyle
Publications: Proceedings of the annual veterinary medical forum (6th 1988); *Journal of veterinary internal medicine*; Membership directory
The College has specialities in Internal Medicine, Cardiology, Oncology and Neurology.

2059   American College of Veterinary Microbiologists, National Animal Disease Center, USDA-ARS, PO Box 70, Ames, Iowa 50010, USA
Tel. (515) 239 8204
Contact point: Secretary-Treasurer – Dr George Lambert
Publication: Directory of diplomates

2060   American College of Veterinary Nutrition, Mark Morris Associates, 5500 SW 7th Street, Topeka, Kansas 66606, USA
Tel. (913) 273 5055
Contact point: Secretary-Treasurer – Dr Michael S. Hand

2061   American College of Veterinary Ophthalmologists, 10661 Ellis Avenue, Suite A, Fountain Valley, California 92708, USA
Tel. (714) 964 4644
Contact point: Secretary-Treasurer – Dr John Dan Lavach
Publications: Directory of diplomates; Newsletter

2062   American College of Veterinary Pathologists, 382 West Street Road, Kennett Square, Pennsylvania 19348, USA
Tel. (215) 444 3432
Contact point: Secretary-Treasurer – Dr Helen M. Acland
Publications: Proceedings of the annual scientific meeting (39th 1988); Membership directory; *Veterinary pathology*

2063   American College of Veterinary Preventive Medicine, 6649 Windson Ct, Columbia, Maryland 21044, USA
Tel. (301) 997 1782
Contact point: Secretary-Treasurer – Dr Lonnie King
Publications: List of diplomates is maintained; *Newsletter*
The College has a speciality section of Epidemiology.

2064   American College of Veterinary Radiology, PO Box 87, Glencoe, Illinois 60022, USA
Tel. (312) 835 1302
Contact point: Executive Secretary – Dr Myron Bernstein
Publications: The College's brochure contains a list of members; *Veterinary radiology*

2065   American College of Veterinary Surgeons, 405 Park Lane Drive, Champaign, Illinois 61820, USA
Contact point: Executive Secretary – Dr A. Schiller
Publications: Veterinary surgery; *Directory of diplomates*

2066   American College of Zoological Medicine, Department of Animal Health, US National Zoological Park, Washington, DC 20008, USA
Tel. (202) 673 4793
Contact point: Secretary – Dr Lyndsay G. Phillips Jr
Publication: Reference guide – a reading list to assist those studying for the College's examination

2067   American Embryo Transfer Association, Association Building, 9th and Minnesota, Hastings, Nebraska 68901, USA
Tel. (402) 462 9032
Contact point: Executive Vice President – Don Ellerbee
Publications: Annual membership roster; *Closer look* (quarterly); special bulletins and updates; Proceedings of the annual convention distributed at the meeting

2068   American Feed Industry Association, 1701 North Fort Myer Drive, Suite 1200, Arlington, Virginia 22209, USA
Tel. (703) 524 0810
Contact point: Corporate Secretary – Rex A. Runyon

Publications: The *AFIA publications catalog* describes the full range. Includes: newsletters (*Safetygram*; *Feedgram*; *Feedline*); Buyer's guide; *FDA inspection manual*; *Feed ingredient guide*; *Farm industry contacts for veterinarians*; *Feed manufacturing technology III* (1985, 608pp.); *Membership directory*; Catalogue of audiovisuals (mostly on safety); *Liquid feed symposia proceedings* and *Nutrition council proceedings*

2069   American Heartworm Society, Executive Office, 808 17th Street NW, Suite 200, Washington, DC 20006, USA
Tel. (202) 223 9669
Contact point: Administrator – Ralph Johnson
Publications: *Proceedings of the heartworm symposium* (triennial – most recent 1989); *AHS bulletin* (quarterly); *Recommended procedures for the treatment and prevention of heartworm disease; Heartworm disease in dogs* (brochure)

2070   American Holistic Veterinary Medical Association, 2214 Old Emmorton Road, Bel Air, Maryland 21014, USA
Tel. (301) 838 7778
Contact point: Executive Secretary – Dr Carvel G. Tiekert
Publications: *Newsletter* (quarterly); Proceedings of annual conference (1988–)

2071   American Humane Association, 9725 East Hampden, Denver, Colorado 80231, USA
Tel. (303) 695 0811
Contact point: Information/Education Coordinator – Carol Moulton
Publications: *The advocate* (quarterly); legislation alerts (occasional); *Animal Humane shoptalk* (bimonthly); *Animal organizations and services directory 1988–89*; *Operational guide for animal care and control agencies*; *Annual report*; educational materials

2072   American Kennel Club, 51 Madison Avenue, New York 10010, USA
Tel. (212) 696 8245
Contact point: Library Director – Roberta Vesley
Library of over 15,000 volumes. The library provides a variety of other information services.

2073   American Pet Products Manufacturers Association, 60 East 42nd Street, New York 10165, USA
Tel. (212) 867 2290
Contact point: Executive Director – Jules Schwimmer
Publication: Survey of attitudes and buying habits of pet owners (1988, 400pp.)

2074   American Society for the Prevention of Cruelty to Animals, 441 East 92nd Street, New York 10128, USA
Tel. (212) 876 7700
Contact point: President – Dr John F. Kullberg
Publications: Report (quarterly); educational material on animal care and welfare; has a library on animal-related information

2075   American Society of Laboratory Animal Practitioners, 182 Grinter Hall, University of Florida, Gainesville, Florida 32611, USA
Tel. (904) 392 9917
Contact point: Secretary-Treasurer – Dr Farol N. Tomson
Publications: Synapse (quarterly); list of members

2076   American Society of Veterinary Ophthalmology, 1528 Shalamar, Stillwater, Oklahoma 74074, USA
Tel. (405) 377 2134
Contact point: Secretary-Treasurer – Dr A. J. Quinn
Publications: Directory (annual); Proceedings of the annual meeting; *Newsletter* (occasional)

2077   American Society of Veterinary Physiologists and Pharmacologists, College of Veterinary Medicine, Virginia Tech Campus, Blacksburg, Virginia 24061, USA
Contact point: Secretary-Treasurer – Dr R. B. Talbot
Publications: Newsletter (bimonthly); roster of members

2078   American Veterinary Computer Society, Drawer V, Mississippi State University, Mississippi State 39762, USA
Tel. (601) 325 3432
Contact point: Secretary-Treasurer – Dr Stephen Waldhalm
Publications: Proceedings of the symposia on computer applications in veterinary medicine (6th symposium 1989); *Newsletter*

2079   American Veterinary Dental College, School of Veterinary Medicine, University of Pennsylvania, 3850 Spruce Street, Philadelphia, Pennsylvania 19104, USA
Tel. (215) 898 3350
Contact point: Secretary – Dr Colin E. Harvey
Publications: Journal of veterinary dentistry; *Directory*; *Proceedings of the 1988 Academy of Veterinary Dentistry meeting*
The meetings of the College are held jointly with those of the Academy of Veterinary Dentistry.

2080   American Veterinary Distributors Association, 106 West 11th Street, Kansas City, Missouri 64105, USA
Tel. (816) 221 5909
Contact point: Executive Director – Mr James Fries
Publication: Schedule of conventions

2081   American Veterinary Epidemiology Society, School of Public Health, University of Texas Health Science Center, Houston, Texas 77225, USA
Tel. (713) 792 4451 or (713) 781 3653
Contact point: President – Dr James H. Steele

2082   American Veterinary Exhibitors Association, PO Box 19006, Birmingham, Alabama 35219, USA
Tel. (205) 979 0830
Contact point: Executive Director – Bob Willis
Publications: Newsletter (quarterly); *Schedule of conventions* (annual)

2083   American Veterinary History Society, Veterinary Microbiology, College of Veterinary Medicine, Iowa State University, Ames, Iowa 50011, USA
Tel. (515) 294 2607
Contact point: Secretary-Treasurer – Dr R. Allen Packer
Publication: Veterinary heritage (two per year), which contains papers given at the annual meeting

2084   American Veterinary Neurology Association, Department of Small Animal Medicine and Surgery, Auburn University, Alabama 36849, USA
Tel. (205) 826 4690
Contact point: Secretary-Treasurer – Dr Donald C. Sorjonen
Publication: Newsletter (biannual)

2085   American Veterinary Society of Animal Behaviour, Department of Physiology, New York State College of Veterinary Medicine, Cornell University, Ithaca, New York 14853, USA
Tel. (607) 253 3450
Contact point: President – Dr Katherine A. Houpt
Publication: Newsletter (occasional)

2086   American Veterinary Society for Computer Medicine, PO Box 1618, Joshua Tree, California 92252, USA
Tel. (619) 365 2221
Contact point: Executive Director – Dr H. A. Carper
Publication: The vet bytes back (monthly)

2087   Animal Air Transportation Association, Inc., PO Box 441110, Fort Washington, Maryland 20744, USA
Tel. (301) 292 1970. Telex: 4997385 AATA. Fax. (301) 292 1787
Contact point: Executive Director – Dale L. Anderson
Publications: International conference (annual, 14th Amsterdam 1988); *AATA newsletter*; *AATA handbook* (with supplements); *Who's who in animal transportation*

2088   Animal Diseases Research Association, Moredun Institute, 408 Gilmerton Road, Edinburgh EH17 7JH, Scotland
Tel. 031–664 3262
Contact point: Secretary – M. J. Mackenzie, or Liaison Officer – Ken Brown
Publications: Report and Accounts (annual); *ADRA newsletter* (at least three per year); leaflets on animal diseases

2089 Animal Health Distributors' Association, 41 Barrack Square, Martlesham Heath, Ipswich, Suffolk IP5 7RF, England
Tel. (0473) 625891. Fax. (0473) 610652
Contact point: Chief Executive – Roger Dawson
Publications: Animal health distributor (quarterly); *Members' circulars* (occasional); *Farmers record book: animal medicine administration record*

2090 Animal Health Institute, PO Box 1417–D50, 119 Oronoco Street, Alexandria, Virginia 22313, USA
Tel. (703) 684 0011. Fax. (703) 684 0125
Contact point: Vice President, Public Information – Mr S. Kimbel
Publications: Animal health letter (formerly *Animal drug news* – bimonthly); *Media resources book*; *Annual report*; *Net sales survey* (annual)

2091 Animal Health Trade Associations Group, PO Box 3, Sheringham, Norfolk NR26 8LZ, England
Tel. (0263) 824948
Contact point: Secretary – Dennis S. Papworth
Publication: Annual report
Maintains a list of qualified persons authorized to sell veterinary drugs not on the general sale list, organizes suitable training courses for such personnel, and maintains and reviews the MAFF *Code of practice for merchants selling or supplying veterinary drugs*.

2092 Animal Health Trust, Lanwades Hall, Kennett, Newmarket, Suffolk CB8 7PN, England
Tel. (0638) 751030. Telex: 265871 84DDS177
Contact point: General Secretary – A. V. Payne
Publications: Animal Health Trust news; *Annual report*; *Equiline*

2093 Animal Welfare Institute, PO Box 3650, Georgetown Station, Washington, DC 20007, USA
Tel. (202) 337 2332
Contact point: John Gleiber or Cathy Liss
Publications: AWI quarterly; a variety of educational items on animal welfare

2094 Association of American Veterinary Medical Colleges, 1522 K Street NW, Suite 834, Washington, DC 20005, USA
Tel. (202) 371 9195
Contact point: Executive Director – Dr Billy E. Hooper
Publication: Journal of veterinary medical education (biannual)

2095 Association of Animal Allergic Veterinarians, Department of Veterinary Microbiology and Preventive Medicine, College of Veterinary Medicine, Iowa State University, Ames, Iowa 50011, USA
Tel. (515) 294 5158
Contact point: Dr Loren A. Will

2096   Association of Avian Veterinarians, PO Box 299, East Northport, New York 11731, USA
Tel. (516) 757 6320
Contact point: Secretary – Dr Robert Irmiger
Publications: Laboratory manual for avian hematology (1984); *AAV today*; Proceedings of the annual seminars and meetings

2097   Association of British Veterinary Acupuncture, East Park Cottage, Handcross, Sussex RH17 6BD, England
Tel. (0444) 400213
Contact point: Secretary – Mrs Jill Hewson
Publication: Newsletter

2098   Association for Comparative Haematology, ICI Central Toxicology Laboratories, Alderley Park, Macclesfield, Cheshire SK10 4TJ, England
Contact point: Secretary – Mrs Sue Howson
Publications: Directory (annual); *Atlas of comparative haematology* (in preparation); *Journal of comparative haematology* (1990–)

2099   Association for Equine Sports Medicine, 176 West Pomona Avenue, Monrovia, California 91016, USA
Tel. (818) 359 3410
Contact point: President – Dr Rick M. Arthur
Publications: AESM quarterly (newsletter); Proceedings of the annual meetings (8th 1988); *Annual report*; *Membership list*
Organizes the international conferences on equine physiology and on equine sports medicine.

2100   Association of Institutes of Tropical Veterinary Medicine, Institute for Parasitology and Tropical Veterinary Medicine, Free University of Berlin, Konigsweg 65, D-1000 Berlin 37, Federal Republic of Germany
Contact point: Secretary – Prof. Dr J. E. Huhn
Publications: Proceedings of the triennial international conferences (6th Wageningen 1989)

2101   Association of Poultry Vaccine Manufacturers UK, 11 Cunningham Avenue, St Albans, Hertfordshire AL1 1JJ, England
Tel. (0727) 53485
Contact point: Secretary General – P. W. Daykin
Holds meetings every few months, hosted by member companies. Permanent working groups have been established in association with MAFF (Weybridge).

2102   Association of Primate Veterinarians, Hazleton Laboratories America, Inc., 9200 Leesburg Turnpike, Vienna, Virginia 22180, USA
Tel. (703) 893 5400 (ext. 381). Telex: 899436 HAZLABS VINA
Contact point: Secretary – Dr Dan W. Delgard
Publication: Newsletter (once or twice yearly)

2103   Association of State Veterinary Officers, MAFF, Block C, Government
Buildings, Whittington Road, Worcester WR5 2LQ, England
Tel. (0905) 763355 (office), (0386) 832258 (home)
Contact point: Honorary Secretary – Mr F. A. Eames
Publication: Forum (two or three times a year)

2104   The Association for the Study of Animal Behaviour, Biology Building,
University of Sussex, Falmer, Brighton BN1 9QG, England
Contact point: Membership Secretary
Publications: Animal behaviour; *ASAB newsletter* (three per year)

2105   Association of Teachers of Veterinary Public Health and Preventive
Medicine, Department of Pathological Sciences, College of Veterinary Medi-
cine, University of Wisconsin, Wisconsin 53706, USA
Contact point: Secretary-Treasurer – Dr Chester Bruce Thomas
Publications: Newsletter; Third and fourth international symposia on veterinary
epidemiology and economics

2106   Association of Veterinarians for Animal Rights, 15 Dutch Street, Suite
500-A, New York 10038, USA
Tel. (212) 962 7055
Contact point: Executive Director – Susan Regan
Publications: Newsletter (bimonthly); position statements on animal welfare issues
(twenty-four currently available)

2107   Association of Veterinarians in Industry (The Horseshoe Club), Hoechst
UK Ltd, Walton Manor, Milton Keynes, Buckinghamshire MK7 7AJ,
England
Tel. (0908) 665050 (work), (0604) 769926 (home)
Contact point: Honorary Secretary – Mr N. J. Everitt
Publications: Biannual symposia (8th – 1987: *Product development in animal health*);
Newsletter (biannual)

2108   Association of Veterinary Anaesthetists of Great Britain and Ireland,
Department of Pharmacology, University of Cambridge, Hills Road, Cam-
bridge CB2 2QD, England
Tel. (0223) 336941
Contact point: Secretary – Dr Andrea M. Nolan
Publication: Journal of the Association of Veterinary Anaesthetists

2109   Association for Veterinary Clinical Pharmacology and Therapeutics,
Department of Clinical Veterinary Medicine, Madingley Road, Cambridge,
CB3 0ES, England
Contact point: Secretary – Dr R. J. Evans
Publications: Proceedings of the meetings; *Journal of veterinary pharmacology and
therapeutics*

2110   Association of Veterinary Students, c/o British Veterinary Association

2111   Association of Veterinary Teachers and Research Workers, AFRC Institute of Animal Physiology and Genetics Research, Babraham Hall, Cambridge CB2 4AT, England
Tel. (0223) 832312 (ext. 423). Fax. (0223) 833676
Contact point: Secretary – Dr F. A. Harrison
Publications: Book of abstracts distributed at the annual conference; *Newsletter* (annual)

2112   Association of Veterinary Technician Educators, Wayne State University – DLAR, 540 East Canfield, Detroit, Michigan 48201, USA
Tel. (313) 577 1156
Contact point: President – Dr Karen Hrapkiewicz
Publications: *Newsletter* (twice a year); biennial symposia on veterinary technician training (latest 1989); slide-tape programme on training and using veterinary technicians

2113   Association for Women Veterinarians, 32205 Allison Drive, Union City, California 94587, USA
Tel. (415) 471 8379
Contact point: Secretary – Dr Chris Stone Payne
Publications: *Roster of women veterinarians*; *Bulletin* (quarterly)
Specializes in information on health issues affecting women veterinarians.

2114   Australian College of Veterinary Scientists, c/o AVA House, PO Box 34, Indooroopilly, Queensland 4068, Australia
Tel. (07) 378 8038. Fax. (07) 878 1048
Contact point: Honorary Secretary – Bryan A. Woolcock
The College holds examinations of professional proficiency in order to determine qualification for membership and fellowship of the College. The College has eleven Chapters and each of these, plus the College, holds meetings and seminars. The College and most of the Chapters also produce newsletters.

2115   Australian Equine Veterinary Association, PO Box 371, Artarmon, New South Wales 2064, Australia
Tel. (02) 411 5342. Fax. (02) 411 5089
Contact point: Administrative Officer – Audrey M. Best
Publications: *Newsletter* (quarterly); Proceedings of the Bain-Fallon lectures (10th 1988); *Guide to examination of horses*

2116   The Blue Cross, The Animals Hospital, 1 Hugh Street, Victoria, London SW1V 1QQ, England
Tel. 01–834 5556 and 4224
Contact point: Secretary – Paul Hannon

2117   British Association of Feed Supplement Manufacturers, Mill House, The
   Hill, Cranbrook, Kent TN17 3AH, England
Tel. (0580) 714204. Telex: 957571 REXENG G
Contact point: Consultant Secretary – W. H. Beaumont
Publication: BAFSM guide to good feed supplement manufacturing practice

2118   British Association of Homeopathic Veterinary Surgeons, Chinham
   House, Stanford in the Vale, Faringdon, Oxon SN7 8NQ, England
Tel. (03677) 324
Contact point: Secretary – C. E. I. Day
Publications: Newsletter (biannual); audiotapes of homeopathy talks/lectures

2119   British Association of Veterinary Homeopathic Surgeons, c/o The British
   Homeopathic Association, 27a Devonshire Street, London W1N 1RJ, England
Tel. 01–925 2163

2120   British Cattle Veterinary Association, Pickworth Lodge, Nr. Sleaford,
   Lincolnshire NE34 0TL, England
Tel. (05297) 495
Contact point: Membership Secretary – Mrs J. S. Watson
Publications: Proceedings (annual); *Newsletters* (quarterly)

2121   British Chelonia Group, 29 Victoria Street, Staple Hill, Bristol BS16 5JP,
   England
Contact point: General Secretary – Mrs Diana Desmond
Publication: Newsletter; *Testudo*

2122   British Equine Veterinary Association, Hartham Park, Corsham,
   Wiltshire SN13 0QB, England
Tel. (0249) 715723. Telex: 44642. Fax. (0249) 715920
Contact point: Administrative Secretary – Mrs Andi E. Ewen
Meetings: Four scientific meetings per year (annual congress in September)
Publications: Equine veterinary journal; *Bulletin*; *Newsletter*; Proceedings of the 1987
   annual congress available on tape

2123   British Goat Society, 34–36 Fore Street, Bovey Tracey, nr. Newton
   Abbot, Devon TQ13 9AD, England
Tel. (0626) 833168
Contact point: Secretary – Susan Knowles
Publications: Herd book; *Year book* (both annual); *Goats today* (formerly *British Goat
   Society journal*, eleven per year)

2124   British Hedgehog Preservation Society, Knowbury House, Knowbury,
   Ludlow, Shropshire SY8 3LQ, England
Tel. (0584) 890287
Contact point: Education Officer – L. H. C. Sharp

Publications: Newsletter (biannual); Leaflets and educational packs (including *Treating sick hedgehogs* (1987, 12pp.) – for veterinary surgeons)

2125   British Horse Society, British Equestrian Centre, Stoneleigh, Kenilworth, Warwickshire CV8 2LR, England
Tel. (0203) 696697. Telex: 311152 BEFKEN. Fax. (0203) 696685
Contact point: Director – Colonel Tim Eastwood; Press/Public Relations Officer – Mrs Ceri S. Burgum
Publications: Members yearbook; *Horseshoe* (three per year); County newsletters and magazines; *The manual of stable management* (Threshold Books, 1988–, 6 vols); Information leaflets

2126   British Laboratory Animals Veterinary Association, Pfizer Central Research, Ramsgate Road, Sandwich, Kent, England
Tel. (0304) 616391
Contact point: Honorary Secretary – Mr A. J. Webb
Publication: Blavanews (biannual)

2127   British Small Animal Veterinary Association, Registration Office, 5 St George's Terrace, Cheltenham, Gloucestershire GL50 3PT, England
Tel. (0242) 584354
Contact point: Honorary Secretary – Mr Fred Nind
Publications: Journal of small animal practice; Congress and membership handbook (annual); *BSAVA news*; BSAVA manuals (each book on a topic of interest to small animal practitioners); *The export and import of dogs and cats: a handbook of regulations* (Edited by C. E. Woodrow, 2nd ed., 1975, 77pp.)
The BSAVA has a network of thirteen active regional groups. There are also specialist groups for the following areas: Neurology (Secretary – G. C. Skeritt. Tel. 051-709 6022 (ext. 3194)), Ophthalmology (Secretary – Dr R. M. Lightfoot. Tel. (0625) 524072), Orthopaedics (Secretary – P. E. Watkins. Tel. (0272) 303030), Quarantine (Secretary – E. R. Strachan. Tel. (0342) 23072)) and Avian (Secretary – A. K. Jones. Tel. (0293) 551158)

2128   British Society of Animal Production, PO Box 3, Penicuik, Midlothian EH26 0RZ, Scotland
Tel. (031) 445 4508
Contact point: Honorary Secretary – Dr R. G. Gunn
Publications: Animal production; BSAP Occasional Publications (proceedings of symposia) – most recent no. 11 *Pig housing and environment*, 1987, 148pp. Publications Series); *Guidelines for the use of animals in research* (1987)

2129   British Veterinary Acupuncture Association, Stockton Close, Woodbridge Road, Guildford, Surrey GU1 1HR, England
Tel. (0483) 61255
Contact point: J. Nicol

2130   British Veterinary Association Animal Welfare Foundation, 7 Mansfield Street, London W1M 0AT, England
Tel. 01–636 6541
Contact point: Director – David A. Paterson
Publications: Symposia: Priorities in animal welfare; Pain relief in animals; Transport of animals; Animals in captivity; Animal diseases

2131   British Veterinary Dental Association, 82 Sketty Road, Enfield, Middlesex EN1 3SF, England
Tel. 01–367 5859
Contact point: Secretary – Lesley A. Johnson
Publications: Newsletter; membership includes associate membership of the American Veterinary Dental College and receipt of its *Journal of veterinary dentistry*

2132   British Veterinary Dermatology Study Group, Faculty of Veterinary Medicine, University College – Dublin, Ballsbridge, Dublin 4, Ireland
Tel. (01) 687988
Contact point: Secretary – Prof. K. P. Baker
Publication: Dermatology news letter (occasional) contains copies of papers presented at the meetings (held at least twice annually, sometimes in collaboration with the European Society of Veterinary Dermatology)

2133   British Veterinary Hospitals Association, 43 The Mall, Ealing, London W5 3TJ, England
Tel. 01–567 2724
Contact point: Secretary – Anthony Young
Publications: Manual of standards for small animal veterinary hospitals; *Manual of standards for equine veterinary hospitals*; *Practice development questionnaire*; *BVHA guide to the Health & Safety at Work Act*; *Newsletter* (contains reports of recent meetings and future programme)

2134   British Veterinary Nursing Association, Unit C3, The Seedbed Centre, Coldharbour Road, Harlow, Essex CM19 5AF, England
Tel. (0279) 450567
Contact point: Public Relations Officer – Mrs J. M. Turner
Publications: The veterinary nursing journal; *Veterinary nursing: the first twenty-five years* (1986)

2135   British Veterinary Poultry Association, Roche Products Ltd, PO Box 7, Welwyn Garden City, Hertfordshire AL7 3AY, England
Tel. (0707) 328128 (ext. 3220)
Contact point: Honorary Secretary – Mr Nigel J. A. Lodge

2136   British Veterinary Radiological Association, Royal Veterinary College, Hawkshead House, Hawkshead Lane, North Mymms, Hatfield, Hertfordshire AL9 7JA, England
Tel. (0707) 55486 (ext. 395)
Contact point: Honorary Secretary – Stephen A. May
Publications: Abstracts of presentations at the meetings – *BVRA abstracts* (1988, **10**); *Newsletter*; *Membership list*

2137   British Veterinary Zoological Society, Penthouse, Braxfield Court, St Anne's Road West, St Anne's on Sea FY8 1LQ, England
Tel. (0253) 720727. Fax. (0253) 32289
Contact point: President – Michael J. Fielding
Publications: Newsletter (twice yearly); Proceedings of the larger symposia (*Proceedings of the 25th anniversary symposium, 18–20th April 1986: Exotic animals in the eighties*. Edited by P. W. Scott and A. G. Greenwood, London: BVA, 1986, 164pp.)

2138   British Wildlife Rehabilitation Council, 1 Pemberton Close, Aylesbury, Buckinghamshire HP21 7NY, England
Tel. (0296) 29860
Contact point: Sue Stocker
Publications: Proceedings of the annual symposia
The Wildlife Hospital Trust is based at the same address and also offers assistance to the veterinary profession on wildlife topics. They take in and treat all species of British wildlife. Publications to date: *Drugs and dosages for use on hedgehogs*; *The care and rehabilitation of injured badgers*; *The complete hedgehog* (By L. Stocker. London: Chatto & Windus, 1987, 176pp.).

2139   Canadian Animal Health Institute, 8 Church Street, PO Box 291, Manotick, Ontario K0A 2N0, Canada
Tel. (613) 692 2861
Contact point: Executive Secretary – Dr Julius F. Frank
Publications: Communiqué (newsletter); informative brochures on the activities of the animal health industry

2140   Canine Eye Registration Foundation, 2025 Lyon Street, San Francisco, California 94115, USA
Tel. (415) 567 2277
Contact point: Secretary-Treasurer – Dolly B. Trauner
Maintains a registry of pure-bred dogs asymptomatic of hereditary eye diseases and promotes and sponsors research into the major hereditary diseases.

2141   Canine Veterinary Group, Copse End, 42 Windsor Road, Bray, Berkshire SL6 2EP, England
Contact point: Secretary – S. P. Dean

2142   Caribbean Veterinary Association, c/o Ministry of Food Production, Marine Exploitation, Forestry and the Environment, St Claire Circle, Port-of-Spain, Trinidad, West Indies
Contact point: Dr E. P. I. Cazabon
The Regional Representative for the Canada/Caribbean Region to the Commonwealth Veterinary Association is Dr J. L. Robinson (Olivers Livestock Station, PO Box 1282, Antigua, West Indies. Tel. 463–1759).

2143   The Cats Protection League, 17 Kings Road, Horsham, West Sussex RH13 5PP, England. Tel. (0403) 65566
Contact point: Director – George Stiller
Publications: The cat (bimonthly); and many brochures and leaflets for cat owners

2144   Centre for Animal Welfare Studies, 84 Hare Lane, Claygate, Esher, Surrey KT10 0QU, England. Tel. (0372) 66560
Contact point: Director – David J. Coffey
Publication: CAWS: Journal of the Centre for Animal Welfare Studies (1988–)

2145   Centre for Tropical Veterinary Medicine, University of Edinburgh, Veterinary Field Station, Easter Bush, Roslin, Midlothian EH25 9RG, Scotland
Tel. 031–445 2001. Telex: 727442 UNIVED G
Contact point: Director
Publications: Tropical animal health and production; *Draught animal news* (biannual); Newsletter (biannual); information leaflets (twenty per year); laboratory handbooks; *Milk production in developing countries* (1985, 555pp.)

2146   Codex Committee on Residues of Veterinary Drugs in Foods, c/o Food and Drug Administration, Center for Veterinary Medicine, 5600 Fishers Lane, Rockville, Maryland 20857, USA
Tel. (301) 443 3450
Contact point: Chairman – Dr Gerald B. Guest
Holds annual meetings attended by representatives of national and international organizations (2nd session 1987; 3rd session 1988; both held in Washington, DC).

2147   Commission of the European Communities, Office for Official Publications, 5 Rue du Commerce, L-2985 Luxembourg
Tel. 49 92 81. Telex: PUBOF LU 1324 B
Publications: Books, statistical works, official publications, conferences and many other documents. These are described in *Publications of the European Communities* (quarterly with annual cumulation)
The Commission has sales and subscription agents in many countries (UK: HMSO; USA: European Community Information Service, 2100 M Street NW, Suite 207, Washington, DC 20037. Tel. (202) 862 9500). There are information offices in each member country (UK: 8 Storey's Gate, Westminster, London SW1P 3AT. Tel. 01–222 8122. Information Office of the European Parliament, 2 Queen Anne's Gate, London SW14 9AA. Tel. 01–222 0411).

2148   Commonwealth Veterinary Association, 35 Lynwood Place, Guelph, Ontario N1G 2V9, Canada
Tel. (519) 824 1304
Contact point: Secretary – Dr J. Archibald (or President – Mr J. T. Blackburn c/o BVA)
Publications: First steps in veterinary science (book); *Commonwealth Veterinary Association news* (biannual); model Veterinary Surgeons Acts and model Association Byelaws

2149   Comparative and Veterinary Immunology Group, AFRC Institute for Animal Health, Compton, Newbury, Berkshire RG16 0NN, England
Tel. (0635) 578411
Contact point: Secretary – Dr Joe Brownlie
Affiliated to the British Society of Immunology. Biannual workshops and meetings are advertised in BSI newsletters. Next major meeting the second international symposium of veterinary immunology (Hanover 1989).

2150   Conference of Public Health Veterinarians, 274 East Torrence Road, Columbus, Ohio 43214, USA
Tel. (614) 447 1420
Contact point: Secretary – Dr Paul C. Bartlett
Publication: Newsletter (quarterly – includes a list of members)

2151   Conference of Research Workers in Animal Disease, Department of Microbiology, College of Veterinary Medicine, Colorado State University, Fort Collins, Colorado 80523, USA
Tel. (303) 491 5740
Contact point: Secretary-Treasurer – Dr Robert P. Ellis
Publication: Abstracts of papers presented at the annual meeting (69th, 1988)

2152   Consultation Mondiale de l'Industrie de la Santé Animale/World Consultation of the Animal Health Industry (COMISA), c/o Sandoz Pharmaceuticals, Sandoz House, Feltham, Middlesex TW13 4EP, England
Tel. 01–890 1366. Telex: 8954032 SDZLON G. Fax. 01–890 1331
Contact point: Secretary – Dr David J. S. Miller (President – Dr James Gillin)

2153   CTA, *see* Technical Centre for Agricultural and Rural Cooperation [2283]

2154   The Delta Society: Interaction of People, Animals, Environment, PO Box 1080, Century Building, Suite 303, 321 Burnett Avenue South, Renton, Washington 98057, USA
Tel. (206) 226 7357
Contact point: Executive Director – Linda M. Hines
Publications: Anthrozoos (quarterly); *Interactions* (semiannual); *People–animals–environment* (biannual)

2155   The Donkey Sanctuary (*and* International Donkey Protection Trust *and* The Slade Centre), Sidmouth, Devon, EX10 0NU, England
Tel. (03955) 6391 and 78222. Telex: 42880 IDPT G
Contact point: Administrator – Mrs E. D. Svendsen MBE

2156   Eastern States Veterinary Association, 2614 NW 34th Street, Suite 4, Gainesville, Florida 32608, USA
Tel. (904) 375 5672
Contact point: Conference Co-ordinator – Dr Colin F. Burrows
Holds an annual veterinary conference (6th, 1989)

2157   Equine Behaviour Study Circle, Grove Cottage, Brinkley, Newmarket, Suffolk, England
Tel. (063) 876 502
Contact point: Secretary – Mrs O. Way
Publication: Equine behaviour (two a year)

2158   Equine Nutrition and Physiology Society, 910 Agricultural Science Building – South, University of Kentucky, Lexington, Kentucky 40383, USA
Contact point: Secretary-Treasurer – Dr Stephen G. Jackson
Publications: Proceedings of the biennial meetings (10th, 1987 – some papers published in *Journal of equine veterinary science* **8** (1988): 237–69)

2159   European Association for Animal Production, Corse Trieste 67, 00198 Rome, Italy
Tel. (06) 830785
Contact point: Secretary General – Prof. Dr J. G. Boyazoglu
Publications: Livestock production science; Proceedings of the annual meetings (40th Dublin 1989) and of various special symposia (available from PUDOC) e.g. *Control of regulation of animal growth* (1988, 200pp., EAAP Publication no. 36)

2160   European Association of Establishments for Veterinary Education, University of Glasgow Veterinary School, Bearsden Road, Glasgow G61 1QH, Scotland
Tel. 041–339 8855 (ext. 5772/3). Fax. 041–942 7215
Contact point: Professor Hugh M. Pirie
Publications: Two books are in preparation: *Register of establishments* (describing the forty-five veterinary schools in Western Europe) and *Curricula* (data on the organization of subjects within the curriculum of each school and data on the hours of teaching)

2161   European Association of Fish Pathologists, Fish Health Service, Eintrachtweg 17, D-3000 Hanover 1, Federal Republic of Germany
Contact point: General Secretary – Dr H-J. Schlotfeldt
Publication: Bulletin of the European Association of Fish Pathologists (quarterly)

2162   European Association of State Veterinary Officers, c/o MAFF, Hook Rise South, Tolworth, Surbiton, Surrey KT6 7NF, England
Tel. 01-337 6611
Contact point: Secretary – Janet M. Bach

2163   European Association of Veterinary Anatomists, c/o Anatomisches Institut der Tierärztlichen Hochschule, Abteilung für Histologie, Bischofsholer Damm 15, D-3000 Hanover, Federal Republic of Germany
Contact point: Secretary General – Prof. Dr R. Shwarz

2164   European Association for Veterinary Pharmacology and Toxicology, Department of Veterinary Pharmacology, Pharmacy and Toxicology, Faculty of Veterinary Medicine, Utrecht, PO Box 80176, 3508 TD Utrecht, The Netherlands
Tel. (030) 733614
Contact point: President – Prof. Dr A. S. J. P. A. M. Van Miert
Publications: *Journal of veterinary pharmacology and therapeutics*; International congresses are held every three years (4th congress, Budapest, 1988) with published proceedings: *Comparative veterinary pharmacology, toxicology and therapy* (MTP Press, 1986), *Veterinary pharmacology and therapeutics* (MTP Press, 1983), *Trends in veterinary pharmacology and therapeutics* (Elsevier, 1980). A workshop devoted to the ruminant forestomach has also been published – *Physiological and pharmacological aspects of the reticulo-rumen* (Martinus Nijhoff, 1987)

2165   European Federation of Manufacturers of Additives in Animal Nutrition (FEFANA), Roonstrasse 5, 5300 Bonn 2, Federal Republic of Germany
Tel. (02 28) 35 24 00. Telex: 886391 AWT D. Fax. (02 28) 36 13 97
Contact point: Secretary General – Dr G. Behm
Publication: 1988 membership directory

2166   European Federation of Parasitologists, The National Swedish Environment Board, Marine Section, Box 584, S-740 71 Oregrund, Sweden
Contact point: Secretary – Jan Thulin
Initiates and organizes a European multicolloquium of parasitology (EMOP V Hungary, 1988).

2167   European Federation of Animal Health (FEDESA), Rue Defacqz 1, Boîte 8, 1050 Brussels, Belgium
Tel. (02) 537 21 25. Telex: 24785. Fax. (02) 537 00 49
Contact point: Administrative Officer – Brigitte Biedermann
Publications: Newsletter; *FEDESA update* (bimonthly) – contains news on the European animal health scene

2168   European Federation of Pharmaceutical Industries' Associations (FEAIP), Avenue Louise 250, Boîte 91, 1050 Brussels, Belgium
Tel. (02) 640 68 15. Telex: 64405 EFPIA B. Fax. (02) 640 19 81
Contact point: Animal Health Committee Chairman – Dr D. J. S. Miller

2169   European Feed Manufacturer's Federation (FEFAC), 223 Rue de la Loi, Boîte 3, B-1040 Brussels, Belgium
Tel. (02) 230 87 15. Telex: 23993. Fax. (322) 230 5722
Contact point: Secretary General – A. P. Namur
Publications: Panorama (occasional newsletter); *Feed and food* (annual compendium of statistics); List of members; *Directory: world feed industry associations* (published by the International Feed Industry Federation); *FEFAC: 25 years at the service of the European compound feed industry* (1984, 45pp.)
The International Feed Industry Federation is based at the same address.

2170   European Society of Veterinary Dermatology, The Royal Veterinary College, Hawkshead House, Hawkshead Lane, North Mymms, Hatfield, Hertfordshire AL9 7TA, England
Tel. (0707) 55199. Fax. (0707) 52090
Contact point: Secretary – Dr David H. Lloyd
Publications: Bulletin (three a year); *Veterinary dermatology* (journal – forthcoming): Proceedings of annual congresses
First World congress of veterinary dermatology to be held in Dijon, France, 27–30 September 1989.

2171   European Society of Veterinary Nephrology and Urology, Department of Veterinary Surgery, University of Bristol, Langford House, Langford, Bristol BS18 7DU, England
Tel. (0934) 852581
Contact point: President – Prof. Peter E. Holt
Publications: Proceedings from the annual meetings have been published in a variety of forms; *Newsletter*

2172   European Society of Veterinary Neurology, Institut für Vergleichende Neurologie, Bremgartenstrasse 109a, Bern 3001, Postfach 2735, Switzerland
Contact point: President – Prof. Marc Vandevelde

2173   European Society for Veterinary Ophthalmology, Animal Health Trust, Lanwades Hall, Kennett, Newmarket, Suffolk CB8 7PN, England
Tel. (0638) 751030. Telex: 265871 84DDS177
Contact point: Membership Secretary – Dr Roger Curtis

2174   European Society of Veterinary Orthopedics and Traumatology, 4 Rue
François 1er, 75008 Paris, France
Tel. 42 89 23 15
Contact point: Dr J. F. Bardet
Publication: Newsletter (twice a year)

2175   European Society of Veterinary Pathology, Institut für Pathologie,
Tierärztliche Hochschule Hannover, Bischofsholer Damm 15, D-3000
Hanover, Federal Republic of Germany
Contact point: Secretary – Prof. Dr S. Überschar

2176   European Society for Veterinary Virology, c/o Central Veterinary
Laboratory, New Haw, Weybridge, Surrey KT15 3NB, England
Tel. (09323) 41111
Contact point: UK Co-ordinator – Mr S. Edwards

2177   European Union of Veterinary Food Hygienists, c/o Directeurs
d'Abattoirs Publics, 54 Avenue des États-Unis, F-78111 Versailles, France
Contact point: President – Dr B. Poulain

2178   European Union of Veterinary Practitioners, c/o Heath Veterinary
Hospital, 7 Queens Road, Haywards Heath, West Sussex RH16 1EH, Eng-
land
Tel. (0444) 413482
Contact point: Secretary – Roger Green

2179   Farm Animal Welfare Council, Block B, Government Buildings, Hook
Rise South, Tolworth, Surbiton, Surrey KT6 7NF, England
Tel. 01–337 4411 (ext. 8031)
Contact point: Secretariat – C. J. Simmons; Chairman – Prof. C. R. W. Spedding
Publications: The Council's structure, activities and membership are outlined in its
handbook (*Background notes on the Council and its work*) and in an article in the *State
veterinary journal* **42** (1988): 11–18

2180   Federation of Asian Veterinary Associations, 16 Jalan Salemba Raya,
Jakarta Pusat 10430, PO Box 402 JKT, Indonesia
Tel. 331180. Telex: 48125 DJP JKT IA
Contact point: Secretary General – Dr Sukobagyo Poedjomartono
Publications: Proceedings of the biennial congresses each held in one of the twelve
member countries (6th Bali 1988)

2181   Federation of European Veterinarians in Industry and Research, Mon-
santo Animal Science, 270 av Tervueren, B-1150 Brussels, Belgium
Contact point: President – Dr W. Vandaele

2182   Federation of Veterinarians of the EEC, 41 Avenue Fonsny, B-1060 Brussels, Belgium
Tel. (032) 2538 2863
Contact point: Permanent Secretary – Mrs Mathilda Herendenz

2183   Feline Advisory Bureau, 350 Upper Richmond Road, Putney, London SW15 6TL, England
Tel. 01–789 9553 (restricted hours)
Contact point: General Secretary – Mrs B. K. Thomas
Publications: FAB bulletin (includes many of the papers presented at the annual conference); leaflets giving advice and information on cat problems and diseases

2184   Food and Agriculture Organization of the United Nations, Via delle Terme di Caracalla, 00100 Rome, Italy
Tel. (06) 57971. Telex: 610181 FAO I. Cables: FOODAGRI ROME
Publications: World animal review; plus a variety of books, statistical works, review papers and reports described in the FAO catalogues

2185   Forensic Zoology Discussion Group, M. J. Chapman and Associates, 351 Kennington Road, London SE11 4QE, England
Tel. 01–735 4320
Contact point: Secretary/Co-ordinator – M. J. Chapman
Publication: Proceedings of meetings (occasional)

2186   Goat Producers Association, Royal Agricultural Society of England, National Agricultural Centre, Stoneleigh, Warwickshire CV8 2LZ, England
Tel. (0203) 555100. Telex: 31697
Contact point: Chairman – Alan Mowlem
Publications: Newsletter (quarterly); Proceedings of the annual conferences (*Developments in goat production*)

2187   Goat Veterinary Society, The Limes, Chalk Street, Rettendon Common, Chelmsford, Essex CM3 5DA, England
Tel. (0245) 353741 (office), (0245) 400618 (home)
Contact point: Honorary Secretary – J. Matthews
Publications: Goat Veterinary Society journal; Annual handbook

2188   Heifer Project International (and Volunteers in Veterinary Assistance), PO Box 808, Little Rock, Arkansas 72203, USA
Tel. (800) 422 0474, (501) 376 6836. Telex: 4949415 HEIFER
Contact point: Director – Lowell Watts
Publications: Sharing life (news magazine); Project lists; *Milk and honey* (volunteer newsletter); Publicity materials
Charitable organization providing livestock to poor families in rural areas worldwide and giving training and help in the care and management of animals. There

is also a UK branch: Heifer (UK) Project, 70 St Marychurch Street, London SE16 4HZ, England. Tel. 01–252 0294.

2189 Home of Rest for Horses, Westcroft Stables, Speen Farm, Speen, Near Aylesbury, Buckinghamshire HP17 0PP, England
Tel. (024028) 464
Publication: Annual report and list of subscribers

2190 The Humane Society of the United States, 2100 L Street NW, Washington, DC 20037, USA
Tel. (202) 452 1100
Contact point: Public Relations Director – Helen L. Mitternight
Publications: HSUS news (quarterly); *Shelter sense* (ten times a year); *Children and animals* (quarterly); *The Humane Society's guide to careers: working with animals*; plus large numbers of printed and audiovisual materials on animal welfare issues

2191 Institute of Animal Technology, Animal Unit, Western General Hospital, Crewe Road South, Edinburgh EH4 2XU, Scotland
Contact point: Honorary Secretary – Mrs Joan S. Robertson
Publications: Bulletin (monthly – includes a suppliers register); *Animal technology*

2192 AFRC Institute for Animal Health, Compton, Newbury, Berkshire RG16 0NN, England
Tel. (0635) 578411. Fax. (0635) 578844
Contact point: Director – Prof. Peter M. Biggs
Publication: Annual report
Apart from the Compton Laboratory the Institute also has staff at the Houghton (Tel. (0480) 64101, Fax. (0480) 67870. Telex: 329154 HPRS) and Pirbright Laboratories (Tel. (0483) 232 442, Fax. (0483) 232448. Telex: 859137 AVRI G) and at Edinburgh (AFRC/MRC Neuropathogenesis Unit. Tel. 031–667 5204, Fax. 031–668 3872)

2193 Institute of Laboratory Animal Resources, c/o National Research Council, 2101 Constitution Avenue, Washington DC 20418, USA
Tel. (202) 334 2590
Contact point: Director – Dr Earl W. Grogan
Publications: ILAR news (quarterly); documents on the care and welfare of laboratory animals

2194 Institute for Wildlife Research, c/o National Wildlife Federation, 1412 16th Street NW, Washington, DC 20036, USA
Tel. (703) 790 4267
Contact point: Director – Maurice N. LeFranc Jr
Publications: Newsletter; bibliographies on wildlife

2195   Interafrican Bureau of Animal Resources of the Organization of African Unity, PO Box 30786, Nairobi, Kenya
Tel. Nairobi 338544/24055/24854
Contact point: Director – Dr W. N. Masiga
Publications: Bulletin of animal health and production in Africa; *IBAR information leaflets* (monthly); publishes the biennial proceedings of the International Scientific Council for Trypanosomiasis Research and Control

2196   International Association for Aquatic Animal Medicine, PO Box 4078, Gulfport, Mississippi 39502, USA
Tel. (601) 868 1235
Contact point: Secretary-Treasurer – Mobashir A. Solangi
Publications: Proceedings of the annual meeting (20th 1989); *Directory* (annual); *Newsletter* (quarterly)

2197   International Association of Milk, Food and Environmental Sanitarians, PO Box 701, Ames, Iowa 50010, USA
Tel. (515) 232 6699
Contact point: Executive Secretary – Kathy R. Hathaway
Publications: Dairy and food sanitation (monthly); *Journal of food protection* (monthly); *Membership directory* (annual)

2198   International Association of Teachers of Veterinary Preventive Medicine, c/o Institut Armand Frappier, PO Box 100, Laval-des-Rapides, Quebec H7V 1B7, Canada
Tel. (514) 687 5010 (ext. 323)
Contact point: Executive Officer – Dr Roger Ruppanner
National member associations meet during the World Veterinary Congress.

2199   International Association for Veterinary Homeopathy and British Veterinary Homeopathy Association, Chinham House, Stanford in the Vale, Faringdon, Oxfordshire SN7 8NQ, England
Tel. (03677) 324
Contact point: President – C. E. I. Day
Publication: International journal for veterinary homeopathy (twice a year)

2200   International Bee Research Association, 18 North Road, Cardiff CF1 3DY, Wales
Tel. (0222) 372409. Telex: 23152 MONREF G 8390
Publications: Apicultural abstracts: Bee world (quarterly); *Journal of apicultural research* (quarterly); *Newsletter for beekeepers in tropical and subtropical countries*; *International book catalogue* (comprehensive stocklist of titles on bees and beekeeping)

2201   International Buffalo Federation, PO Box 102, Dokki, Guiza, Egypt
Tel. 701211. Telex: 94022 NAREC UN
Contact point: President – Prof. Dr M. R. Shalash

2202   International Buffalo Information Center, Kasetsart University Library, Bangkhen, Bangkok 10900, Thailand
Tel. 5790113
Contact point: Director – Mrs Piboonsin Watanapongse
Publications: Bibliographies, directories and newsletters.
Maintains an extensive library and provides an enquiry and referral service.

2203   International Commission on Trichinellosis, Veterinary Medical Research Institute, Iowa State University, Ames, Iowa 50011, USA
Contact point: Secretary General – Dr Miroslav Stankiewicz
Publications: List of members; Proceedings of quadrennial conferences; Proceedings of other meetings are published in *Widomosci parazytologiezne*

2204   International Committee on Equine Exercise Physiology, Animal Health Trust, Physiology Unit, PO Box 5, Balaton Lodge, Snailwell Road, Newmarket, Suffolk CB8 7DW, England
Tel. (0638) 661111. Telex: 265871 84MNU267
Contact point: Dr David H. Snow
Publications: *Equine exercise physiology 2: proceedings of the second international conference on equine exercise physiology* (Edited by J. R. Gillespie and N. E. Robinson. Davis, California: ICEEP Publications, 1987, 810pp.); *Equine exercise physiology: proceedings of the first international conference* (Cambridge: Granta Editions, 1983, 543pp.); next meeting 1990

2205   International Committee on Veterinary Anatomical Nomenclature, Winterthurerstrasse 260, CH-8057 Zurich, Switzerland
Contact point: Secretary – Dr Josef Frewein
Publications: *Nomina anatomica avium; Nomina anatomica veterinaria; Nomina histologica*
An umbrella organization of the following International Committees: Veterinary Gross Anatomical Nomenclature; Veterinary Histological Nomenclature; Veterinary Embryological Nomenclature; Avian Nomenclature. They meet every two or three years in connection with the World Association of Veterinary Anatomists (next Rio de Janeiro, August 1989).

2206   International Congress on Animal Reproduction and Artificial Insemination – Executive Committee, Department of Obstetrics and Gynaecology, Box 7039, Swedish University of Agricultural Sciences, S-750 07 Uppsala, Sweden
Contact point: Secretary General – Prof. Stig Einarsson
Publications: Proceedings of the congresses (quadrennial – next The Hague 1992)

2207   International Dairy Federation and IDF Group of Experts on Mastitis, Square Vergote 41, B-1040 Brussels, Belgium
Tel. 733 98 88. Telex: 63818
Contact point: Secretary General – M. Staal

Publications: Mastitis newsletter (free); *Bulletin of the IDF*; IDF standards; *Mastitis research index* (4th ed., 1987); International Mastitis Symposium, August 14–15, 1987 (next symposium to be held in Austria in 1989). The Chairman of the IDF Group of Experts on Mastitis is James M. Booth (for address see [2278])

2208 International Embryo Transfer Society, 309 W. Clark Street, Champaign, Illinois 61820, USA
Tel. (217) 356 3182
Contact point: Executive Secretary – Sarah Seidel
Publications: Manual of the International Embryo Transfer Society (Recommendations for the sanitary handling of embryos) (updated annually); Proceedings of the annual conference (15th 1988); *Membership directory* (annual); *International embryo movement* (Edited by W. C. D. Hare and S. M. Seidel, 1988, 198pp.) – proceedings of a meeting held in 1987

2209 International Goat Association, Department of Animal, Dairy and Veterinary Sciences, Utah State University, Logan, Utah 84322, USA
Contact point: Secretary-Treasurer – Dr Warren C. Foote
Publications: Small ruminant research; Proceedings of the international conferences on goats (4th Brazil 1987, 5th India 1992)

2210 International Group of Specialist Racing Veterinarians (IGSRV), Equine Hospital, Royal Hong Kong Jockey Club, Sha Tin Racecourse, New Territories, Hong Kong
Telex: 65581 RHKJC HX
Contact point: Honorary Secretary/Treasurer – D. K. Mason
Publications: General meetings are held with those of the International Conference of Racing Analysts and Veterinarians and are published in the proceedings (biannual)

2211 International Llama Association, Administrative Office, PO Box 37505, Denver, Colorado 80237, USA
Tel. (303) 699 9545
Contact point: General Manager – Sandy Chapman
Publications: ILA newsletter (bimonthly); *Membership directory* and *Llama catalog* (annual)

2212 International Pig Veterinary Society, R. do Ouvidor, 60/164, Centro 20040, Rio de Janeiro, Brazil
Tel. (021) 224 6080. Telex: (021) 32891 CERT BR
Contact point: President – Luciano Roppa
Publications: Proceedings of the biennial conference (10th Rio de Janeiro 1988, next Lucerne 1990)

2213   International Primatological Society, Monell Chemical Senses Center, 3500 Market Street, Philadelphia, Pennsylvania 19104, USA
Contact point: Secretary General – Dr Gisela Epple
Publication: IPVS news (occasional)

2214   International Society of Animal Clinical Biochemistry, École Nationale Vétérinaire, 23 Chemin des Capelles, 31706 Toulouse, France
Tel. (061) 49 11 40
Contact point: Prof. J. P. Braun
Publication: Third international congress held in Cambridge in 1988 (*Animal clinical biochemistry: the future*, Edited by D. J. Blackmore, Cambridge: CUP, 1988, 386pp.)

2215   International Society for Animal Hygiene, Faculty of Veterinary Medicine, Swedish University of Agricultural Sciences, POB 345, S-532 00 Skara, Sweden
Tel. (0) 511 30000
Contact point: President – Prof. Ingvar Ekesbo
Publications: Proceedings of triennial congresses (High Tatra 1982, Hannover 1985 and 6th, Skara, 1988, *Environment and health*, 2 vols, 926pp.)

2216   International Society for Human and Animal Mycology, Mycological Reference Laboratory, Central Public Health Laboratory, 61 Colindale Avenue, London NW9 5HT, England
Tel. 01-200 4400 (ext. 3508 and 3511)
Contact point: General Secretary – Dr D. W. R. Mackenzie
Publications: Journal of medical and veterinary mycology; Newsletter (twice yearly); Holds quadrennial congresses (last Barcelona 1988)

2217   International Society for the Study of the Human–Companion Animal Bond, *see* Delta Society [2154]

2218   International Society for Veterinary Epidemiology and Economics, Royal Veterinary and Agricultural University, Bulowsvej 13, DK-1870 Copenhagen V, Denmark
Tel. (01) 35 17 88
Contact point: Prof. Preben Willeberg
Publications: Proceedings of the international symposia on veterinary epidemiology and economics (4th Singapore 1984, 480pp.; 5th Copenhagen 1988 (in: *Acta veterinaria Scandinavica* **supplement 84** (1988)); 6th Ottawa 1991); *Newsletter* (annual)

2219   International Society of Veterinary Ophthalmology, École Nationale Vétérinaire de Lyon, BP 31, Marcy l'Étoile, 69752 Charbonnières-les-Bains, France
Tel. 78 87 00 84
Contact point: Secretary – Dr Bernard Clerc

2220   International Society of Veterinary Perinatology, Alternate Care Division, Baxter Healthcare Corporation, One Parkway North Suite 430, PO Box 840, Deerfield, Illinois 60015, USA
Tel. (312) 940 1638
Contact point: Executive Director – Dr Michael V. Ward
Publication: ISVP newsbulletin

2221   International Technical Consultation on Veterinary Drug Registration, Ministry of Agriculture and Fisheries, PO Box 20401, 2500 EK's Gravenhage, The Netherlands
Contact point: Chairman of Standing Committee – Dr J. Frens
Publications: Proceedings of the biannual meetings (4th 1988); *Veterinary drug registration newsletter*

2222   International Veterinary Academy on Disaster Medicine, 1918 George Allen Drive, Ames, Iowa 50010, USA
Tel. (515) 232 1982
Contact point: Secretary – Dr O. H. V. Stalheim
Publication: The disaster newsletter

2223   International Veterinary Acupuncture Society, RD 4, PO Box 216, Chester Springs, Pennsylvania 19425, USA
Tel. (215) 827 7742
Contact point: Executive Director – Dr Meredith L. Snader
Publications: Membership directory; *Newsletter* (quarterly); Proceedings of the annual meetings; *Acupuncture points and meridians in the dog* (by L. A. A. Janssens)

2224   International Veterinary Association for Animal Production, Avenue de Broqueville 198, B-1200 Brussels, Belgium
Tel. (32 2) 770 19 46
Contact point: President – Dr Guiseppe Enne
Publications: Zootechnia (quarterly); World Congresses (bi- or triannual, last Madrid 1985)

2225   International Veterinary Auxiliary, Dr Eleodoro Lobos 254, 1405 Buenos Aires, Argentina
Contact point: President – Sra. Ines R. de Descamps
Publication: Bulletin (annual)
Formerly known as the International Women's Auxiliary to the veterinary profession. Membership is now open to spouses of veterinarians of both sexes.

2226   International Veterinary Ear, Nose and Throat Association, VHUP 2044, 3850 Spruce Street, Philadelphia, Pennsylvania 19104–6010, USA
Tel. (215) 898 3350
Contact point: Dr C. E. Harvey

2227   International Veterinary Radiology Association, Department of Veterinary Clinical Sciences, University of Sydney, New South Wales 2006, Australia
Contact point: Secretary – Dr A. K. W. Wood
Publication: Veterinary radiology
Holds world triennial veterinary radiology conferences (8th Sydney 1988, 9th Utrecht 1991).

2228   International Veterinary Students Association, Höfergasse 3/12, 1090 Vienna, Austria
Tel. (222) 4816192
Contact point: President – Dietmar Gerstner
Publications: IVSA newsletter (three a year)

2229   International Working Group on *Trypanosoma evansi* Infections, 228 Boulevard du Président Wilson, 33000 Bordeaux, France
Contact point: Secretary of the Group – Dr Louis Touratier
Publications: Accounts of the Group's meetings are noted in *Revue scientifique et technique de l'OIE*. The Group meets at OIE headquarters and at relevant international events

2230   The Kennel Club, 1 Clarges Street, Piccadilly, London W1Y 8AB, England
Tel. 01–493 6651
Contact point: Senior Executive and General Secretary
Publications: Year book Part 1: Members, associates and councils. Part II: Canine breed clubs and societies. Part III: Rules and regulations.

2231   Laboratory Animal Science Association, 20 Queensberry Place, London SW7 2D7, England
Tel. 01–581 8333
Contact point: Information Officer – G. Curry
Publications: Laboratory animals; *LASA newsletter* (quarterly); *Buyers Guide*

2232   The Latham Foundation, Latham Plaza, Clement & Schiller Streets, Alameda, California 94501–1397, USA
Tel. (415) 521 0920
Contact point: President – Hugh H. Tebault
Publication: Dynamic relationships in practice: animals in the helping professions (1984, 500pp.)

2233   Meat and Livestock Commission, PO Box 44, Winterhill House, Snowdon Drive, Winterhill, Milton Keynes MK6 1AX, England
Tel. (0908) 677577. Telex: 82227. Fax. (0908) 609221
Publications: Annual report; Beef, Sheep and *Pig yearbooks*;

2234   Milk Marketing Board, Thames Ditton, Surrey KT7 0EL, England
Tel. 01-398 4101. Telex: 8956671. Fax. 01-398 8485
Contact point: Administration Manager/Public Relations – Mrs C. A. Carter
Publications: Milk producer (monthly); *Dairy facts and figures* (UK and EEC editions); *Better management; Better breeding*; Farm Management Service Information Unit reports

2235   Morris Animal Foundation, 45 Inverness Drive East, Englewood, Colorado 80112, USA
Tel. (303) 790 2345
Contact point: Director of Information – Carole Williams
Publication: Companion animal news (three times a year)

2236   National Animal Control Association, PO Box 321, Indianola, Washington 98342, USA
Tel. (206) 297 3293
Contact point: Executive Secretary – Mike Burgwin
Publications: NACA news (bimonthly); NACA policy statements; videos on *Rabies* and *Raptor capture and restraint*

2237   National Association of Federal Veterinarians, 1023 15th Street NW, Third Floor, Washington, DC 20005, USA
Tel. (202) 223 3590
Contact point: Executive Vice President – Dr Edward L. Menning
Publications: The federal veterinarian (monthly); *Directory*; video and audio cassette library

2238   National Association for Veterinary Acupuncture, 951 W Bastanchury Road, Fullerton, California 92635, USA
Contact point: Dr Richard Glassberg
Publication: A compendium of human and veterinary acupuncture and equine acupuncture

2239   National Mastitis Council, 1840 Wilson Boulevard, Arlington, Virginia 22201, USA
Tel. (703) 243 8268
Contact point: Director of Operations and Membership Services – Ann Saeman
Publications: Udder topics (newsletter – bimonthly); available from Nasco are: *Current concepts of bovine mastitis; National Mastitis Council proceedings* (annual); NMC fact sheets; *Recommended milking procedures barn card; The modern way to efficient milking; Milking procedures checklist;* NMC slide set (586 slides and printed

scripts and tape cassette naratives); *Microbiological procedures for use in the diagnosis of bovine mastitis* (2nd ed., 1981); *Laboratory and field handbook on bovine mastitis* (1987, 208pp.)

2240   National Office of Animal Health, 3 Crossfield Chambers, Gladbeck Way, Enfield, Middlesex EN2 7HF, England
Tel. 01-367 3131. Telex: 298916. Fax. 01-363 1155
Contact point: Public Relations Executive – Mrs Alison M. Glennon
Publications: Annual symposium on effective registration of animal health products; *Animal health matters*; *Veterinary service sheets*; compendium of data sheets on veterinary products; variety of other services to members

2241   National Sheep Association, The Sheep Centre, Malvern, Worcestershire WR13 6PH, England
Tel. (0684) 892661
Contact point: Secretary – Mr John Thorley
Publications: The sheep farmer (ten a year); *Annual report and accounts*

2242   National Wildlife Rehabilitators Association, RR 1 Box 125E, Brighton, Illinois 62012, USA
Contact point: Membership Chair – Elaine M. Thrune
Publications: List of wildlife related internships; *Wildlife rehabilitation* (1982–) proceedings or selected papers from the annual national symposia; *Manual of wildlife medicine*; *Introduction to wildlife rehabilitation*; *Wildlife rehabilitation minimum standards and accreditation program*; *Membership directory* (annual); *MWRA newsletter*

2243   North American Veterinary Technician Association, Purdue University, Lynn Hall, LAC, West Lafayette, Indiana 47907, USA
Tel. (317) 494 1107
Contact point: A. Patrick Navarre, RVT

2244   Office International des Épizooties, 12 Rue de Prony, 75017 Paris, France
Tel. (1) 42 27 45 74. Telex: 642285 EPIZOTI F. Fax. (1) 42 67 09 87
Contact point: Director General – Dr L. Blajan
Publications: A wide range of periodicals, technical reviews, conference proceedings and statistical works. Described in an annual *Publications catalogue*

2245   Orthopedic Foundation for Animals, 2300 Nifong Boulevard, Columbia, Missouri 65201, USA
Tel. (314) 442 0418
Contact point: Director – Dr E. A. Corley
Publications: Library of canine pelvic radiographs; operates a dysplasia control registry to evaluate radiographs of purebred dogs to certify the dogs are free of orthopaedic problems; Proceedings of the canine hip dysplasia meetings; *Hip dysplasia: a monograph for dog breeders and owners* (pamphlet, 1983)

2246   Pan American Foot and Mouth Disease Center, Caixa Postal 589-ZC-00, 20001 Rio de Janeiro, Brazil
Tel. 771 3128. Telex: (021) 30253 CPFA BR
Contact point: Director – Raul Casas Olascoaga
Publication: Boletín del Centro Panamericano de Fiebre Aftosa (includes research papers and a bibliography of papers on vesicular diseases)

2247   Pan American Association of Veterinary Sciences, c/o Inter-American Institute for Cooperation on Agriculture [1785]
Contact point: Executive Director – Dr Hector Campos
Organize the Panamerican congress of veterinary sciences (11th Lima 1988).

2248   Pan American Health Organization (WHO Regional Office for the Americas), 525 Twenty Third Street NW, Washington, DC 20037, USA
Tel. (202) 861 3200. Telex: OFSANPAN WASHINGTON 248338
Contact point: Director – Dr Carlyle Guerro de Macedo
Publications: Bulletin of the Pan American Health Organization (quarterly); a variety of monographs on animal health

2249   Pedigree Petfoods Education Centre, National Office, Waltham-on-the-Wolds, Melton Mowbray, Leicestershire LE14 4RS, England
Tel. (0664) 410000. Telex: 34675. Fax. (0664) 60804
Contact point: External Relations Co-ordinator – Mrs Christine Greaves
Publications: Wide range of leaflets and other educational materials for pet owners; *Pedigree digest* (quarterly); operate a film and video library; sponsor the Waltham Symposia, published in the *Journal of small animal practice*, and the *Catlopaedia*, the *Doglopaedia*, and *The Waltham book of dog and cat nutrition*

2250   People's Dispensary for Sick Animals, PDSA House, South Street, Dorking, Surrey RH4 2LB, England
Tel. (0306) 888291
Contact point: Press and Public Relations Officer – Marilyn Marchant
Publications: Annual report; leaflets on pet care for owners; educational materials

2251   Pet Food Institute, 1101 Connecticut Avenue NW, Suite 700, Washington, DC 20036, USA
Tel. (202) 857 1120
Contact point: Director of Regulatory Affairs – Mr Timothy R. Rugh

2252   The Pet Food Manufacturers' Association, 6 Catherine Street, London WC2B 5JJ, England
Tel. 01–836 2460. Telex: 299388. Fax. 01–836 0580
Contact point: Executive Secretary – Miss L. Archer

2253   Pet Health Council, 4 Bedford Square, London WC1B 3RA, England
Tel. 01–255 2424
Publications: Leaflets, posters and background papers for pet owners, teachers,
breeders, doctors and environmental health officers

2254   Pet Information Bureau/PIJAC, 1710 Rhode Island Avenue NW,
Washington, DC 20036, USA
Tel. (202) 452 1525
Contact point: Marshall Meyers

2255   Pet Trade and Industry Association, 6th Floor, 60–66 Saffron Hill,
London EC1N 8QX, England
Tel. 01–242 4380. Telex: 27969
Contact point: Secretary – M. G. Colle
Publication: Pet trade yearbook and buyers' guide

2256   Pig Health Control Association, Madingley, Cambridge CB3 8AH,
England
Tel. (0954) 210434
Contact point: Secretary-Treasurer – Mrs E. A. Ross
*Publication: Annual report: abstracts of publications and herd lists; The work and benefits of
the PHCA* and *Aims and achievements* (both pamphlets)
Operates health control schemes for six diseases and publishes lists of herds free
from the diseases and veterinary regulations for the checking of the herds.

2257   Pig Veterinary Society, 16 Wood End Lane, Little Horwood, Buckinghamshire MK17 0PE, England
Tel. (0908) 665050 (office), (029671) 3595 (home)
Contact point: Secretary – Simon E. G. Smith
Publications: Pig veterinary journal (formerly *The Pig Veterinary Society proceedings*)
(1977–, twice a year) contains papers presented at the two technical meetings
held each year; *PVS newsletter* (occasional)

2258   Post-Graduate Committee in Veterinary Science, (The University of
Sydney), PO Box A561, Sydney South, New South Wales 2000, Australia
Tel. (02) 264 2122. Fax. (02) 261 4620
Contact point: Associate Director – Douglas I. Bryden
Publications: A wide range of printed and audiovisual materials in the field of con-
tinuing education

2259   Primate Society of Great Britain, Department of Biology, The Open
University, Walton Hall, Milton Keynes MK7 6AA, England
Tel. (0908) 652506
Contact point: Secretary – Dr Robert Hubrecht

Publications: Primate eye (three per year) includes an annual *Current field studies supplement; The welfare of pet marmosets* (published jointly with UFAW) compiled by the Captive Care Working Party; there is also a Conservation Working Party

2260 Ralston Purina Company, Checkerboard Square, St Louis 63164, Missouri, USA
Tel. (800) 222 8387, (314) 982 1000. Telex: 447620
Publications: A variety of handbooks, manuals and information sheets for small animal practitioners. Titles include: *Handbook of canine and feline urinalysis* (1981), *Handbook of veterinary cytology* (1978), *Bone marrow evaluation in veterinary practice* (1979), *The morphology of canine and feline blood cells* (1974), *Diagnosis of gastrointestinal parasitism in dogs and cats* (1980)

2261 Raptor Research Foundation, 4718 Dunn Drive, Sarasota, Florida 33583, USA
Contact point: President – Jeffrey L. Lincer
Publications: Journal of raptor research (quarterly); Directory (biennial)

2262 Registry of Veterinary Pathology, Armed Forces Institute of Pathology, Washington, DC 20306, USA
Tel. (202) 576 2452
Contact point: Registrar – John M. Plelcher
Publications: Comparative pathology bulletin; Animal models of human disease (handbook); *Resources of biomedical and zoological specimens* (biennial)

2263 Royal Agricultural Society of England, National Agricultural Centre, Stoneleigh, Kenilworth, Warwickshire CV8 2LZ, England
Tel. (0203) 696969. Telex: 31697. Fax. (0203) 696900
Contact point: Press office
Publications: Profile (directory and guide to the Society and to other organizations at the Centre); *National calendar of events*

2264 Royal Society for the Prevention of Cruelty to Animals, Causeway, Horsham, West Sussex RH12 1HG, England
Tel. (0403) 64181
Contact point: Executive Director – Andrew Richmond
Publications: Film and video catalogue; Educational sources; *Journal* (quarterly); *Animal world* (bimonthly); *First aid for stranded Cetaceans* (1988, 20pp.)
The European Conference Group on the Protection of Food Animals is based at the RSPCA (Secretary/Treasurer – David B. Wilkins). The Group is to stage a Fifth European Conference in 1991.

2265 Scientists' Center for Animal Welfare, 4805 St Elmo Avenue, Bethesda, Maryland 20814, USA
Tel. (301) 654 6390
Contact point: Co-ordinator – Lee Krulisch

Publications: Newsletter (quarterly); *Effective animal care and use committees* (Edited by F. B. Orlans, R. C. Simmonds and W. J. Dodds, 1987); *Scientific perspectives on animal welfare* (Edited by W. J. Dodds and F. B. Orlans. New York: Academic Press, 1982); Technical papers and audiotapes; *Laboratory animal welfare bibliography* (1988)

2266   Sheep and Beef Cattle Society of the New Zealand Veterinary Association, PO Box 524, Wellington, New Zealand
Publications: Proceedings of the annual seminar (17th, 1987); *Ectoparasites of sheep in New Zealand and their control* (Edited by W. A. G. Charleston, 1985, 79pp.)
The Dairy Cattle Society of the NZVA also publishes its proceedings

2267   Sheep Veterinary Society, Moredun Research Institute, 408 Gilmerton Road, Edinburgh EH17 7JH, Scotland
Tel. 031-664 3262 (office), 062-082 2532 (home)
Contact point: Secretary – C. J. Lewis
Publication: Proceedings of the Sheep Veterinary Society

2268   Society of Aquatic Veterinary Medicine, 4250 East Chapman Avenue, Orange, California 92669, USA
Contact point: President – Dr Robert Jack
Publication: Newsletter (quarterly) – alerts members to proposed diving trips and continuing education events

2269   Society for Companion Animal Studies, 23 Glengall Road, London SE15 6NJ, England
Tel. 01–639 5140
Contact point: Administrator – Nikki Holmyard
Publications: Newsletter (quarterly); *Guidelines for the introduction of pets in nursing homes and similar institutions*

2270   Society of Comparative Oncology, Department of Clinical Veterinary Medicine, University of Cambridge, Madingley Road, Cambridge CB3 0ES, England
Tel. (0223) 37637
Contact point: Secretary – Mr D. E. Bostock

2271   Society of Feed Technologists, 85 St Peter's Road, Reading, Berkshire RG6 1PD, England
Tel. (0734) 65130
Contact point: Secretary – S. H. C. Foye
Publications: Proceedings of the meetings (four a year)

2272   Society of Greyhound Veterinarians, Beech House, Queens Road, Hersham, Walton on Thames, Surrey KT12 5NH, England
Tel. (0932) 228691
Contact point: President – Mr A. J. Westaway

2273   Society for International Veterinary Symposia, College of Veterinary Medicine, University of Illinois, 1008 West Hazelwood Drive, Urbana, Illinois 61801, USA

Tel. (217) 333 5300

Contact point: Executive Secretary – Prof. Erwin Small

Organizes continuing education meetings in countries around the world (Twenty-third meeting India and Nepal 1988). These are designed to foster better international relations and understanding among veterinarians.

2274   Society of Practising Veterinary Surgeons, Green Farm, Shordley, Hope, Wrexham, Clywd LL12 9RT, Wales

Tel. (0244) 570364 (office), (0978) 761039 (home)

Contact point: Honorary Secretary – D. Brian Edwards

Holds regional seminars throughout the United Kingdom; weekend meetings for young graduates on management and financial problems in practice; three day vacational course for undergraduates (September); annual weekend meeting for members (May).

2275   Society for the Study of Animal Breeding, Scobells Farm, Boast Lane, Barcombe, Lewes, East Sussex BN8 5DY, England

Tel. (0273) 400393

Contact point: Honorary Secretary – Mr R. T. Pepper

Publications: Scientific proceedings of the three meetings per year are distributed to members; *Newsletter* (three times a year)

2276   The Society for the Study of Reproduction, 309 West Clark Street, Champaign, Illinois 61820, USA

Tel. (217) 356 3182

Contact point: Executive Secretary – Carl D. Johnson

Publication: Biology of reproduction (monthly)

2277   Society for Theriogenology, Association Building, 9th and Minnesota, Hastings, Nebraska 68901, USA

Tel. (402) 463 0392

Contact point: Executive Director – Don Ellerbee

Publications: Newsletter (bimonthly); *Proceedings of the annual fall conference*; manuals; videotape library

2278   Society for Veterinary Epidemiology and Preventive Medicine, Milk Marketing Board Veterinary Laboratory, Cleeve House, Lower Wick, Worcester WR2 4NS, England

Tel. (0905) 424940. Fax. (0905) 429476

Contact point: Secretary – James M. Booth

Publications: Proceedings of the annual meetings (available from M. V. Thrusfield – Royal (Dick) School of Veterinary Studies)

2279   Society for Veterinary Ethology, APAD (The Edinburgh School of
Agriculture), Bush Estate, Penicuik, Midlothian EH26 0QE, Scotland
Tel. 031–445 5353
Contact point: Honorary Secretary – Dr Alistair B. Lawrence
Publications: Newsletter (twice a year); The proceedings of the meetings are
published in *Applied animal behaviour science*; The honorary librarian has a file of
reprints in a computer database; *Membership list*

2280   Society of Veterinary Urology, College of Veterinary Medicine,
University of Minnesota, Room C-325, 1352 Boyd Avenue, St Paul,
Minnesota 55108, USA
Tel. (612) 625 4254
Contact point: Secretary-Treasurer – Dr David J. Polzin

2281   The Society of Women Veterinary Surgeons, 39 Fairway Road,
Shepshed, Loughborough, Leicestershire LE12 9DS, England
Tel. (0509) 508224
Contact point: President – Mrs N. D. Lewis

2282   Student American Veterinary Medical Association, 930 North Meacham
Road, Schaumberg, Illinois 60196, USA
Tel. (312) 885 8070
Contact point: SAVMA Advisor – Dr Karen M. Wernette
Publication: INTERVET (six times a year, September through May)

2283   Technical Centre for Agricultural and Rural Cooperation, Postbus 380,
6700 AJ Wageningen, The Netherlands
Tel. (8380) 20484. Telex: 30169 CTA NL. Fax. (8380) 31052
Contact point: Documentalist – Thiendou Niang
Publications: Annual report; Spore (bimonthly); *Pigs and poultry production in the tropics;
Primary animal healthcare in Africa* (seminar report); *Manual of poultry production in
the tropics* (with CAB International and IEMVT); *Matching ruminant production
systems with available resources in the tropics and sub-tropics*; other publications
designed to foster collaboration between the EEC and African, Caribbean and
Pacific countries

2284   The Tortoise Trust, BM Tortoise, London WC1N 3XX, England
Tel. (0249) 720114. Telex: 265871 MONREF G Ref 72:MAG32237
Contact point: Jill Hewson
Publications: Variety of technical bulletins and guides; *Newsletter*

2285   Tropical Agriculture Association, Marydene, Old Litten Lane, Froxfield,
Petersfield, Hampshire GU32 1BG, England
Tel. (0730) 84430
Contact point: General Secretary – L. J. Foster

Publications: Newsletter (contains reports of the association's meetings); *Directory of members available for employment or consultation* (annual); a *Register of tropical agriculturalists for charitable developments* is being compiled; *Tropical agriculturalists – future prospects* (British Council, 1987, 108pp.) reviews the supply and demand of veterinarians

2286   United Kingdom Agricultural Supply Trade Association (UKASTA), 3 Whitehall Court, London SW1A 2EQ, England
Tel. 01–930 3611. Telex: 917868. Fax. 01–930 3952
Contact point: Director General – H. V. Willshaw
Publications: The benefits of membership; *AgriTrade* (monthly); *UKASTA yearbook*; *Report and accounts* (annual); *Feed facts* (annual); *UKASTA digest* (bimonthly).
UKASTA no longer represents distributors of packaged animal health products.
This role is now served by the Animal Health Distributors Association.

2287   United States Animal Health Association, 6924 Lakeside Avenue, PO Box 28176, Suite 205, Richmond, Virginia 23228, USA
Tel. (804) 266 3275
Contact point: Executive Director – Ella R. Blanton
Publications: Proceedings of the annual meeting (formerly the *Proceedings of the United States Livestock Sanitary Association*) (92nd 1988); *Foreign animal diseases: their prevention, diagnosis and control* (4th ed., 1984)

2288   Universities Federation for Animal Welfare, 8 Hamilton Close, South Mimms, Potters Bar, Hertfordshire EN6 3QD, England
Tel. (0707) 58202
Publications: Annual symposia from 1968; *Report and accounts* (annual); *News-sheet* (April); Publication list describes many items of interest including: *Guidelines for the recognition and assessment of pain in animals* (1989), *A summary of statute law relating to animal welfare in England and Wales Parts I–III* (1987), *Humane killing of animals* (4th ed., 1988), *Euthanasia of amphibians and reptiles* (1989)

2289   Vétérinaires sans Frontières, 12 rue Mulet, 69001 Lyon, France
Tel. 78 27 77 76. Telex: CCP LYON 151807F
Contact point: Executive Secretary – A. de Biran
Publication: Habbanae (quarterly newsletter)

2290   Veterinarians for Amnesty International, 20 Mont Street, Guelph, Ontario N1W 2W1, Canada
Tel. (519) 823 5013
Contact point: Co-ordinator – Dr John Prescott
Publication: Newsletter (monthly)

2291   Veterinary Cancer Society, 2015 Linden Drive West, Madison, Wisconsin 53706, USA
Tel. (608) 263 7600
Contact point: Corresponding Secretary – Robert C. Rosenthal
Publications: Newsletter; Proceedings of annual conference (9th 1989)

2292   Veterinary Cardiovascular Society, 193 Campkin Road, Cambridge CB4 2LE, England
Tel. 01–273 3854 (office), (0223) 312703 (home)
Contact point: Secretary – Mrs S. E. Matic

2293   Veterinary Christian Fellowship, 36 St John's Street, Huntingdon, Cambridgeshire PE18 8JL, England
Tel. (0480) 52601
Contact point: Secretary – John Brown
Publication: Newsletter (bimonthly)

2294   Veterinary Deer Society, 27 Hereford Close, off Victoria Road, Beverley, North Humberside HU17 8PT, England. Also available c/o BVA
Tel. (0482) 867093 (office), (0482) 867093 (home)
Contact point: Secretary – T. L. Alexander
Publication: Publication of the Veterinary Deer Society (biannual)

2295   Veterinary Emergency and Critical Care Society, 177 Grove Park, Fort Dix, New Jersey 08640, USA
Contact point: President – Dr Gary Stamp
Publications: Proceedings of the 1st international veterinary emergency and critical care symposium (San Antonio, Texas, 1988); *Journal of veterinary emergency and critical care* (1985–)

2296   Veterinary Hemoparasite Research Workers, Office of the Dean, School of Veterinary Medicine, Louisiana State University, Baton Rouge, Louisiana 70803, USA
Tel. (504) 346 3200
Contact point: Chairman – Richard J. Hidalgo
Publication: Proceedings of the national veterinary hemoparasite disease conference (8th 1989)

2297   Veterinary History Society, 14 Huntingdon Road, Cambridge CB3 0HH, England
Tel. 01–216 7219 (office), (0223) 351308 (home)
Contact point: Secretary – S. A. Hall
Publication: Veterinary history (contains papers presented at the meetings)

2298   Veterinary Medical Data Program, South Campus Courts, Building C, Purdue University, West Lafayette, Indiana 47907, USA
Tel. (317) 494 8179
Contact point: Office Manager – Marlene Moore
Publication: Databases with clinical data on cases seen by collaborating hospitals and on inheritable eye problems in dogs

2299   Veterinary Orthopedic Society, PO Box 6129, Salt Lake City, Utah 84109, USA
Tel. (801) 484 8912
Contact point: Executive Secretary – Nancy Bunker
Publications: Abstracts of the annual meeting; *Newsletter* (annual); Membership list

2300   Veterinary Public Health Association, Springfield Lodge, 6 Summer-heath Road, Hailsham, East Sussex BN27 3DS, England
Tel. (0323) 841922 (office), (0323) 840688 (home)
Contact point: Honorary Secretary – Mrs E. Thomas
Publications: Two-day scientific meetings are held twice a year and the papers distributed to attendees

2301   Veterinary Working Group for Osteosyntesis, AO-VET Center, C/o Institut Strauman, CH-4437 Waldenburg, Switzerland
Tel. (061) 97 80 80

2302   Vets for the World (VETAID), Centre for Tropical Veterinary Medicine, Easter Bush, Roslin, Midlothian EH25 9RG, Scotland
Tel. 031–667 7347. Telex: 727442 UNIVED G
Contact point: Secretary – N. R. M. Short
Publication: Newsletter
Charitable trust involved in improving animal health and production in the developing world.

2303   The Wellcome Trust, 1 Park Square West, London NW1 4LJ, England
Tel. 01–486 4902. Fax. 01–935 0359
Contact point: External Relations
Publications: Biennial report; *Grants and support for research*; *Fifty years of the Wellcome Trust 1936–86*

2304   Western Poultry Disease Conference, Division of Agriculture, Arizona State University, Tempe, Arizona 85287, USA
Contact point: Executive Secretary – Dr Richard Chalquest
Publication: Proceedings of the annual conference (37th 1988)

2305 Western Veterinary Conference, Suite 210, 2235 East Flamingo Road, Las Vegas, Nevada 89119, USA
Tel. (702) 794 0626
Contact point: Executive Director – Dr Kenneth D. Weide
Publication: Directory (annual)
Holds an annual continuing education conference (61st 1989).

2306 Western World Pet Supply Association, PO Box 1337, 1445 Hintington Drive, Suite 101, South Pasadena, California 1030, USA
Tel. (818) 799 7182
Contact point: Executive Vice President – Thomas H. McLaughlin
Publication: Pet news (quarterly)
Holds trade shows semiannually.

2307 Wildlife Disease Association, PO Box 886, Ames, Iowa 50010, USA
Publications: Journal of wildlife disease; *Wildlife disease newsletter* (quarterly); slide sets

2308 Winrock International, Winrock International Institute for Agricultural Development, Petit Jean Mountain, Morrilton, Arkansas 72110, USA
Tel. (501) 727 5435. Telex: 910720 6616 WIHQUD. Fax: (501) 727 5242
Publications: OCIAC updates (nine times a year) – newsletter on agricultural communication; the *Catalog of publications and videotapes* describes many reports, monographs, proceedings, factsheets, videotapes and occasional papers on agricultural development and animal health, husbandry and management. The catalogue includes the International Stockmen's School Handbooks (available from Westview Press), titles currently available are: *Beef cattle science handbook* (**20** 1984), *Dairy science handbook* (**16** 1984), *Sheep and goat handbook* (**4** 1984), *Stud managers' handbook* (**19** 1984) and *Emerging technology and management for ruminants* (1985)

2309 World Association for the Advancement of Veterinary Parasitology, SmithKline Beckman AHP, Applebrook Center, 1600 Paoli Pike, Westchester, Pennsylvania 19380, USA
Tel. (215) 251 7400
Contact point: Secretary-Treasurer – Dr V. J. Theodorides
Publications: The Association meets every two years (13th Conference East Berlin August 1989) and publishes its proceedings. The plenary lectures appear in *Veterinary parasitology. Newsletter*; *Guidelines for evaluating the efficacy of anthelmintics*: in ruminants (bovine and ovine) *Veterinary parasitology* **10** (1982): 265–84; in swine **21** (1986) 69–82; in horses **30** (1988) 57–72; *Standardized nomenclature of animal parasitic diseases* (SNOPAD): *Veterinary parasitology* **29** (1988) 299–306

2310   World Association for Animal Production, Corso Trieste 67, 00198 Rome, Italy
Tel. (06) 860785
Contact point: Secretary General – Dr K. Kállay
Publications: News items (twice a year); world conferences Tokyo (1983), Helsinki (1988), 7th Canada 1992

2311   World Association for Buiatrics, Rinderklinik, Bischofsholer Damm 15, D-3000 Hanover 1, Federal Republic of Germany
Tel. (0511) 856 243
Contact point: Secretary General – Prof. Dr M. Stöber
Publications: Proceedings of world congresses on diseases in cattle – 14th Dublin (1986), 15th Palma de Mallorca, Spain, (1988), next Brasilia (1990); *List of WAB-associated corporative members*

2312   World Association for the History of Veterinary Medicine, Tierärztliche Hochschule Hannover, Bischofsholer Damn 15, D-3000 Hanover 1, Federal Republic of Germany
Tel. (0511) 85 65 03. Telex: 22034 TIHO D
Contact point: Prof. Dr E-H. Lochmann
Publications: International symposia held every one or two years (23rd 1989). A booklet of abstracts of the lectures is published

2313   World Association of Veterinarians Specialized in Fish Diseases, Institut für Zoologie und Hydrobiologie, Tierärztliche Fakultät der Universität München, Kaulbachstrasse 37, 8000 Munich 22, Federal Republic of Germany
Tel. (89) 21 80 26 87
Contact point: Prof. Dr R. Hoffmann

2314   World Association of Veterinary Anatomists, Department of Veterinary Anatomy, Cornell University, Ithaca, New York 14853, USA
Tel. (607) 253 3554
Contact point: Secretary General – Prof. W. O. Sack
Publications: Anatomia, histologia, embryologia (Zentralblatt für Veterinärmedizin, Section C) (quarterly); *WAVA news*
General Assembly meets at the International Congress of Anatomy or the World Veterinary Congress. Meetings every two or three years.

2315   World Association of Veterinary Educators, Department d'Anatomie et Physiologie Animales, Faculté de Médecine Vétérinaire, Université de Montréal, C.P. 5000, Saint Hyacinthe, Quebec J2S 7C6, Canada
Tel. (514) 773 8521 (ext. 295)
Contact point: Prof. Dr Jean Piérard

2316   World Association of Veterinary Food Hygienists, Box 22067, S-104 22
Stockholm, Sweden
Tel. (08) 785 50 50 (office), (08) 800 500 (home). Telex: 11803. Fax. (08) 50 55 00
Contact point: Secretary – Dr K. G. Linderholm
Publications: Symposia proceedings (10th Stockholm 1989)

2317   World Association of Veterinary Laboratory Diagnosticians, Inter-
American Institute for Cooperation on Agriculture, Caixa Postal 09–1070,
SHIS-Q15 – Blaco D, Commercial Local, 71600 Brasilia D.F., Brasil
Contact point: Secretary-Treasurer – Dr Michael Bedoya
Publications: Proceedings of international symposia (triennial – 5th Guelph 1989)

2318   World Association of Veterinary Microbiologists, Immunologists and
Specialists in Infectious Diseases, École Nationale Vétérinaire d'Alfort, 7
Avenue du Général de Gaulle, 94704 Maisons Alfort, France
Tel. (1) 48 93 71 31
Contact point: President – Prof. Ch. Pilet
Publication: Proceedings of the international symposia (9th Perugia 1986); First
world congress held in Lyon in 1988

2319   World Association of Veterinary Pathologists, École Nationale Vétéri-
naire d'Alfort, 7 Avenue du Général de Gaulle, 94704 Maisons Alfort,
France
Tel. (1) 43 53 35 36. Telex: ECALFOR 213863 F
Contact point: President – Prof. A-L. Parodi
Publication: WAVP newsletter (irregular)

2320   World Association of Veterinary Physiologists, Pharmacologists and
Biochemists, Département d'Anatomie et Physiologie Animale, Faculté de
Médecine Vétérinaire, Université de Montréal, CP 5000, Saint Hyacinthe,
Quebec J2S 7C6, Canada
Tel. (514) 773 8521
Contact point: Prof. L. P. Phaneuf

2321   World Association of Wildlife Veterinarians, PO Box 358, Sabie 1260,
Republic of South Africa
Tel. (013142) 1440
Contact point: Corresponding Secretary – Dr B. H. Pappin
Inaugural meeting to be held in 1990.

2322   World Equine Veterinary Association, 7762 Roberts Road, Hilliard,
Ohio 43026, USA
Tel. (614) 878 4136
Contact point: Secretary/Treasurer – Dr Vernon L. Tharp

Publications: Symposia proceedings – most recent – *The horse in international commerce* (1987) published in *Journal of equine veterinary science* **8** (1988): (2) and (3)

2323   World Federation of Parasitologists, National Institute of Public Health and Environmental Hygiene, PO Box 1, NL-3720 BA Bilthoven, The Netherlands
Contact point: Secretary – Dr F. van Knapen
Publications: *WFP newsletter* (twice a year); *Membership list*; Proceedings of the quadrennial international congress for parasitology (last Brisbane 1986, next Paris 1990 – ICOPA VII)

2324   World Health Organization, Avenue Appia, 1211 Geneva 27, Switzerland
Tel. (022) 91 21 11. Telex: UNISANTE GENEVA 27821
Publications: *World health* (ten times a year); *World health forum* (quarterly); *Bulletin of the World Health Organization*; plus a variety of monographs, reports, recommendations, guidelines, statistics

2325   World Rabbit Science Association, Tyning House, Shurdington, Cheltenham, Gloucestershire GL51 5XF, England
Tel. (0242) 862387
Contact point: Secretary – Peter Horne
Publications: Proceedings of the quadrennial world congresses (4th Budapest 1988)

2326   World Small Animal Veterinary Association, Royal Veterinary College, Hawkshead Lane, Hatfield, Hertfordshire AL9 7TA, England
Tel. (0707) 55486
Contact point: Honorary Secretary – Dr P. G. C. Bedford
Publications: *Journal of small animal practice*; *Proceedings* (536pp.) and *Abstracts* (395pp.) from the 13th WSAVA conference, Barcelona, 1987

2327   World Society for the Protection of Animals, 106 Jermyn Street, London SW1Y 6EE, England
Tel. 01–839 3066
Contact point: Director General – Trevor H. Scott
Publications: *Animals international* (quarterly); leaflets, posters and fact sheets on current issues in animal welfare
The society has 40,000 individual members and links with 300 member humane societies around the world.

2328   World Veterinary Association/Association Mondiale Vétérinaire, Isabel la Católica 12, Madrid 28013, Spain
Tel. (01) 247 18 38. Telex: 41805 UCVET
Contact point: Secretary-Treasurer – Prof. Dr C. L. de Cuenca
Publications: *Bulletin* (three times a year – free to those with an interest in veterinary information); *World catalogue of veterinary films/video tapes and films/video*

tapes of veterinary interest; *Directory of veterinary schools and faculties*; *List of WVA members*; *Short history of the WVA*; *Exchange of veterinary medical personnel between schools and faculties in WVA member countries. Possibilities of postgraduate studies*; the proceedings of the World Veterinary Congresses are issued by the Organizing Committees (23rd Congress, Montreal, 1987, *Proceedings* (2 vols, 1,120pp. Contains the presentations and discussions at the plenary sessions) and *Abstracts* (494pp. Containing abstracts of all the presentations))

2329 World Veterinary Poultry Association, c/o AFRC Institute for Animal Health, Houghton Laboratory, Huntingdon, Cambridgeshire PE17 2DA, England
Tel. (0480) 64101
Contact point: Dr L. N. Payne
Publications: Avian pathology; Proceedings of the quadrennial conferences (9th Brighton 1989)

2330 World's Poultry Science Association, Meadfoot, Chalkside Road, Terrick, Aylesbury, Buckinghamshire HP17 0TJ, England
Tel. (029661) 3302
Contact point: British branch – Miss M. C. French at above address; Secretary: Prof. Dr R-M. Wagner, Institut für Kleintierzucht, 3100 Celle, Dornbergstr. 25/27, Federal Republic of Germany
Publications: The proceedings of the poultry science symposia of the British branch (now held annually – 21st 1988) are published by Butterworths; European poultry congress (7th Paris 1986); *World's poultry science journal*
The World's Association organizes a World's Poultry Congress tri- or quadrennially (23rd Japan 1988).

2331 World's Women's Veterinary Association, 74 Janefield Avenue, Ste. 88, Guelph, Ontario, Canada
Contact point: President – Dr Elizabeth McGregor

ONLINE SYSTEMS

The international headquarters are listed. Contacts are given for the most important of the systems based outside the UK or USA and with representatives in either of those countries.

2332 AGNET, University of Nebraska, Lincoln, Nebraska 68583, USA. Tel. (402) 472 1892

2333 BLAISE (BLAISE-LINK and BLAISE-LINE), The British Library, Bibliographic Services Division, 2 Sheraton Street, London W1V 4BH, England. Tel. 01–323 7074, 01–323 7070 (help desk). Telex: 21462 BELREF G. Fax. 01–323–7039

2334 BRS Information Technologies, 1200 Route 7, Latham, New York 12100, USA. Tel. (800) 345 4277, (518) 783 1161

2335 CAN/OLE (Canadian Online Enquiry Service), *see* CISTI

2336 CISTI, National Research Council of Canada, Institute for Scientific and Technical Information, Montreal Road, Ottawa, Ontario K1A 0S2, Canada. Tel. (613) 993 1210. Telex: 0533115 CA

2337 COMPU-MARK, New Premier House, Suite 3, 150 Southampton Row, London WC1B 5AL, England. Tel. 01–278 4646

2338 COMPUSERVE, PO Box 20212, Columbus, Ohio 43220, USA. Tel. (800) 848 8199, (614) 457 0802

2339 DATACENTRALEN, DC Host Centre, I/S Datacentralen af 1959, Landlystvej 40, DK-2650 Hvidovre, Copenhagen, Denmark. Tel. (01) 75 81 22. Telex: 27122 DC DK. Fax. (01) 75 05 50

2340 DATA-STAR, Plaza Suite, 114 Jermyn Street, London SW1Y 6HJ, England. Tel. 01–930 5503. Telex: 94012671 STAR G. Fax. 01–930 2581

DATA-STAR, Radio-Suisse Ltd, Laupenstrasse 18a, CH-3008 Berne, Switzerland. Tel. (031) 50 95 00. Telex: 912972 RSAG CH. Fax. (031) 50 96 75

D-S Marketing, Suite 110, 485 Devon Park Drive, Wayne, Pennsylvania 19087, USA. Tel. (800) 221 7754, (215) 687 6777. Fax. (215) 687 0984

2341 DIALCOM, 6120 Executive Boulevard, Rockville, Maryland 20852, USA. Tel. (301) 881 9020, (800) 435 7342

2342 DIALOG Information Services, 3460 Hillview Avenue, Palo Alto, California 94304, USA. Tel. (800) 334 2564, (415) 858 3810. Telex: 334499 (DIALOG)

DIALOG Information Services, PO Box 188, Oxford OX1 5AX, England. Tel. (0865) 730275. Telex: 837704 INFORM G. Fax: (0865) 736354

2343 DIMDI (Deutsches Institut für Medizinische Dokumentation und Information), Weisshausstrasse 27, Postfach 420580, D-5000 Cologne 41, Federal Republic of Germany. Tel. (0221) 47 241. Telex: 8881364

2344 DUN & BRADSTREET, 26–32 Clifton Street, London EC2P 2LY, England. Tel. 01–377 4377. Telex: 886697 DEANBE G. Fax. 01–247 3836

2345 ESA-IRS, ESRIN, Via Galileo Galilei, PO Box 64, 00044 Frascati (Rome), Italy. Tel. (06) 941801, Help Desk (06) 94180300. Telex: 610637 ESRIN I. Fax: (06) 94180361

IRS-DIALTECH, Department of Trade and Industry, Room 392, Ashdown House, 123 Victoria Street, London SW1E 6RB. Tel. 01–212 6578, 01–212 6582

2346 FARAD, c/o Dr S. F. Sundlof, Department of Physiological Sciences, College of Veterinary Medicine, Box J-137, University of Florida, Gainesville, Florida 32610, USA. Tel. (904) 392 4085.

2347 IMSBASE, IMS International, 364 Euston Road, London NW1 3BL, England. Tel. 01–387 8434. Telex: 8954520 IDSLDN G. Fax. 01–388 9391

IMSBASE, IMS International Executive Campus, 660 West Germantown Pike, Plymouth Meeting, Pennsylvania 19462, USA. Tel. (215) 834 5076. Telex: 6851007. Fax. (215) 834 5100

2348 IMSMARQ, PO Box 917, London NW1 3BU, England. Tel. 01–387 8434. Telex: 8954520. Fax. 01–388 9391

2349 JICST (Japan Information Center of Science and Technology), 5–2, Nagatacho 2-Chome, Chiyoda-ku, Tokyo 100, Japan. Tel. (03) 581 6411. Telex: 02223604 J. Fax. (03) 581 6446

2350 MAXWELL ONLINE, 8000 Westpark Drive, McLean, Virginia 22102, USA. Tel. (800) 45-ORBIT, (703) 442 0900. Fax: (703) 893 4632

MAXWELL ONLINE, Achilles House, Western Avenue, London W3 0UA, England. Tel. 01–992 3456, 01–993 7333 (help desk). Telex: 8814614. Fax. 01–993 7335

2351 MiCIS (Microbial Culture Information Service), Laboratory of the Government Chemist, Queen's Road, Teddington, Middlesex TW11 0LY, England. Tel. 01–943 7612

2352 NATIONAL LIBRARY OF MEDICINE, Medlars Management Section, 8600 Rockville Pike, Bethesda, Maryland 20894, USA. Tel. (301) 496 6193

2353 ORBIT SEARCH SERVICE, *see* MAXWELL ONLINE

2354 PERGAMON FINANCIAL DATA SERVICES, *see* MAXWELL ONLINE

2355   PROFILE INFORMATION, Sunbury House, 79 Staines Road West, Sunbury on Thames, Middlesex TW16 7AH, England. Tel. (0932) 787231. Fax. (0932) 787231

2356   STN INTERNATIONAL, Postfach 2465, D-7500 Karlsruhe 1, Federal Republic of Germany. Tel. (07247) 808–555. Telex: 17724710 + . Fax. (07247) 808–666.

STN INTERNATIONAL, The Royal Society of Chemistry, Thomas Graham House, Science Park, Milton Road, Cambridge CB4 4WF, England. Tel. (0223) 420237 (help desk), (0223) 420066. Telex: 818293 ROYAL. Fax. (0223) 423623

STN INTERNATIONAL, 2540 Olentangy River Road, PO Box 02228, Columbus, Ohio 43202, USA. Tel. (614) 421 3600, (800) 848 6533. Telex: 6842086 CHMAB. Fax. (614) 421 3713

2357   TELESYSTEMES-QUESTEL, 83–85 Boulevard Vincent-Auriol, 75013 Paris, France. Tel. (01) 45 82 64 64

2358   TEXTLINE and NEWSLINE, Reuter Textline, 85 Fleet Street, London EC4P 4AJ, England. Tel. 01–324 8022. Telex: 23222

Reuters Information Services, 40 East 52nd Street, New York 10022, USA. Tel. (800) 426 4318, (212) 593 5532

2359   TSUKUBA DAIGAKU, Gakujutsu Joho Shori Center, Tennodai, Sakura-Mura, Niihari-gun, Ibaraki, Japan. Tel. (0298) 53 2450

2360   VETERINARY NETWORK, 600 University Avenue, Los Gatos, California 95030, USA. Tel. (408) 354 3477

2361   VETERINARY COMPUTERISED INFORMATION SYSTEM (VCIS), The Veterinary Information Company, Suite 108–110, Langmuir Laboratory, Brown Road, Ithaca, New York 14850, USA. Tel. (607) 257 4303. Fax. (607) 257 2445

2362   VETERINARY SERVICES DATA BANK (VSDB), c/o Dr E. I. Pilchard, USDA, APHIS, US, 740 Federal Building, 6505 Belarest Road, Hyattsville, Maryland 20782, USA. Tel. (301) 436 8069

ONLINE DATABASES

The international headquarters are listed. Details of representatives within the UK and USA are given for the most important databases.

2363   AGDEX, Edinburgh School of Agriculture, West Mains Road, Edinburgh EH9 3JG, Scotland. Tel. 031–668 3471. Telex: 727617. Fax. 031–667 2601

2364   AGREP (AGricultural REsearch Projects), Commission of the European Communities, DG XIII, Bâtiment Jean Monnet, Plateau du Kirchberg, BP 1907, Luxembourg. Tel. (352) 243011. Telex: 2752 EURDOC LU

2365   AGRIBUSINESS U.S.A., Pioneer Hi-Bred International, 5608 Merle Hay Road, PO Box 183, Johnston, Iowa 50131, USA. Tel. (800) 826 5944, (515) 270 3925

2366   AGRICOLA, Head – Automated Retrieval Section, Room 300, National Agricultural Library Building, Beltsville, Maryland 20705, USA. Tel. (301) 344 3704

2367   AGRIS, Head – AGRIS Coordinating Centre, Library and Documentation Systems Division, Food and Agriculture Organization, Via delle Terme di Caracalla, 00100 Rome, Italy. Tel. (06) 57971 (ext. 4993). Telex: 610181 FAO I

2368   BIOBUSINESS, *see* BIOSIS

2369   BIOSIS, BioSciences Information Service, Education and Training Group, 2100 Arch Street, Philadelphia, Pennsylvania 19103, USA. Tel. (800) 523 4806, (215) 587 4847. Telex: 831739. Fax. (215) 587 2016

BIOSIS Help Desk, Vital Information Limited, 30 Hockliffe Street, Leighton Buzzard, Bedfordshire LU7 8HP, England. Tel. (0525) 382897. Telex: 82671 MONREF G quoting MAG95829. Fax. (0525) 382308

2370   BRITISH TRADE MARKS, The Patent Office, State House, 66–71 High Holborn, London WC1R 4TP, England. Tel. 01–831 2525

2371   CAB ABSTRACTS, CAB International, Wallingford, Oxfordshire OX10 8DE, England. Tel. (0491) 32111. Fax. (0491) 33508. Telex: 847964 COMAGG G

CAB International North American Office, 845 North Park Avenue, Tucson, Arizona 85719, USA. Tel. (800) 528 4841, (602) 621 7897. Telex: 910 952 1143 AZU TUC

2372   CABS (CURRENT AWARENESS IN BIOLOGICAL SCIENCES), *see* MAXWELL ONLINE in previous section

2373   CAMBRIDGE SCIENTIFIC ABSTRACTS, 7200 Wisconsin Avenue, Bethesda, Maryland 20814, USA. Tel. (301) 961 6700

2374   CARIS, Head – CARIS Coordinating Centre, Library and Documentation Systems Division, Food and Agriculture Organization, *see* AGRIS. Tel. (06) 57971 (ext. 3190). Telex: 610181 FAO I

2375   CHEMICAL ABSTRACTS files, *see* STN INTERNATIONAL in previous section

2376   CHEMICAL BUSINESS NEWSBASE, *see* STN INTERNATIONAL in previous section

2377   CHEMICAL INDUSTRY NOTES, *see* STN INTERNATIONAL in previous section

2378   CONFERENCE PROCEEDINGS INDEX, *see* BLAISE in previous section

2379   CRIS/USDA, Current Research Information System, US Department of Agriculture, Science and Education Administration/TIS, National Agricultural Library Building, Beltsville, Maryland 20705, USA. Tel. (301) 344 3850

2380   CURRENT BIOTECHNOLOGY ABSTRACTS, *see* STN INTER-NATIONAL in previous section

2381   CURRENT CONTENTS SEARCH, *see* SCISEARCH

2382   DVJB, The Danish Veterinary and Agricultural Library, The Royal Veterinary and Agricultural University, Bulowsvej 13, DK-1870 Frederiksberg C, Denmark. Tel. (01) 35 17 88 (ext. 2217)

2383   EMBASE PLUS, Excerpta Medica Publishing Group, Molenwerf 1, 1014 AG Amsterdam, The Netherlands. Tel. (020) 5803 535. Telex: 18582 ESPA NL. Fax. (020) 5803 429

2384   FEDERAL RESEARCH IN PROGRESS, *see* NTIS. Tel. (703) 487 4929

2385   INFOMAT INTERNATIONAL BUSINESS, *see* PROMT

2386   INPADOC, International Patent Documentation Centre, Moellwald-platz 4, A-1040 Vienna, Austria. Tel. (0222) 658784. Telex: 136337 INPA A

2387   MEDLINE, *see* NATIONAL LIBRARY OF MEDICINE in previous section

2388   MINE (Microbial Information Network Europe), Rhonda Platt (UK MINE Project Administrator), Culture Collection and Industrial Services, CAB International Mycological Institute, Ferry Lane, Kew, Surrey TW9 3AF, England. Tel. 01–940 4086. Telex: 265871 MONREF G. Fax. 01–581 1671 (indicate 'for CMI')

2389   NTIS, US Department of Commerce, National Technical Information Service, 5285 Port Royal Road, Springfield, Virginia 22161, USA. Tel. (703) 487 4600

2390   PASCAL, Centre National de la Recherche Scientifique, Centre de Documentation Scientifique et Technique, 26 Rue Boyer, 75971 Paris Cedex 20, France. Tel. (1) 43 58 35 59. Telex: 220880 CNRSDOC F. Fax. (1) 43 58 03

2391   PATOLIS, *see* INPADOC

2392   PHARMACEUTICAL NEWS INDEX, Customer Services Department, UMI/Data Courier, 620 South Firth Street, Louisville, Kentucky 40202, USA. Tel. (502) 582 4111, (800) 626 2823

2393   PHARMACONTACTS, *see* PHIND

2394   PHARMAPROJECTS, *see* PHIND

2395   PHIND (Pharmaceutical and Health Care Industries News Database) – PHID/PHIC/PHIN, PJB Publications Ltd, 18/20 Hill Rise, Richmond, Surrey TW10 6UA, England. Tel. 01–948 3262. Telex: 263124 PJBB G. Fax. 01–948 5598

2396   RINGDOC, *see* VETDOC

2397   PROMT, Predicasts, 11001 Cedar Avenue, Cleveland, Ohio 44106, USA. Tel. (800) 321 6388, (216) 795 3000. Telex: 985604. Fax. (216) 229 9944

Predicasts Europe, 8–10 Denman Street, London W1V 7RF, England. Tel. 01–494 3817/01–434 2954. Telex: 296276 CLSI UK. Fax: 01–734 5935

2398   RTECS (Registry of Toxic Effects of Chemical Substances), US Department of Health and Human Services, Public Health Service National Institute for Occupational Safety and Health, 4676 Columbia Parkway, Cincinnati, Ohio 45226, USA

2399   SCISEARCH, Institute for Scientific Information, 3501 Market Street, Philadelphia 19104, USA. Tel. (800) 523 1857, (215) 386 0100. Telex: 845305. Fax. (215) 386 6362

SCISEARCH, Institute for Scientific Information, 132 High Street, Uxbridge, Middlesex UB8 1DP, England. Tel. (0895) 70016. Telex: 933693 UKISI

2400   SIGLE, *see* BLAISE in previous section

2401   TOXLINE and TOXNET, *see* NATIONAL LIBRARY OF MEDICINE in previous section

2402   TRADEMARKSCAN-FEDERAL   and   TRADEMARKSCAN-STATE, Thomson & Thomson, 500 Victory Road, North Quincy, Massachusetts 02171, USA. Tel. (800) 692 8833, (617) 479 1600. Telex: 6971430. Fax. (617) 786 8273

2403   VETDOC, Derwent Publications Ltd, Rochdale House, 128 Theobalds Road, London WC1X 8RP, England. Tel. 01–242 5823. Telex: 267487 DERPUB G. Fax. 01–405 3630

Derwent Inc., 1313 Dolley Madison Boulevard, Suite 303, McLean, Virginia 22101, USA. Tel. (800) 451 3451, (703) 790 0400. Fax. (703) 790 1426

2404   WORLD PATENTS INDEX (WPI), *see* VETDOC

2405   ZOOLOGICAL RECORD, *see* BIOSIS

PUBLISHERS AND BOOKSELLERS

The head office for each of the major publishers is listed. Their UK and USA distributors or agents are noted where this may be particularly useful. Addresses for editorial and sales offices of these publishers and for local offices of other publishers represented in the UK can be found in *British books in print* [48] or *Whitaker's book list* [59]. American publishing houses are similarly listed in *Books in print* [46].

2406   Academic Press (Harcourt Brace Jovanovich), 24/28 Oval Road, London NW1 7DX, England. Tel. 01–267 4466. Telex: 25775 ACPRES G. Fax. 01–482 2293

Academic Press, Orlando, Florida 32887, USA. Tel. (305) 345 4100. Telex: ACP ORL 568364

2407   Akademie-Verlag Berlin, Leipziger Str. 3/4, Postfach 1233, 1086 Berlin, Democratic Republic of Germany. Tel. 223 62 29. Telex: 114420

2408 J. A. Allen, 1 Lower Grosvenor Place, London SW1W 0EL, England. Tel. 01–834 5606. Telex: 28905/3810

2409 American Veterinary Publications, 5782 Thornwood Drive, Goleta, California 93117, USA. Tel. (805) 967 5988

2410 Angus & Robertson Publishers, PO Box 290, Unit 4, Eden Park, 31 Waterloo Road, North Ryde, New South Wales 2113, Australia. Tel. (02) 888 4111. Telex: 26452 ARPUB AA

2411 Edward Arnold, 41 Bedford Square, London WC1B 3DQ, England. Tel. 01–637 7161. Telex: 265806 EDWARD G. Fax. 01–436 5776

2412 The AVI Publishing Company, PO Box 831, 250 Post Road East, Westport, Connecticut 06881, USA. Tel. (203) 226 0738

2413 Baillière Tindall (UK: Academic Press. USA: W. B. Saunders)

2414 MTP Press Limited, *see* Kluwer

2415 Birkhäuser Verlag, PO Box 133, CH-4010 Basel, Switzerland. Tel. (061) 735300. Telex: 963475 BIRKH CH. Fax. (061) 731427

2416 Blackwell Scientific Publications, Osney Mead, Oxford OX2 0EL, England. Tel. (0865) 240201. Telex: 83355 MEDBOK G. Fax. (0865) 721205

2417 Blandford Press, *see* Cassell

2418 R. R. Bowker, 245 West 17th Street, New York 10011, USA. Tel. (212) 645 9700. Telex: 127703. (UK: Butterworth)

2419 Butterworth & Co. (Publishers), Borough Green, Sevenoaks, Kent TN15 8PH, England. Tel. (0732) 884567. Telex: 95678

2420 Cambridge University Press, Edinburgh Building, Shaftesbury Road, Cambridge CB2 2RU, England. Tel. (0223) 312393. Telex: 817256

2421 Cassell, Artillery House, Artillery Row, London SW1P 1RT, England. Tel. 01–222 7676. Telex: 9413701 CASPUB G. Fax. 01–799 1514

2422 Chalcombe Publications, Honey Lane, Hurley, Maidenhead, Berkshire SL6 5LR, England. Tel. (062882) 6868. Telex: 847159 MARLOW G. Fax. (062882) 3630

2423 Churchill Livingstone, 1560 Broadway, New York 10036, USA. Tel. (212) 819 5400. Telex: 662266. (UK: Longman)

2424   Clarendon Press, *see* Oxford University Press

2425   William Collins Sons & Co., 8 Grafton Street, London W1X 3LA, England. Tel. 01–493 7070. Telex: 25611 COLLINS G. Fax. 01–493 3061

2426   Cornell University Press, Box 250, 124 Roberts Place, Ithaca, New York 14851, USA. Tel. (607) 257 7000. Telex: WUI 6713054

2427   CRC Press Inc., 2000 Corporate Boulevard NW, Boca Raton, Florida 33431, USA. Tel. (305) 994 0555. Telex: 568689. (UK: Wolfe Publishing)

2428   Dairy Goat Journal Publishing Company, c/o Kent Leach, PO Box 1908, Scottsdale, Arizona 85252, USA. Tel. (602) 991 4628

2429   B. C. Decker, 3228 South Service Road, Suite 205, Burlington, Ontario L7N 3H8, Canada. Tel. (416) 639 6215. Telex: 0618009. (UK: Blackwell. USA: C. V. Mosby)

2430   Marcel Dekker Inc., 270 Madison Avenue, New York 10016, USA. Tel. (212) 696 9000. Telex: 421419. Fax. (212) 685 4540

2431   Antonio Delfino Editore, Via Udine 32140, 00161 Rome, Italy. Tel. (06) 865490

2432   Deutsche Gesellschaft für technische Zusammenarbeit (GTZ), Postfach 5180, D-6236 Eschborn/Taunus 1, Federal Republic of Germany. Tel. (06196) 79–0. Telex: 41523–0

2433   Diamond Farm Book Publishers, PO Box 537, Alexandria Bay, New York 13607, USA

2434   Edagricole, Casella Postale 2202, Via Emilia Levante 31, 40139 Bologna, Italy. Tel. (051) 49 22 11

2435   Editorial Hemisferio Sur, Pasteur 743, 1028 Buenos Aires, Argentina

2436   Editorial Inter-Medica, Casilla de Correo 4625, 1113 Buenos Aires, Argentina. Tel. 833234

2437   Ellis Horwood, Market Cross House, Cooper Street, Chichester, West Sussex PO19 1EB, England. Tel. (0243) 789942. Telex: 86516 ELWOOD G. Fax. (0243) 778855

2438   Elsevier Science Publishers, PO Box 211, 1000 AE Amsterdam, The Netherlands. Tel. (020) 5803 911. Telex: 18582 ESPA NL

2439 Verlag Eugen Ulmer, Wollgrasweg 41, Postfach 700561, D-7000 Stuttgart 70, Federal Republic of Germany. Tel. (0711) 4507-0. Telex: 23634 ULMER D. Fax. (0711) 4507120

2440 Farming Press, Wharfedale Road, Ipswich, Suffolk IP1 4LG, England. Tel. (0473) 43011. Fax. (0473) 240501. (USA: Diamond Farm Book Publishers)

2441 Ferdinand Enke Verlag, Postfach 1304, D-7000 Stuttgart 1, Federal Republic of Germany. Tel. (0711) 8931-0. Telex: 07252275 GTV D. Fax. (0711) 8931-298

2442 VEB Gustav Fischer Verlag, *see* VEB Verlage für Medizin und Biologie

2443 Gustav Fischer Verlag, Wollgrasweg 49, Postfach 72 01 43, D-7000 Stuttgart 70, Federal Republic of Germany. Tel. (0711) 45 50 38, (0711) 45 10 00. Telex: 7111488 FIBUCH. Fax. (0711) 455 03 34

2444 Fishing News Books, 1 Long Garden Walk, Farnham, Surrey GU9 7HX, England. Tel. (0252) 726868. Telex: 859500 SHARET G. (USA: UNIPUB)

2445 FN-Verlag, Postfach 640, D-4410 Warendorf, Federal Republic of Germany. Tel. (025) 81 76 96. Telex: 89950 FNGER D

2446 Gakusosha Company, 2-16-28 Nishikata, Bunkyo-ku, Tokyo 113, Japan. Tel. (03) 818 8701. Fax. (03) 818 8704

2447 Gower Publishing Company, Gower House, Croft Road, Aldershot, Hampshire GU11 3HR, England. Tel. (0252) 331551. Telex: 858001 GOWER G

2448 Grafton Books *and* Granada Publishing, *see* William Collins

2449 Grune & Stratton, PO Box 6280, Duluth, Minnesota 55806, USA. (UK: Academic Press)

2450 Harper & Row, Middlesex House, 32-42 Cleveland Street, London W1P 5FB, England. Tel. 01-631 8300. Telex: 21736. Fax. 01-631 3594

2451 Heffers, 20 Trinity Street, Cambridge CB2 3NG, England. Tel. (0223) 358351. Telex: 81298. Fax: (0223) 410464

2452 Henston, Friary Court, 13-21 High Street, Guildford, Surrey GU1 3DX, England. Tel. (0483) 502125

2453   HMSO (Her Majesty's Stationery Office) Publications Centre, PO Box 276, London SW8 5DT, England. Tel. 01–873 0022 (enquiries), 01–873 9090 (orders). Telex: 297138. Fax. 01–873 8463. (US: UNIPUB)

2454   S. Hirzel Verlag, Sternwartenstr. 8, Postfach 506, 7010 Leipzig, Democratic Republic of Germany. Tel. (041) 282263

2455   Holt-Saunders, *see* W. B. Saunders

2456   Institut National de la Recherche Agronomique (INRA), Service des Publications, Route de St-Cyr, 78026 Versailles, France. Tel. (01) 30 83 34 06. Telex: INRAPUB 699 368F

2457   Institute of Aquaculture, Book Department, University of Stirling, Stirling FK9 4LA, Scotland. Tel. (0786) 73171 (ext. 2189)

2458   Interpharm Press, PO Box 530, Prairie View, Illinois 60069, USA. Tel. (312) 459 8480. Telex: 499–5880 INTPHARM. Fax. (312) 459 4536

2459   The Interstate Printers and Publishers, PO Box 50, Danville, Illinois, 61834, USA. Tel. (217) 446 0500

2460   Iowa State University Press, 2121 S. State Avenue, Ames, Iowa 50010, USA. Tel. (515) 292 0140. (UK: Baillière Tindall/W. B. Saunders)

2461   S. Karger, Allschwilerstrasse 10, PO Box, CH-4009 Basel, Switzerland. Tel. (061) 38 08 80. Telex: 962652 CH. Fax. (061) 385 383. (UK: John Wiley & Sons)

2462   Kendall/Hunt Publishing Company, 2460 Kerper Boulevard, Dubuque, Iowa 52001, USA. Tel. (319) 588 1451. Telex: 468541

2463   Kimpton's Medical Bookshop, 205 Great Portland Street, London W1N 6LR, England. Tel. 01–580 6833. Telex: 295441 KMB

2464   Kluwer Academic Publishers, PO Box 17, 3300 AA Dordrecht, The Netherlands. Tel. (078) 334200. Telex: 29245 KAPG NL. Fax. (078) 334254

2465   Lea & Febiger, 600 Washington Square, Philadelphia, Pennsylvania 19106, USA. Tel. (800) 433 3850, (215) 922 1330

Lea & Febiger, 145a Croydon Road, Beckenham, Kent BR3 3RB, England. Tel. 01–650 4929. Telex: 8951182 GECOMS G. Fax. 01–658 0077

2466   H. K. Lewis, 136 Gower Street, London WC1E 6BS, England. Tel. 01–387 4282. Telex: 22607 HKLMED G

2467   Librairie de la Nouvelle Faculté, 10 Rue Casimir Slavigne, 75006 Paris, France. Tel. (01) 43 25 47 11

2468   Librairie Zoothèque, 38 Avenue Général de Gaulle, 94704 Maisons Alfort, BP 234, France. Tel. 43 68 61 74

2469   Librería Agrícola, Fernando VI, 2, 28004 Madrid, Spain. Tel. 419 13 79.

2470   J. B. Lippincott, PO Box 1430, East Washington Square, Philadelphia, Pennsylvania 19105, USA. Tel. (215) 238 4200. (UK: Harper & Row)

2471   Liverpool University Press, PO Box 147, Liverpool L69 3BX, England. Tel. 051–709 6022. Telex: 627095 UNIPL G

2472   Longman Group, Longman House, Burnt Mill, Harlow, Essex CM20 2JE, England. Tel. (0279) 26721. Telex: 81259 LONGMN G. Fax. (0279) 31059. (USA: John Wiley & Sons)

2473   Maloine SA, 27 Rue de l'École de Médecine, 75006 Paris, France. Tel. (01) 43 25 60 45. Telex: 203215 F

2474   Martinus Nijhoff, *see* Kluwer

2475   Masson et Cie, 120 Boulevard St Germain, 75280 Paris Cedex 06, France. Tel. (01) 46 34 21 60. Telex: 260946

2476   McGraw-Hill/Interamericana de Mexico, Apartado Postal 26370, Cedro 512, Cd. Atlampa 06450 Mexico, D.F. Tel. 541 3155. Telex: 1771196 NEISME. Fax. (905) 541 1603

2478   Microinfo, PO Box 3, Alton, Hampshire GU34 2PG, England. Tel. (0420) 86848. Telex: 858431 MINFO G. Fax. (0420) 89889

2479   MAFF Publications, Lion House, Willowburn Estate, Alnwick, Northumberland NE66 2PF, England. Tel. (0665) 602881

2480   Misset International, PO Box 4, 7000 BA Doetinchem, The Netherlands. Tel. (08340) 49562. Telex: 45481 MSSET NL. Fax. (08340) 40515

2481   A. E. Morgan, Stanley House, 9 West Street, Epsom, Ewell, Surrey KT18 7RL, England. Tel. (03727) 41411. Fax. (03727) 44493

2482   Morgan-Grampian, 30 Calderwood Street, London SE18 6QH, England. Tel. 01-355 7777. Telex: 896238

2483 C. V. Mosby Co., 11830 Westline Industrial Drive, St Louis, Missouri 63146, USA. Tel. (314) 872 8370. Telex: 62935642. Fax. (314) 432 1380. (UK: Williams & Wilkins)

2484 MTP Press, *see* Kluwer

2485 Nasco, 901 Janesville Avenue, Fort Atkinson, Wisconsin 53538, USA. Tel. (414) 563 2446

2486 National Academy Press, 2101 Constitution Avenue NW, Washington, DC 20418, USA. Tel. (202) 334 3318. Telex: 248664 (UK: John Wiley & Sons)

2487 Nicolás Moya – Librería Médica Carretas 29, 28012 Madrid, Spain. Tel. 522 52 94

2488 Noyes Data Corporation, Mill Road, Grand Avenue, Park Ridge, New Jersey 07656, USA. Tel. (201) 391 8484

2489 Oliver & Boyd, Robert Stevenson House, 1–3 Baxter's Place, Leith Walk, Edinburgh EH1 3BB, Scotland. Tel. 031–556 2424. Telex: 727511. Fax. 031–558 1278

2490 Organizzazione Editoriale Medico Farmaceutica srl, Via Edolo 42, PO Box 10434, 20125 Milan, Italy. Tel. (02) 66 91 344. Telex: 323598 OEMF MI I. Fax: (02) 66 97 191

2491 Oxford University Press, Walton Street, Oxford OX2 6DP, England. Tel. (0865) 56767. Telex: 837330. Fax. (0865) 56646

2492 Paul Parey Scientific Publishers, Spitalerstr. 12, Postfach 106304, D-2000 Hamburg 1, Federal Republic of Germany. Tel. (040) 321511. Telex: 2161391 PARV D

2493 Pergamon Press, Headington Hill Hall, Oxford OX3 0BW, England. Tel. (0865) 64881. Telex: 83177. Fax. (0865) 60285

2494 The Pharmaceutical Press, 1 Lambeth High Street, London SE1 7JN, England. Tel. 01–735 9141. (USA: Rittenhouse Book Distributors)

2495 Piccin Nuova Libraria, Via Altinate 107, 35121 Padua, Italy. Tel. (049) 65 55 66. Telex: 432074 PICCIN I

2496 Plenum Press, 233 Spring Street, New York 10013, USA. Tel. (212) 620 8000. Telex: 23/421139

2497   Éditions du Point Vétérinaire, 25 rue Bourgelat, 94700 Maisons-Alfort, France. Tel. 43 53 20 01. Telex: 231616

2498   PUDOC (Centre for Agricultural Publishing and Documentation), PO Box 4, 6700 AA Wageningen, The Netherlands. Tel. (08370) 84541. Telex: 45015 BLUWG NL. Fax. (08370) 84761

2499   Rittenhouse Book Distributors, 511 Feheley Drive, King of Prussia, Pennsylvania 19406, USA

2500   W. B. Saunders, 210 West Washington Square, Philadelphia, Pennsylvania 19105, USA. Tel. (215) 574 4700. Telex: 834795. (UK: Academic Press)

2501   K. G. Saur, Heilmanstr. 17, Postfach 711009, D-8000 Munich 71, Federal Republic of Germany. Tel. (089) 79104–0. Telex: 5212067. Fax. (089) 7914469. (UK and USA: Bowker)

2502   Verlag M. & H. Schaper, Postfach 810669, Grazer Str. 20, D-3000 Hannover 81, Federal Republic of Germany. Tel. (0511) 83 00 18

2503   F. K. Schattauer Publishers, PO Box 2945, D-7000 Stuttgart, Federal Republic of Germany. Tel: (0711) 221733. Telex: 17111402 FKS. Fax. (0711) 221735

2504   Schlütersche Verlagsanstalt und Druckerei, Postfach 5440, Georgswall 4, D-3000 Hannover 1, Federal Republic of Germany. Tel. (0511) 1236–0. Telex: 923978

2505   Scientechnica, *see* John Wright

2506   Shin-Suisan Shimbun-Sha Ltd., 3–16–12 Roppongi, Minato-ku, Tokyo, Japan

2507   Springer-Verlag, Heidelberger Platz 3, D-1000 Berlin 33, Federal Republic of Germany. Tel. (030) 8207–1. Telex: 183319 SPBLN D. Fax. (030) 8214091

2508   Superintendent of Documents, Government Printing Office, Washington, DC 20402, USA

2509   George Thieme Verlag, Postfach 732, Rudigesstr. 14, D-7000 Stuttgart 30, Federal Republic of Germany. Tel. (0711) 8931–0. Telex: 7252275 GTV D

2510   VEB George Thieme Verlag, *see* VEB Verlage für Medizin und Biologie

2511   C. C. Thomas, 2600 South First Street, Springfield, Illinois 62794, USA. Tel. (217) 789 8980

2512   TFH (Tropical Fish Hobbyist) Publications, One TFH Plaza, Third and Union Avenues, Neptune City, New Jersey 07753, USA. Tel. (201) 988 8400. Telex: 132468. Fax. (201) 988 5466

2513   UNIPUB, 4611-F Assembly Drive, Lanham, Maryland 20706, USA. Tel. (301) 459 7666

2514   USDA-APHIS (US Department of Agriculture – Animal and Plant Health Inspection Service), Printing and Distribution Management Branch, Room G-186, Federal Building, 6505 Belcrest Road, Hyattsville, Maryland 20782, USA. Tel. (301) 436 8413

2515   VEB Verlage für Medizin und Biologie, Villengang 2, Postfach 176, Jena 6900, Democratic Republic of Germany. Tel. 273 32. Telex: 058886176. (UK: Blackwell)

2516   Veterinary Book Guild, *see* American Veterinary Publications

2517   Veterinary Learning Systems, 2936 Brunswick Pike, PO Box 5818, Lawrenceville, New Jersey 08648, USA. Tel. (609) 882 5600. Fax. (609) 882 6357

2518   Veterinary Medicine Publishing, 9073 Lenexa Drive, Lenexa, Kansas 66215, USA. Tel. (800) 255 6864, (913) 492 4300

2519   Veterinary Practice Publishing, PO Box 4457, Santa Barbara, California 93140, USA. Tel. (805) 965 1028

2520   Veterinary Textbooks, 36 Woodcrest Avenue, Ithaca, New York 14850, USA. Tel. (607) 272 1860

2521   Éditions Vigot, 23 Rue de l'École de Médecine, 75006 Paris, France. Tel. (01) 43 29 54 50. Telex: VIGOT 201708 F

2522   Watt Publishing, Sandstone Building, Mount Morris, Illinois 61054, USA. Tel. (815) 734 4171. Fax. (815) 734 4201

2523   Westport Publications, 3 Henrietta Street, London WC2E 8LT, England. Tel. 01–240 1003

2524   Westview Press, 5500 Central Avenue, Boulder, Colorado 80301, USA. Tel. (303) 444 3541. Telex: 239479

2525   John Wiley & Sons, 605 3rd Avenue, New York 10158, USA. Tel. (212) 850 6000. Telex: 127063

John Wiley & Sons, Baffins Lane, Chichester, West Sussex PO19 1UD, England. Tel. (0243) 779777. Telex: 86290 WIBOOK G. Fax. (0243) 775878

2526   Williams & Wilkins, 428 East Preston Street, Baltimore, Maryland 21202, USA. Tel. (800) 638 0672, (301) 528 4221. Telex: 87669 WILCO. Fax. (301) 528 8550

Williams & Wilkins, The Broadway Centre, 2–6 Fulham Broadway, London SW6 1AA, England. Tel. 01–385 2357. Telex: 919891 WAVERLY G. Fax. 01–385 2922

2527   Williamson Publishing, Church Hill Road, Charlotte, Vermont 05445, USA. Tel. (802) 425 2102

2528   Wolfe Publishing, Brook House, 2–16 Torrington Place, London WC1E 7LT, England. Tel: 01–636 4622. Telex: 8814230. Fax. 01–637 3021

2529   John Wright, PO Box 63, Westbury House, Bury Street, Guildford, Surrey GU2 5BH, England. Tel. (0483) 300966. Telex: 859556 SCITEC G. Fax. (0483) 301563

2530   Verlag Zahnärztlich-medizinisches Schrifttum, Insterburgerstrasse 2, Postfach 81 05 09, D-8000 Munich 81, Federal Republic of Germany

Index

Numbers in square brackets refer to items in Parts II and III. Numbers without brackets refer to pages in Part I.

In general, items in Part II have been placed in a section devoted to a particular species where it was feasible to do so. Thus, when looking for material on a specific subject, e.g. ophthalmology, it is advisable to examine the section devoted to the species of interest, as well as using the more general texts in the relevant Specialities section.

Most of the organizations listed in Part III have not been indexed by name since within each section in Part III entries are listed in alphabetical order. Organizations have, however, been indexed by subject.

AAV today, [1083]
ABPI data sheet compendium, [253]
The ABPI guide to acronyms and abbreviations, [186]
Abs, M., [1040]
abstracting services, 53–62, 73–5; [12]–[28]
Abstracts of Bulgarian scientific literature, [12]
Abstracts on hygiene and communicable diseases, [1607]
ACAROLOGY VI, [1533]
Acha, P.N., [1609]
Acker, D., [1244]
Ackerman, N., [777], [789]
Acta veterinaria (Beograd), [87]
Acta veterinaria (Brno), [88]
Acta veterinaria Hungarica, [89]
Acta veterinaria Japonica, [36]
Acta veterinaria Scandinavica, [90]
acupuncture, societies, [2097], [2129], [2223], [2238]
Adam, W.S., [898]
Adams, D.R., [899]
Adams, R.J., [1671]
Advances in animal welfare science, [1755]
Advances in carriers and adjuvants for veterinary biologics, [1391]
Advances in clinical chemistry, [1302]
Advances in disease vector research, [1480]

Advances in Medical and Veterinary Virology, [1739]
Advances in parasitology, [1481]
Advances in small animal practice, 73; [773]
Advances in veterinary medicine, [118]
Advances in veterinary science and comparative medicine, 73; [60]
Advisory Committee for the Coordination of Information Systems, [1]
Agar, N.S., [1305]
AGDEX, 78; [37], [2363]
AGLINET, 34
Union list of serials, 34; [76]
AGRA EUROPE, [297]
AGREP, 45; [274]
AGRICOLA, 74; [2366]
Agricultural and Food Research Council, 43; [275], [276], [2025]; *see also*, [2192]
Agricultural and veterinary chemicals, [320]
Agricultural & veterinary sciences international who's who, 39; [188]
The agricultural budgeting and costing book, [293]
Agricultural compendium for rural development in the tropics and subtropics, [1717]
The agricultural notebook, [1256]
Agricultural research centres, [187]
Agricultural statistics, [286]

Agricultural statistics: United Kingdom, [286]
Agricultural supply industry, [319]
Agrindex, 74; [29]
Agri-practice, [494]
AGRIS, 74, 92; [2367]
Agroselekt. Reihe 4. Veterinärmedizin, 73; [13]
AGROVOC: a multilingual thesaurus of agricultural terminology, 74; [167]
Aguirre, G., [1469]
Ainsworth, G. C., [1397]–[1399]
Ainsworth and Bisby's Dictionary of the fungi, [1397]
Alamargot, J., [388]
Alcock, J., [900]
Alden, C. L., [778]
Alexander, F., [1677]
Alexander, J. O., [1485]
Alexander, J. W., [828]
Alexander, T. L., [512]
Algers, B., [1279]
Ali, T. M., [707]
Allan White Memorial Video Library, 99; [348]
Allen, A. R., [1668]
Allen, D., [419]
Allen, D. Jr, [717]
Allen, D. G., [779]
Allen, E., [870]
Allen, W. E., [695]
allergy, societies, [2023], [2095]
Allsop, C. E., [1525]
Altman, N. H., [981], [983]
Altman, P. L., [978]
American Animal Hospital Association, [2033]
American Association of Avian Pathologists, [2036]
American book publishing record, [43]
American doctoral dissertations, [152]
American journal of veterinary research, 82; [91]
American Kennel Club, [901], [2072]
American Veterinary Medical Association, 17, 39, 99–100; [2013]
Directory, 39–40; [211]
Amlacher, E., [1158]
Amman, K., [902]
amphibians and reptiles, [1090]–[1103]
societies, [2121]
see also exotic pets, zoo and wild animals
Amstutz, H. E., [420]
Amtsberg, G., [1264]
anaesthesia, [1215]–[1225]

societies, [2055], [2108]
Anaesthesia, [1215], [1223]
Analytical toxicology methods manual, [1704]
anatomy and histology, [1226]–[1243]
societies, [2044], [2163], [2205], [2314]
The anatomy of the domestic animals, [1227]
ancillary personnel, 12–13; [386]–[401]
societies, [2112], [2134], [2243]
Anders, K., [1176]
Andersen, A. C., [903], [904]
Anderson, D. P., [1201]
Anderson, N., [1534]
Anderson, N. V., [1417]
Anderson, O. R., [1593]
Anderson, R. C., [1119], [1120]
Anderson, R. S., [863]
Andrewes' Viruses of vertebrates, [1751]
Andrews, A. H., [421], [422]
Andrews, E. J., [983]
Animal Air Transportation Association, [1358]
Animal and human health, [1624]
Animal behaviour, [1282]
Animal breeding abstracts, 60; [1636]
Animal disease occurrence, 53, 55, 98–9; [284]
Animal disease thesaurus, 86; [156]
Animal Diseases Research Association, [2088]
Animal drug analytical manual, [1678]
Animal feed science and technology, [1454]
Animal genetics, [1660]
Animal health and nutrition service, [301]
Animal health facts and figures, 50; [316]
Animal health in Australia, [367]
Animal health international, [321]
'*Animal health international*' directory, 46, 98; [214]
Animal health news and index, 87; [249]
Animal Health Trust, [2092]
Animal health yearbook, 98; [285]
animal husbandry and production, [1244]–[1262]
societies, [2128], [2159], [2224], [2233], [2234], [2263], [2275]–[2277], [2308], [2310]
Animal pharm, 46-9; [322]
Animal pharm bookshop, [316]
Animal production, [92]
Animal production: quarterly statistics, [286]
Animal reproduction science, [1661]
Animal salmonellosis, [287]
Animal technology, [1030]

animal welfare, *see* behaviour; welfare of animals

Annales de médecine vétérinaire, [93]

Annales de recherches vétérinaires, [94]

Annual book of ASTM standards, [334]

Annual register of merchants' premises, [250]

Annual review of . . ., [61]

The anthelmintic index, [1486]

Anthelmintics for cattle, sheep, pigs, horses and poultry, [251]

Antigua, national association, [1845]

Antimicrobials and agriculture, [1696]

The antimicrobials annual, [1675]

Apicultural abstracts, [1206]

Appel, M.J., [1740]

Applebe, G.E., [1362]

Applied animal behaviour science, [1283]

aquatic animals, societies, [2196], [2268]; *see also* amphibians and reptiles; fish

Archer, R.K., [1306]

Archibald, J., [780], [905]

Archiv für experimentelle Veterinärmedizin, [95]

Archives of animal nutrition, [1455]

Argentina
    directory, [226]
    national associations, [1846]–[1849]

Armour, J., [423], [1527]

Arnoczky, S.P., [783]

Arora, B.M., [510]

Arrington, L.R., [953]

Arthur, G.H., [1641]

Article summaries, 58, 60; [14]

Ashdown, R.R., [402], [696]

Ashford, R.W., [1602]

Aspinall, K.W., [376]

associations
    audiovisual materials, 90–100; [338]–[359]
    directories, 40–1
    national, 6, 17–18; [1845]–[2022]
    specialist, [2023]–[2331]

Atwell, R.B., [908]

Audio Veterinary Medicine, [355]

audiovisual materials, 99–100; [338]–[359]

Augustine, G., [1563]

Auriol, P., [1720]

Austin, B., [1159], [1160]

Austin, C.R., [1638]

Austin, D.A., [1159], [1160]

Australia
    directories, 40; [194], [227], [228]
    journals, [96], [864]

    libraries, [1789]–[1794]
    national association, [1850]
    societies, 40; [2114], [2115]
    trade association, [2027]

Australian standard diagnostic techniques for animal diseases, [1352]

Australian Veterinary Association, [1850]
    Yearbook, [194]

Australian veterinary journal, [96]

Australian veterinary practitioner, [864]

Austria
    journal, [144]
    libraries, [1795],
    national associations, [1851]–[1853]

Austwick, P.K.C., [1399]

Avens, J.S., [1060]

Avian biology, [1037]

Avian diseases, [1084]

Avian immunology: proceedings of the second international conference, [1079]

Avian pathology, [1085]

Axelrod, H.R., [1155]

Bachmann, P.A., [1744]

bacteriology, [1263]–[1269]; *see also* microbiology

Bade, D.H., [1247]

Badgers and bovine tuberculosis – a review of policy, [424]

Baggott, J.D., [1679], [1691]

The Bahamas, national association, [1854]

Bailey, L., [1208]

Bailie, J.H., [442]

Baillière's comprehensive veterinary dictionary, 86; [158]

Baillière's veterinary diary, [325]

Baker, H.J., [984]

Baker, J., [1776]

Baker, J.K., [377]

Baker, J.R., [1522], [1598]

Baker, K.P., [781]

Balk, M.W., [1026]

Ball, J.G., [1196]

Ball, P.J.H., [469]

Banco de Información en Medicina Veterinaria y Zootecnia, 32

Bangladesh, national association, [1855]

Banks, W.J., [1229]

Barbados, national association, [1856]

Bargai, U., [425]

Barlow, R.M., [530]

Barnes, H.J., [1054]

Barnes, M., [1245]
Barnett, K.C., [1468]
Barone, R., [954]
Barré, N., [1266]
Barron, N.S., [621]
Barta, O., [1340]
Bartlett, T., [968]
Basu, S.B., [501]
Bath, D.L., [426]
Batik, G., [1469]
Batt, R.M., [1448]
Baxter, S., [622], [629]
Beattie, C.P., [1595]
Beaver, B.G., [849]
Beaver, B.V.G., [707], [871]
Becht, J.L., [764]
Beck, A.M., [906]
Bedford, P.G.C., [907]
Beef yearbook, [288]
Beer, J.V., [1112]
behaviour, [1270]-[1283]
   societies, [2085], [2104], [2157], [2279]
Belgium
   directory, [229]
   journal, [143]
   libraries, [1796], [1797]
   national associations, [1857]-[1859]
Belize, national association, [1860]
Bell, J.C., [1610]
Belschner, H.G., [427], [531], [623],
   [697]
Benirschke, K., [985]
Bennett, B., [595]
Bergey's Manual of systematic bacteriology,
   [1263]
*Berliner und Münchener tierärztliche
   Wochenschrift*, [97]
Berman, E., [869]
Berrier, H.H., [1288]
Beveridge, M.C.M., [1161]
Bezuidenhout, A.J., [681]
Bhide, S., [1565]
bibliographies, 71-2; [43]-[59]
Bibliography of agriculture, 74; [30]
Bibliography of reproduction, [1635]
Bibliography of the history of medicine, [1318]
Bibliography on swamp buffalo 1976-85,
   [499]
biographical information, *see* directories
Biological abstracts, 74; [15]
*Biological abstracts/RRM (reports, reviews,
   meetings)*, [31]
*Biological substances: international standards
   and reference reagents*, [215]
Biologische Tiermedizin, [1697]
*Biologizace a chemizace živočisné
   výroby - veterinaria*, [98]
Biology and management of the Cervidae, [524]
Biology Databook Editorial Board, [978]
*Biology of deer production: proceedings of the
   international conference . . .*, [523]
Biology of the Reptilia, [1090]
BIOSIS, 78; [2369]
BIOSIS/CAS Selects, 66
Biotechnology in growth regulation, [1568]
birds, *see* poultry and cage birds
Bishop, G., [896]
Bisping, W., [1264]
Bistner, S.I., [360], [1469]
Black's veterinary dictionary, [157]
Blackmore, D.J., [698]
Blake, P.W., [1246]
Blakely, J., [1247]
Blakeslee, J.R. Jr, [1750]
Blanchard, J.R., [2]
Blaxter, Sir K.L., [513]
Bleby, J., [896]
Blin, P.C., [954]
Bliss, D.E., [1209]
Block, S.S., [1687]
Blodinger, J., [1680]
Blogg, J.R., [1470]
Blood, D.C., [158], [403], [1294], [1359]
Blowey, R.W., [428]
Blunt, M.H., [532]
Board, P.G., [1305]
Boch, J., [1113]
Boever, W.J., [1143]
Bogan, J.A., [404]
Bohensky, F., [872]
Bojrab, M.J., [782]-[784]
Bolivia, national associations,
   [1861]-[1863]
Bondi, A.A., [1418]
Bonning, L., [870]
books, 23-4
   general texts, 87-8; [376]-[385]
   multivolume works and series,
      [364]-[375]
   newly published, 66-7
   reference books, 85-7; [360]-[363]
Books at Boston Spa, [44]
Books in English, [45]
Books in print, 72; [46]
Books in the Science Reference Library, [47]
booksellers, *see* publishers and booksellers

Booth, E.S., [873]
Booth, N.H., [1681]
Boreham, P.F.L., [908]
Bosman, H.G., [615]
Bosset, R., [1114]
Bostock, D.E., [1460]
Botkin, M.P., [533]
Botswana, national association, [1864]
Bovee, K.C., [909]
Bovine respiratory disease, [492]
Brack, M., [1611]
Brander, G.C., [1682], [1683]
Brasmer, T.H., [785]
Braund, K.G., [786]
Brazil
    directory, [230]
    libraries, [1798], [1799]
    national associations, [1865]-[1867]
Breeding and management in birds of prey,
    [1146]
Breeding management and foal development,
    [699]
Bremner, A.S., [1612]
Brent, G., [624], [625]
Brick, J.O., [1016]
Briggs, D.M., [164]
Briggs, H.M., [164]
Brigstocke, T.D.A., [491], [1445], [1446]
Brinker, W.O., [787], [788]
*The Bristol veterinary handbook of antimicrobial
    therapy*, [1684]
British approved names 1986, [252]
British book news, 67; [38]
British books in print, [48]
British cattle, [429]
British Film Institute, [349]
British Institute of Regulatory Affairs, 94
British journal of nutrition, [1456]
British Library, 30-1, 34
British Library Document Supply Centre,
    [1783]
The British Mastitis Conference, [493]
British medical journal, [146]
British national bibliography, 72; [49]
British pharmacopoeia 1988, [252]
British pharmacopoeia (veterinary) 1985, [252]
British poultry science, [1086]
British reports, translations and theses, 85;
    [149]
British sheep, [534]
British Small Animal Veterinary
    Association, 12, 70, 88; [2127]
British Standards Institution, [335]

BRITISH TRADE MARKS, 96; [2370]
British union catalogue of periodicals, 84; [78]
British Universities Film and Video
    Council, [350]
British Veterinary Association, 17, 68-9,
    93; [2011]
British veterinary codex, [252]
British Veterinary Hospitals Association,
    [2133]
British veterinary index, [309]
British veterinary journal, 82-3; [99]
British Veterinary Nursing Association,
    12-13; [2134]
British Virgin Islands, national
    association, [1868]
Broce, A.B., [1530]
Brobst, D., [698]
Bromage, N.R., [1186]
Bromiley, M., [700]
Broster, W.H., [430]
Brothwell, D., [1776]
Brown, C.M., [701]
Brown, E.M., [1231]
Brown, J.H., [702]
Brown, R., [968]
brucellosis, [1265]
Bryson, T., [535]
BSI standards catalogue, 94; [335]
Buck, W.B., [1712]
Buckner, R., [917]
Budras, K-D., [910]
Buffalo bulletin, [507]
Buffalo journal, [508]
buffaloes, [499]-[509]
    societies, [2201], [2202]
Bulgaria
    library, [1800]
    national associations, [1869], [1870]
Bulletin de l'Academie Vétérinaire de France,
    [100]
Bulletin de l'Office International des Épizooties,
    [289]
*Bulletin of animal health and production in
    Africa*, [1732]
Bulletin of the World Veterinary Association,
    69; [326]
Bundy, C.E., [437], [438], [626]
Burch, R.L., [1771]
Burk, R.L., [789]
Burke, T.J., [790]
Burkholder, C.R., [791]
Burns, M., [586]
Burr, E.W., [1041], [1042]

Burton, N.R., [389]
Bush, B., [792], [911]
Bush, B.M., [912]
Bush, E.A.R., [3]
Butler, D., [703]
Butterworth, B.B., [878]
Butterworth, M.H., [431]
Buxton, A., [1380]
Bywater, R.J., [1683], [1690]

CAB ABSTRACTS, 53-5, 62, 76-8;
    [2371]
CAB International, [2371]
    abstracting journals, 53-6, 60, 62
    bibliographies, 72
    serials checklist, 84; [79]
CAB thesaurus, 53-5, 86; [159]
cage birds, *see* poultry and cage birds
Calabrese, E.J., [986]
Calf rearing, [432]
Calhoun, M.L., [898]
Calnek, B.W., [1054]
Cambridge Scientific Abstracts, [16]
camelids, [672]-[686]
    societies, [2211]
Campbell, J.R., [1248]
Campbell, T.W., [1043]
Campbell, W.C., [1487]
Campbell, W.E., [793], [913]
Camus, E., [1266]
Canada
    directories, [195], [231], [232]
    journals, [101], [102], [323]
    libraries, [1801], [1802]
    national association, [1871]
    trade association, [2139]
Canadian journal of veterinary research, [101]
Canadian vet supplies, [323]
Canadian veterinary journal, [102]
Canning, E.U., [1594]
Cantwell, G.E., [1210]
Cantwell, H.D., [738]
cardiology, societies, [2024], [2292]
Caribbean Veterinary Association, [2142]
CARIS, 45; [2374]
Carles, A.B., [536]
Carrasco, C., [168]
Carroll, E.J., [475]
Carroll, W.E., [638]
Carson, T.L., [1712]
Carter, G.R., [1353], [1381], [1382]
CAS BioTech updates, 66
CAS selects, 66

*Casarett and Doull's Toxicology: the basic
    science of poisons*, [1705]
Cass J.S., [976]
Cassell, D., [704]
Castelló, J.A., [169]
Castle, M.E., [433]
Catalog of American national standards, 94;
    [336]
*A catalogue of audio visual programmes for
    veterinary nurses, June 1987*, [401]
*Catalogue of British Official Publications not
    published by HMSO*, [39]
*Catalogue of Lewis's medical, scientific and
    technical lending library*, 72; [50]
Catcott, E.J., [780], [914]
cats, [869]-[893]
    societies [2143], [2183]
    see also small animals
cattle, [417]-[498]
    societies, [2120], [2207], [2266], [2311]
The cattle industry and welfare in Great Britain,
    [434]
Cayman Islands, national association,
    [1872]
Caywood, D.D., [794]
CD-ROM technology, 79-80
Central African Republic, national
    association, [1873]
Centro Internacional de Agricultura
    Tropical, [1786]
Chandler, E.A., [773], [874], [915]
Chaplin, R.E., [514]
charitable organizations, *see* voluntary
    organizations; welfare of animals
Chastain, C.B., [795]
Chatelain, E., [584]
Cheeke, P.R., [955], [956], [1706]
Chemical abstracts, 74, 96; [17]
Chemical patents index, 95-6; [18]
*Chemical regulation of immunity in veterinary
    medicine*, [1347]
Cheng, T.C., [1488]
Cheville, N.F., [1550], [1551]
Chheda, H.R., [1721]
Chiasson, R.B., [965], [987]
Chile, national associations, [1874]-[1876]
China, national association, [1877]
Chirurgia veterinaria, [19]
Chivers, D.J., [1023]
Chrisman, C.L., [796]
Christensen, F.C., [923]
Christensen, V.W., [437], [438], [626]
Christiansen, I.J., [797]

Christie, W.W., [1419]
Christoph, H-J., [916]
Church, D.C., [1420], [1421]
Churchill, P., [705]
CIH keys to the nematode parasites of vertebrates, [1483]
citation analysis, 28, 75
Clarke, E.G.C., [1707]
Clarke, K.W., [1218], [1690]
Clarke, R.D., [917]
Clarkson, M.J., [444], [537]
classification schemes, 33-4
clinical chemistry, *see* haematology; pathology
Clinical chemistry: reference edition, [1314]
Clinical insight, 55, 68; [103]
Clinical toxicology of commercial products, [1702]
Cockrill, W. Ross, [502], [503], [672], [684]
Code of Federal Regulations. Title 21, 93; [262]
Code of practice: the hygienic production of goats' milk [585]
Code of practice for merchants selling or supplying veterinary drugs, [2091]
Code of practice for the housing and care of animals used in scientific procedures, [1756]
Code of practice for the storage and dispensing of medicines . . ., [1360]
Code of recommendations for the welfare of livestock, [1757]
Coetzer, J.A.W., [1711]
Coffman, J.R., [706]
Cohen, B.J., [996]
Cole, D.J.A., [663], [1414], [1415]
Cole, W.C., [1022]
Coles, B.H., [1044]
Coles, E.H., [1307]
Collier, G.M., [746]
Collins, B.C., [935]
Collins, C.H., [1383], [1384]
Colloquium on recognition and alleviation of animal pain and distress, [1758]
Colombia
   directory, [233]
   library, [1786]
   national association, [1878]
Colours and markings of horses, [707]
COMISA, 46; [2152]
Commercial rabbit production, [957]
Commission of the European

Communities, 92-4; [170], [364], [2147]
Committee on infectious diseases of mice and rats, [988]
Committee on the Care and Use of Laboratory Animals, [979]
Commonwealth Veterinary Association, 16; [2148]
Companion animal practice, [865]
companion animals, 8; *see* small animals, cats, dogs etc. *See also* welfare of animals
Comparative Animal Nutrition, [1413]
Comparative immunology, microbiology and infectious diseases, [104]
Comparative pathology bulletin, [1560]
Compendium of data sheets for veterinary products, 87; [253]
Compendium on continuing education for the practicing veterinarian, 73; [62]
The complete book of cat health, [875]
The complete handbook of approved new animal drug applications in the United States, [263]
Compound evaluation and analytical capability national residue program plan, [270]
Comprehensive dissertations index, [153]
COMPUMARK, 98; [2337]
computerized information systems, 29, 49, 64-6, 75-81
   current awareness services, 66
   online databases, [2363]-[2405]
   online systems, [2332]-[2362]
   societies, [2078], [2086]
Concise veterinary dictionary, 86; [160]
conferences, 68-70; [325]-[333]
Congo People's Republic, national association, [1879]
Connell, J., [1759]
Conrad, J.H., [638]
CONSULTANT, 75
Contemporary issues in small animal practice, 73; [774]
continuing education, 69-70
Controlled vocabulary (of CBAH), 53-5; [161]
Cooper, J.E., [1091], [1115]-[1117], [1147]
Cooper, M.E., [1361]
Cooper, M.J., [442]
Cooper, M.R., [1708]
Cooper, N. McG., [435], [538]
Cornelius, L.M., [830]

Cornell Research Foundation, [264]
Cornell veterinarian, [105]
Corsi, P., [1316]
Cosgrove, G. E., [1000]
Costa Rica
    library, [1785]
    national association, [1880]
Cottral, G. E., [1385]
Council of Europe, [216]
County NatWest Securities Limited, [301]
Coutts, G. S., [1045]
Cowey, C. B., [1196]
Cox, J. E., [405], [1237]
Cox, N. A., [1613]
Craig, J. V., [1272]
Craigie, E. H., [958]
Crandall, L. S., [1118]
Crane, S. W., [783]
Crane, T. D., [1701]
Crawford, L. M., [1369]
CRC Handbook Series in Zoonoses, [1608]
Crispens, C. G. Jr, [989]
critical care and emergency medicine,
    society, [2295]
Croft, P. G., [918]
Crompton, D. W. T., [1535]
Crop protection chemicals reference, [265]
Croston, D., [539]
Crow, S. E., [798]
Crowder, L. V., [1721]
Cuba, national association, [1881]
Cullison, A. E., [1422]
Cumulative book index, [51]
Cunha, T. J., [627], [708]
Cuni-sciences: éditions de synthèses scientifiques,
    [973]
Cunningham, E. P., [1642]
Cunningham, F. E., [1613]
Cunningham, J. M. M., [519], [548]
Cuq, P., [954]
Current awareness in . . ., [40]
current awareness services, 52–66;
    [36]–[42]
Current contents, 62–3; [41]
Current primate references, [975]
Current research in Britain: biological sciences,
    45; [277]
Current serials received, [80]
Current therapy in equine medicine – 2, [709]
Current therapy in theriogenology 2, [1643]
*Current Topics in Veterinary Medicine and
    Animal Science*, [365]
Current veterinary therapy: food animal
    practice – 2, [406]
*Current veterinary therapy IX: small animal
    practice*, [799]
Current work in the history of medicine, [1336]
Curtis, P., [1046]
Curtis, S. E., [1249]
Cyprus, national associations, [1882],
    [1883]
Czechoslovakia
    journals, [88], [98]
    national associations, [1884], [1885]
Czerkawski, J. W., [1423]

Daelemans, J., [1255]
Dagg, A. I., [676]
Dairy farmer, [495]
Dairy herd fertility, [436]
Dairy science abstracts, 60; [417]
Dale, J. R., [1362]
Dalling, Sir T., [361]
Dallman, M. J., [882]
Dalton, C., [1280]
Dalton, D. C., [1644]
Dangerous properties of industrial materials,
    [1703]
Dansk veterinærtidsskrift, [106]
Darke, P. G. G., [919]
Dasmann, W., [515]
Davidson, W. R., [516]
Davies, A. S., [540]
Davis, J. W., [1119]–[1121], [1129]
Davis, L. E., [800]
Davis, R. B., [1071]
Dawkins, M., [1273]
Dawkins, M. S., [1760]
Day, C., [801]
Day, G., [541]
de Bairacli Levy, J., [1688]
de Groot, E. C. B. M., [1555]
De La Plain, S., [456]
de Lahunta, A., [924], [1230], [1240],
    [1407]
de Nahlik, A. J., [517]
Decision making in veterinary medicine series,
    [366]
deer, [510]–[528]
    society, [2294]
Deer, [527]
Deer farming, [528]
Della-Porta, A. J., [1730]
Dellmann, H-D., [1231]
Denmark
    directory, [234]

journals, [90], [106], [122]
library, [1803]
national association, [1886]
Dennett, T.B., [1309]
Denny, H.R., [710], [920]
dentistry, [1284]-[1288]
    societies, [2056], [2079], [2131]
dermatology, societies, [2029], [2057],
    [2132], [2170]
Deutsche tierärztliche Wochenschift, [107]
Developments in Animal and Veterinary Science,
    [368]
Developments in Biological Standardization,
    [369]
Developments in Veterinary Virology, [1741]
Devendra, C., [586], [587]
Dewey decimal classification, 33
dictionaries, 85-6, 103; [156]-[185]
Dictionary of argiculture in six languages, [171]
Dictionary of animal production terminology,
    [175]
Dictionary of dairy terminology, [176]
Dieterich, R.A., [511]
Dietz, O., [711]
Diggins, R.V., [437], [438], [626]
Dik, K.J., [712]
directories, 37-50; [186]-[283]
    general and biographical, 37-41;
        [186]-[213]
    of individuals, 38-40
    of industry and drugs, 45-50; [214]
        [273]
    of organizations, 40-1
    of research, 44-5; [274]-[283]
Directory: caring for animals, 39-40; [211]
*Directory of animal rights/animal welfare
    organizations*, [1754]
Directory of current research on sheep and goats,
    [529]
*Directory of names in buffalo studies and
    research*, [500]
Directory of research grants, [278]
Directory of research workers in agriculture,
    [190]
Directory of UK animal health companies,
    [254]
disaster medicine, societies, [2222]
Disease information, [289]
Diseases of aquatic organisms, [1203]
Diseases of fishes, [1155]
Diseases of marine animals, [1109]
*Diseases of zoo animals. Proceedings of the 30th
    international symposium*, [1148]

Disinfection, sterilization and preservation,
    [1687]
*Disorders of the ruminant digit (Fifth
    international symposium)*, [414]
Dissertation abstracts international, 85; [148],
    [154]
Dobberstein, J., [1549]
Dobson, A., [1449], [1450]
Dobson, H., [1354]
Dobson, M.J., [1449]
Dodds, W.J., [1773]
dogs, [894]-[952]
    societies, [2072], [2140], [2141], [2230]
    see also small animals
Dolling, C.H.S., [542]
Domestic animal endocrinology, [1575]
Dominica, national association, [1887]
Dominican Republic, national
    association, [1888]
Done, S.H., [402], [696]
donkeys, societies, [2155]
Donnersberger, A.B., [876]
The Dooley letter, [1582]
Dorian, A.F., [173]
Dougherty, R.W., [1664]
Douglas, S.W., [1628]
Dowell, V.R. Jr, [1048]
Downing, E., [543], [588]
Doyle, M.P., [1614]
Drazner, F.H., [802]
Drochner, W., [628]
drugs
    directories [214]-[273]
    societies, [2221]
    see also legislation and regulatory
        matters; therapeutics, pharmacology
        and pharmaceutics
Drummond, R.O., [1489]
Dubey, J.P., [544], [1595], [1596]
Dubiski, S., [959]
Ducks and geese, [1047]
Dufty, J.H., [477]
Duke's Physiology of the domestic animals,
    [1562]
Dulin, M.P., [1162]
Duncan, I.J.H., [1078]
Duncan, J.L., [742], [1527]
Duncan, J.R., [1308]
Dunn, A.M., [1490], [1527]
Dunn, P., [589]
Duwel, D., [1505]
*DVM: the news magazine of veterinary
    medicine*, [1584]

DVM management consultants' report, [1583]
Dyce, K. M., [1232]
Dykova, I., [1594]

Eadie, J., [513]
Eales, F. A., [545]
Easter Schools in Agricultural Science, [370]
Eastern States Veterinary Association,
    [2156]
EASYVET, [309]
Eckert, R., [1563]
The ecology and control of feral cats, [892]
Ecuador, national association, [1889]
Edgson, F. A., [921]
Edington, N., [1752]
Edney, A. T. B., [803], [804]
education, 5, 18–20
    societies, [2094], [2105], [2110], [2111],
        [2112], [2160], [2198], [2228],
        [2273], [2274], [2282], [2315]
Edwards, E. H., [713]
Edwards, M. J., [427]
Edwards, N. J., [805]
Edwards, R. A., [1428]
Efficient sheep production from grass, [573]
Egusa, S., [1172]
Egypt, national association, [1890]
Eisenmenger, E., [1284]
Eissner, G., [1343]
Ekesbo, I., [1279]
Eklund, M. W., [1048]
El Salvador, national association, [1891]
Eley, J. T., [1116]
Elkan, E., [1099]–[1163]
Ellis, A. E., [1164], [1197]
Ellis, P. R., [378]
*Elsevier's dictionary of pharmaceutical science
    and techniques*, [172]
*Elsevier's encyclopaedic dictionary of medicine in
    five languages*, [173]
*Elsevier's lexicon of parasites and diseases in
    livestock*, [174]
Elsley, F. W. H., [660]
The encyclopaedia of pet rabbits, [960]
*Energy allowances and feeding systems for
    ruminants*, [1424]
England, R. B., [439]
English, P. R., [629], [630]
Ensminger, M. E., [440], [441], [546],
    [631], [1049], [1250], [1251]
Enz, H., [1068]
Epidemiology and infection, [1393]
epidemiology and preventive medicine,

    [1288]–[1301]
    societies, [2032], [2063], [208], [2218],
        [2198], [2278]
The equine athlete, [765]
Equine exercise physiology, [2204]
Equine infectious diseases V, [764a]
Equine practice, [766]
Equine veterinary data, [767]
Equine veterinary journal, [768]
Erickson, H. H., [1774]
Erlerwein, D. L., [1576]
Escobar, R. C., [675]
Espinasse, J., [407]
Esslemont, R. J., [442]
Etgen, W. M., [443]
Ethiopia
    library, [1788]
    national association, [1892]
Ettinger, S. J., [806], [922]
European Association for Animal
    Production, [175], [2159]
European pharmacopoeia, [216]
European research centres, [189]
European Union of Veterinary
    Practitioners, [2178]
Eusebio, J. A., [632]
Evans, G., [1645]
Evans, H. E., [923], [924]
Evans, J. M., [877], [925]
Ewer, T. K., [1252]
Ewing, W., [255]
Excerpta medica, 74; [20]
exotic pets, zoo and wild animals,
    [1104]–[1154]
    societies, [2049], [2050], [2066], [2137],
        [2138], [2194], [2242], [2284],
        [2307], [2321]
Experimental and applied acarology, [1538]
Experimental parasitology, [1539]

Faccini, J. M., [999]
Fackelman, G. E., [714]
FAO Animal Production and Health Papers,
    [371]
FAO Animal Production and Health Series,
    [372]
FAO production yearbook, [291]
FAO trade yearbook, [292]
FARAD, 79; [2346]
*FARAD – the food animal residue avoidance
    databank trade name file*, [266]
Farid, M. F. A., [673]
Farm Animal Welfare Council, [2179]

Farm diary, 69; [331]
Farm management pocketbook, [293]
Farmers weekly, [1261]
FARM-TRAK, [300]
Farrell, L., [2]
Farrow, C. S., [807]
Faull, W. B., [444], [537]
Favre, D. S., [1363]
Fayer, R., [1596]
FDA veterinarian, [1372]
FEDERAL RESEARCH IN
    PROGRESS, 45; [2384]
Federation of Asian Veterinary
    Association, 16; [2180]
Federation of Veterinarians of the EEC,
    16; [2182]
FEDESA, 49; [2167]
Feed additive compendium, [267]
feed and feedstuffs,
    companies, [2260], [2249]
    societies, [2271]
    trade associations, [2068], [2117],
        [2165], [2169], [2251], [2252],
        [2255], [2286]
    see also nutrition and digestion
*Feed composition: UK tables of feed
    composition*, [1432]
Feed compounder, [1457]
Feed international, [1458]
Feedstuffs, 69; [1459]
FEFAC, 46; [2169]
FEFANA, 46; [2165]
Feldman, D. B., [990]
Feldman, E. C., [808]
Feline health topics for veterinarians, [893]
Felius, M., [445]
Fell, H. R., [547]
Fellowship of the Royal College of
    Veterinary Surgeons, 20
Fenner, F., [961], [1744], [1745]
Fenner, W. R., [809]
The ferret, [1031]
Field, H. E., [878]
Field, R. A., [533]
Field guide to wildlife diseases, [1123]
Fiennes, R. N. T-W-, [1122], [1461]
Fiji, national association, [1893]
Finco, D. R., [840]
Finland
    directory, [235]
    library [1804]
    national associations, [1894], [1895]
fish, [1155]-[1205]

societies, [2161], [2313]
    see also aquatic animals
Fish pathology, [1204]
Fish physiology, [1156]
Fisher, R., [744]
Flatt, R. E., [971]
Flecknell, P. A., [991]
Fletcher, A. M., [947]
Fletcher, J., [518]
Flo, G. L., [788]
Flynn, R. J., [992]
Fogh, J., [993]
Fogle, B., [810]
Foley, C. W., [1646]
Folsch, D. W., [1761]
Food and agricultural legislation, [1373]
Food and Agriculture Organization of the
    United Nations, 91-2, 99; [1874],
    [2184]
Food and chemical toxicology, [1715]
Food chemical news, [1374]
Food Safety and Inspection Service, [270]
Food science and technology abstracts, [1412]
Foot and mouth disease: ageing of lesions,
    [1746]
Foot and mouth disease bulletin, [1738]
Footrot in ruminants, [574]
Forbes, J. M., [1425]
Ford, E. H. R., [1023]
Ford, R. B., [811]
Foreign animal disease report, [1300]
Fortschritte der Veterinärmedizin, [118]
Foster, H. L., [994]
Foundation for Continuing Education of
    the New Zealand Veterinary
    Association, 70; [63]
Foundation grants index, [279]
Fowler, M. E., [1124], [1217]
Fowler, V. R., [629], [1568]
Fox, J. G., [994]-[996]
Fox, M. W., [926]-[928], [1755], [1762],
    [1763]
Fox, P. R., [812]
France
    directories, [196], [197], [236]
    journals, [93], [94], [100], [124], [126],
        [128], [129]
    libraries, [1805]-[1807]
    national associations, [1896]-[1901]
Frandson, R. D., [1233]
Franti, C. E., [1297]
Frape, D. L., [715]
Fraser, A., [548], [736]

Fraser, A. F., [1274], [1275]
Fraser, G., [1380]
FRCVS, *see* Fellowship of the Royal
    College of Veterinary Surgeons
Freed, D. L. J., [1623]
Freudiger, U. D., [824]
Fricke, W., [910]
Frith, C. H., [997], [998]
Frohne, D., [1709]
Fry, P. D., [1577]
Frye, F. L., [1092], [1093]
Fudin, C. E., [822]
Fuller, R., [446]

Gabrisch, K., [1125[, [1126]
Gall, C., [590]
The Gambia, national association, [1902]
Ganjam, V. K., [795]
Gans, G., [1090]
Garden, K. L., [540]
Garner, F. M., [985]
Garrett, P. D., [591], [882]
Gaskell, C. J., [874], [825]
Gatenby, R. M., [549]
Gauthier-Pilters, H., [676]
Gay, W. I., [1669]
Gelatt, K. N., [1471]
general veterinary books, [376]–[385]
genetics, *see* reproduction and genetics
George, J. E., [1489]
Georgi, J. R., [1491]
German books in print, [52]
German Democratic Republic
    directory, [237]
    journals, [95], [120]
Germany, Federal Republic
    directories, [198]–[201], [238]
    journals, [97], [107], [118], [125], [133]
    libraries, [1808], [1809]
    national associations, [1903]–[1906]
Ghana, national association, [1907]
Ghittino, P., [1171]
Ghoshal, N. G., [1234]
Gibbons, L. M., [1492]
Gibbs, A., [1745]
Gibbs, E. P. J., [1743], [1744]
Gibson, T. E., [1493]
Gil, J. I., [1615]
Gilbert, S. G., [633]
Gill, H. S., [1194]
Gill, J. L., [1777]
Ginther, O. J., [716]
Giovanella, B. C., [994]

Giovannetti, J. F., [4]
Glock, R. D., [639]
Glover, H., [929]
Goat health and production, [617]
Goat production and research in the tropics,
    [609]
Goat Veterinary Society journal, [616]
goats, [584]–[618]
    societies, [2042], [2123], [2186], [2187],
    [2209]
Godbolt, S., [7]
Gomez, J. A., [1631]
*Goodman and Gilman's The pharmacological
    basis of therapeutics*, [1685]
Goodwin, D. H., [550], [634]
Gordon, B. J., [717]
Gordon, I., [1647]
Gordon, R. F., [1050]
Gorman, N. T., [1341]
Gosselin, R. E., [1702]
Gourley, I. M., [813]
government publications, 89–91
Graber, M., [1494]
Gracey, J. F., [1616]
Grange, J. M., [1384]
Grant, D. I., [814]
Grants register, 46; [280]
Graves, W., [595]
Gray, D. E., [53]
Gray, E. A., [1323]
*Grazing plans for the control of stomach and
    intestinal worms in sheep and in cattle*,
    [1495]
Great Britain, *see* United Kingdom
Greaves, P., [999]
Greece, national associations, [1908],
    [1909]
Greeley, R. G., [842]
Greene, C. E., [815]
Greenhalgh, J. F. D., [1428]
Greenough, P. R., [447]
Greenwood, A. G., [1147]
Greer, W. J., [377]
Grenada, national association, [1910]
Grey, R. M., [822]
greyhounds, society, [2272]
Grigson, C., [1286]
Grimm, F., [1051]
Grimshaw, A., [691]
Griner, L. A., [1127]
Gross, L., [1462]
Grovum, W. L., [1450]
Guatemala, national association, [1911]

Gude, W. D., [1000]
Guerts, R., [707]
Guidance notes for the protection of persons against ionising radiations arising from veterinary use, [1626]
Guide to good pharmaceutical manufacturing practice, [1364]
Guide to infectious diseases of mice and rats, [988]
Guide to the care and use of experimental animals, [980]
A guide to veterinary pesticides, [256]
Guidelines for radiology service in veterinary medicine, [1625]
Guidelines on the use of living animals in scientific investigations, [1764]
Gunsser, I., [712]
Guss, S. B., [592]
Guyana, national association, [1912]
Gwynne-Jones, O., [921]
Gyles, C. L., [1267]
Gylstorff, I., [1051]

Haan, C. de, [1722]
Habel, R. E., [750], [1230], [1235]
Haberkamp de Antón, G., [171]
Hacker, J. B., [1426]
haematology, cytology and clinical chemistry, [1302]–[1315]
  societies, [2098], [2214]
Haensch, G., [171]
Hafez, E. S. E., [1276], [1648]
Hagan and Bruner's Microbiology and infectious diseases of domestic animals, [1387]
Hagstad, H. V., [1617]
Hails, M. R., [1701]
Hair, J. A., [1514]
Hall, D. E., [930]
Hall, G. E., [1202]
Hall, H. T. B., [1723]
Hall, L. W., [383], [1218], [1690], [1778]
Hall, R. D., [1530]
Halliday, J., [593]
Halliwell, R. E. W., [1341]
Hallows, B., [481]
Halver, J. E., [1166]
Hamilton, W. J., [513]
Hamm, T. E. Jr, [1024]
Hammond's Farm animals, [1253]
Hand, M. S., [829]
Handbook of medicinal feed additives, [257]
Handbook of pharmaceutical excipients, [217]
Handbook of tropical veterinary laboratory diagnosis, [1719]
Handbook of veterinary procedures and emergency treatment, [360]
Handbook on animal diseases in the tropics, [1718]
Handbuch der speziellen pathologischen Anatomie der Haustiere, [1549]
Handbuch der Zootierkrankheiten, [1110]
Handy-Marchello, B., [386]
Hanrahan, J. P., [1564]
Hanson, M. G., [1290]
Hanson, R. P., [1290]
Hardy, R., [448]
Haresign, W., [255], [663], [1414], [1415]
Harkness, J. E., [962]
Harris, R. S., [1025]
Harrison, G. J., [1052]
Harrison, L. R., [1052]
Harrison, R. J., [1139]
Harrison, R. M., [1779]
Hart, B. L., [816], [879], [931], [1277]
Hart, E., [551], [968]
Hart, L. A., [816]
Harthoorn, A. M., [1219]
Harvey, C. E., [1285]
Hawken, M. L., [1355]
Hawkey, C. M., [1309]
Hawksworth, D., [1059]
Hawksworth, D. L., [1397]
Hay, J. B., [1342]
Hayes, F. A., [516]
Hayes, M. H., [718]
Haynes, H. D., [917]
Heady, E. O., [1565]
Health management information pack, [1289]
Health science books 1876–1982, [56]
heartworm, societies, [2069]
Heath, E., [1724]
Heath, J. S., [390]
Hebel, R., [1001]
Hecker, J. F., [552]
hedgehogs, societies, [2124], [2138]
Heep, R. B., [1568]
Helminthological abstracts, 62; [1476]
Henderson, D., [553]
The Henston veterinary vade mecum, [258], [259]
Hepburn, J., [597]
Herman, H. A., [1649]
Herpetological journal, [1103]
Herrtage, M. E., [1628]
Herwig, N., [1167]

Hetherington, L., [594]
Heymer, A., [1270]
Hickman, J., [719]-[721], [1665]
Higgins, A.J., [677]
higher qualifications, 19-20
Hilbery, A.D.R., [817], [874]
Hill, D., [449]
Hill, D.A., [1128]
Hime, J.M., [1002]
Hine, R.S., [160]
Hinks, W., [450]
Hird, J.F.R., [861], [862]
Hirsch, G.P., [1000]
histology, *see* anatomy and histology
Historia medicinae veterinariae, [1335]
history of veterinary medicine, 3-7;
      [1316]-[1337]
   societies, [2083], [2297], [2312]
HMSO (Her Majesty's Stationery
      Office), 90; [2453]
Hoar, W.S., [1156]
Hoard's dairyman, [496]
Hobson, P.N., [1427]
Hodges, R.D., [1053]
Hoerlein, B.F., [1409]
Hoff, G.L., [1093], [1129]
Hoffman, G.L., [1168]
Hofmeyr, C.F.B., [1667]
Hofstad, M.S., [1054]
Hohn, R.B., [787]
Holmes, D.D., [1003]
Holmes, J.R., [722]
Holzworth, J., [880]
homeopathy and holistic medicine,
      societies, [2070], [2118], [2119],
      [2199]; *see also* acupuncture;
      therapeutics, pharmacology and
      pharmaceutics
Honduras, national association, [1913]
Hong Kong, national association, [1914]
Hoogstraal, H., [1482]
horses, [687]-[769]
   societies, [2099], [2122], [2125], [2157],
      [2158], [2189], [2204], [2210], [2322]
Houlton, J.E.F., [818]
Houpt, K.A., [645], [1278]
Howard, D.H., [1400]
Howard, E.B., [1130]
Howard, J.L., [406]
Huang, H.K., [652]
Hubbard, G.B., [1141]
Hubbell, J.A.E., [1221]
Hubbert, W.T., [1617], [1618]

Hudson, P.J., [1131]
Huet, M., [1169]
Hughes, I., [819]
Hughes, I.B., [804]
Hughes, J.W., [444]
Hughes, P.E., [635]
Hugo, W.B., [1687]
Humphrey, M., [721]
Humphreys, D.J., [1710]
Hungary
   journal, [89]
   libraries, [1810]
   national association, [1915]
Hungate, R.E., [1427]
Hungerford, T.G., [379]
*The T.G. Hungerford Vade Mecum Series for
      Domestic Animals*, [1676]
Hunt, R.D., [1006], [1552]
Hunter, R.H.F., [1650]
Hurnik, J.F., [1271]
Hurov, L., [1666]
Huser, H-J., [1004]
Hutchison, M.F., [1117]
Hutner, S.H., [1592]
Hutt, F.B., [932]
Huxtable, C.R.R., [1556]
Hvass, H., [1094]
hygiene, *see* public health

*ICAR: inventory of Canadian agricultural
      research*, [281]
Iceland, national association, [1916]
ILAR news, [1032]
Immunoassays for veterinary and food analysis,
      [1392]
*Immunogenetic approaches to the control of
      endoparasites*, [575]
Immunological reviews, [1338]
immunology, [1338]-[1351]
   societies, [2046], [2149], [2318]
IMSMARQ, 98; [2348]
In practice, 73; [64]
In practice: the small animal book, [820]
*Index-catalogue of medical and veterinary
      zoology*, 74; [1477]
Index medicus, 74; [32]
Index of agricultural and food research, [275]
Index of current research on pigs, [620]
*Index of equine research in the British Isles and
      Ireland*, [694]
Index of veterinary specialities, 87; [260]
Index to conference proceedings received, [333]
Index to theses with abstracts, 85; [150]

Index veterinarius, 53–6; [33]
indexing services, 53–6, 60, 62–3, 73–5;
    [29]–[35]
India
    directories, [239]
    journal, [108]
    national association, [1917]
Indian veterinary journal, [108]
Indonesia, national association, [1918]
industry, 45–50
    European associations, [2165],
        [2167]–[2169], [2181], [2182]
    societies for veterinarians in, [2040],
        [2107], [2181]
    world association of the veterinary
        industry, [2152]
    see also trade
Infection and immunity, [1394]
Information sources on tropical agriculture,
    [191]
Ingermann, R.L., [1080]
Inglis, J.K., [1005]
Ingram, D.G., [1291]
Ingram, D.L., [640]
INPADOC, 96; [2386]
insects, *see* invertebrates
Institute for Animal Health, [2192]
Institute of Laboratory Animal
        Resources, [2193]
Institute for Scientific Information, [2399]
Integrated tse-tse fly control, [1536]
Inter-American Institute for Cooperation
        in Agriculture, [1785]
Intercontinental Medical Statistics (IMS),
    51; [309]
intergovernmental publications, 91–3
interlibrary lending, 34
International Air Transportation
        Association, [1365]
International animal health directory, 46; [218]
International Association of Agricultural
        Librarians and Documentalists
        (IAALD), 32–3
International books in print, [54]
International Buffalo Association newsletter,
    [509]
*International congress on animal reproduction
    and artificial insemination*, [1658]
International Dairy Federation, [176]
*International directory of market research
    organisations*, 51
International encyclopedia of veterinary medicine,
    [361]

International index of laboratory animals, [977]
International journal for parasitology, 69;
    [1540]
International journal for veterinary homeopathy,
    [2199]
International Laboratory for Research on
        Animal Diseases, 44; [1787]
International Livestock Centre for Africa,
    [1788]
International Organization for
        Standardization, 94; [337]
The international pharmacopoeia, [219]
International pigletter, [666]
International Veterinary Auxiliary, [2225]
International Veterinary Pathology Slide
        Bank, [356]
International zoo yearbook, [1108]
International zoo-sanitary code, 15; [1366]
Intravartolo, C.S., [391]
invertebrates, [1206]–[1214]
    society, [2200]
Iran, national association, [1919]
Iraq, national association, [1920]
Ireland
    directory, [202]
    journal, [109]
    library, [1811]
    national associations, [1921]–[1923]
Irish veterinary journal, [109]
ISO catalogue, 94; [337]
Israel, national associations, [1924],
    [1925]
Italy
    directory, [240]
    libraries, [1784], [1812]
    national associations, [1926]–[1928]
Ivens, V., [1600]
Ivermectin and abamectin, [1487]

Jablonski, S., [162]
Jackson, O.F., [1091]
Jacobs, D.E., [723]
Jacobson, E.R., [1093]
Jahresbericht Veterinärmedizin, 74; [21]
Jain, N.C., [475]
Jainudeen, M.R., [1731]
Jamaica, national association, [1929]
Janssens, P.G., [1528]
Japan
    journals, [36], [110], [111], [115]
    library, [1813]
    national associations, [1930], [1931]
Japanese journal of veterinary research, [110]

444   INDEX

Japanese journal of veterinary science, [111]
Jeffcott, L. B., [1306]
Jenkins, T. W., [933]
Jennings, F. W., [1527]
Jennings, P. B., [408]
Jensen, P., [1279]
Jensen, R., [451]
Jesspu, J., [541]
Johnson, A. W., [1708]
Johnson, C. L., [430], [533]
Johnson, D. J., [1022]
Johnson, G., [636]
Johnson, P. T., [1207]
Johnston, A. M., [724]
Johnston, D. E., [1684]
Johnston, J. H., [1668]
Johnston, O. M., [724]
Johnston, R. G., [554]
Jones, B. D., [821]
Jones, D. E., [934]
Jones, E. G., [895]
Jones, E. W., [1220]
Jones, H. G., [935]
Jones, K., [827]
Jones, T. C., [985], [1006], [1552]
Jones, W. E., [725], [726]
Jones's animal nursing, [392]
Jordan, A. M., [1597]
Jordan, F. T. W., [1050]
Jordan, national association, [1932]
Jørgensen, R. J., [452]
Joshwa, J. D., [934]
Journal of animal science, [113]
Journal of applied rabbit research, [974]
Journal of comparative haematology, [2098]
Journal of comparative pathology, [114]
Journal of controlled release, [1698]
Journal of dairy research, [497]
Journal of dairy science, [498]
Journal of equine veterinary science, [769]
Journal of fish diseases, [1205]
Journal of helminthology, [1541]
Journal of invertebrate pathology, [1214]
Journal of medical and veterinary mycology, [1406]
Journal of microencapsulation, [1698]
Journal of parasitology, [1542]
Journal of reproduction and fertility, [1662]
Journal of small animal practice, [867]
Journal of the American Animal Hospital Association, [866]
Journal of the American Veterinary Medical Association, 69, 82; [112]

Journal of the Association of Veterinary Anaesthetists, [1224]
Journal of the Japan Veterinary Medical Association, [115]
Journal of the South African Veterinary Association, [116]
Journal of veterinary dentistry, [2079], [2121]
Journal of veterinary diagnostic investigation, [2047]
Journal of veterinary emergency and critical care, [2295]
Journal of veterinary medical education, [2094]
Journal of veterinary medicine, [118]
Journal of veterinary parasitology, [1543]
Journal of veterinary pharmacology and therapeutics, [1699]
Journal of wildlife diseases, [1153]
Journal of zoo animal medicine, [1154]
journals, 23-4, 82-4; [87]-[147]
    lists of, 83-4; [76]-[86]
Jubb, K. V. F., [1553]
Juergenson, E. M., [453], [454], [555]
Jungerman, P. F., [1401]

Kabata, Z., [1170]
Kahrs, R. F., [455]
Kaneko, J. J., [1310]
Kaplan, H. M., [963]
Karstad, L. H., [1107], [1120], [1121]
Katic, I., [1324]
Kavanagh, M., [1132]
Kay, R. N. B., [513]
Kay, W. J., [822]
Kealy, J. K., [823]
Keller, P. D., [824]
Kellerman, T. S., [1711]
Kelley, K. C., [953]
Kellogg, B., [595]
Kellogg, F. E., [516]
Kellogg, R., [595]
Kellon, E. M., [727]
Kelly, D. F., [825]
Kelly, W. R., [380]
Kemp, R. L., [1519]
Kennedy, P. C., [1553]
Kenya
    libraries, [1787], [1814], [1815]
    national associations, [1933], [1934]
Kerker, A. E., [5]
Kerr, M. G., [1311]
Kersjes, A. W., [409]
Kettle, D. S., [1496]
Key-word index of wildlife research, [1104]

Kidder, D.E., [637]
Kiley-Worthington, M., [456], [728]
Kilgour, R., [1280]
Kilkenny, B., [419]
Killick-Kendrick, R., [1603]
Kim, K.C., [1497], [1498]
Kimberling, C.V., [556]
King, A.S., [1038], [1055], [1236], [1238], [1408]
King, J.W.B., [1659]
Kinkelin, P. de, [1171]
Kirk, R.W., [360], [799], [834]
Kirkbride, C.A., [381]
Kirkness, J.M., [186]
Kitchell, R.L., [1774]
Klaassen, C.D., [1705]
Klemm, W.R., [1780]
Klette, H., [1068]
Klide, A.M., [1686]
Klös, H-G., [1133]
Knapp, E.J., [1578]
Knecht, C.D., [844], [1668]
Koch, T., [1234]
Korea, national association, [1935]
Kozlovsky, V.G., [177]
Krakowka, S., [1750]
Kraus, A.L., [971]
Kreier, J.P., [1591], [1598]
Krider, J.L., [638]
Kruesi, W.K., [595]
Kruse, G.O.W., [1511]
Kruth, S.A., [779]
Kubota, S.S., [1172]
Kuhns, L., [1576]
Kung, S.H., [1686]
Kunz, S.E., [1489]
Kutscher, A.H., [822]

Laboratory animal science, [1034]
Laboratory Animal Science Association, [2231]
laboratory animals, [975]–[1034]
  societies, [2034], [2041], [2053], [2075], [2126], [2191], [2193], [2231], [2265], [2288]
Laboratory animals, [1033]
laboratory diagnosticians, societies, [2047], [2317]
laboratory manuals, [1352]–[1357]
Ladds, P.W., [457]
Laing, J.A., [1651]
Laird, L.M., [1173]
Laird, M., [1499], [1500]

Lambrecht, J., [1255]
Lamming, G.E., [1568], [1639]
Lampson, S.M., [948]
Lancaster, J.L., [1501]
Land, R.B., [576]
Lane, D.R., [392]
Lane, J.G., [826]
Lang, E.M., [1133]
language problems, 101–3; *see also* dictionaries
Lanting, F.L., [936]
Large animal veterinarian: covering health and nutrition, [416]
large animals, [402]–[416], *see also* cattle, sheep etc.
Larson, B.L., [1566]
Lasley, J.F., [1248], [1646]
Latshaw, W.K., [1239]
law, *see* legislation
Lawrence, K., [1102]
Lawrence, T.L.J., [1448], [1567], [1568]
Lean, I., [458]
Leatherdale, D., [167]
Leaver, J.D., [459]
Lebanon, national association, [1936]
Leech, F.B., [1292]
Lees, P., [404]
legislation, 13–4, 93–4; [1358]–[1378]
  societies, [2221]
Legislation affecting the veterinary profession in the United Kingdom, [1367]
Lehrbuch der Anatomie der Haustiere, [1227]
Leighton, R.L., [827]
Leman, A.D., [639]
Leonard's Orthopedic surgery of the dog and cat, [828]
Lesak, A.E., [876]
Lesotho, national association, [1937]
Levandowsky, M., [1592]
Leverett, B., [964]
Levi, W.M., [1056]
Levine, N.D., [1502], [1599], [1600]
Lewi, P.J., [1007]
Lewis, B.P., [268]
Lewis, D., [729]
Lewis, H.K. & Co., 67; [50], [2466]
Lewis, L.D., [829]
Lewis, R.J.Sr, [1703]
Lewis's quarterly list, [42]
Leyhausen, P., [881]
libraries, 30–4: [1783]–[1844]
Library of Congress classification, 33
Liddle, C.G., [869]

Lightfoot, R.J., [580]
Lightner, D.V., [1187]
Lilley, G.P., [6]
Lindsay, D.R., [577]
Lindsey, J.R., [984]
Linton, A.H., [1687]
Lipowitz, A.J., [794]
Liska, W.D., [821]
List of FDA approved animal drug products, [269]
List of research workers 1981 in the agricultural sciences in the Commonwealth, [190]
List of serials abstracted (by CBAH), 84; [81]
Lister, D., [1569]
Livestock manual for the tropics, [1725]
Livestock production and diseases in the tropics, [1731]
Livestock production science, [1262]
Llama medicine workshop for veterinarians, [685]
llamas, societies, [2211]
Lloyd, D.H., [1405]
Loeb, W.F., [1008]
Loew, F.M., [996]
Logan's Medical and scientific abbreviations, [163]
Lom, J., [1594]
Long, P.L., [1601]
Lord, P.F., [852]
Lorenz, M.D., [830], [1410]
Loring, M., [1363]
Losos, G.J., [1726]
Love, R.J., [623]
Lovell, T., [1174]
Low, D.G., [840]
Low, R., [1057]
Lowrey, R.S., [1422]
Lucke, V.M., [825]
Lukefahr, S.D., [956]
Lumb, W.V., [1220]
Lusby, K.S., [461]
Luttmann, G., [595]
Luxembourg, national association, [1938]
Lyubashenko, S.Ya., [1134]

McAllister, E.S., [737]
McBane, S., [730], [731]
MacCallum, F.J., [447]
McCarthy, G., [732]
McClure, R.C., [882]
McCulloch, W.F., [1618]
McCurnin, D.M., [393], [1579]

McDonald, L.E., [1652], [1681]
McDonald, P., [1428]
McDowell, L.R., [1429], [1430]
MacEwen, E.G., [1466]
McIlwraith, C.W., [412], [733], [734]
Mack, R., [166], [167], [178], [179]
Mackay, D.R., [451]
McKay, F.W., [1464]
McKay, J.C., [1659]
McKeever, K., [1135]
Mackenzie, D., [596]
Mackie, A.M., [1196]
McLaughlin, C.A., [965]
MacLean, A., [630]
McLelland, J., [1038], [1055], [1243]
MacLeod, G., [1688]
McLeroy, G.B., [587]
McNitt, J.I., [956], [1254]
McPherson, C.W., [1019]
Madden, F.W., [1649]
Madewell, B.R., [1465]
Madigan, J.E., [735]
MAFF Publications, 90; [2479]
Maghreb Veterinary Associations Group, 16
Magrane, W.G., [937], [1467]
Mahy, B.W.J., [1747]
MAIL: Medicines Act information letter, [1375]
Maintenance and reproduction of reptiles in captivity, [1095]
Les maladies de la chèvre: colloque international, [610]
Malawi, national association, [1939]
Malaysia, national associations, [1940], [1941]
Malta, national association, [1942]
management, see practice management
The management and diseases of sheep, [578]
Management and welfare of farm animals: the UFAW handbook, [1765]
Mander, C., [1245]
Maner, J.H., [646]
Manipulating pig production, [664]
Manners, M.J., [637]
Manning, M.J., [1198]
Manning, P.J., [1020]
Manolson, F., [736]
Mansmann, R.A., [737]
Manual for animal health auxiliary personnel, [394]
Manual of poultry production in the tropics, [1058]

Manual of small animal . . ., [775]
Manual of veterinary investigation laboratory techniques, [1356]
Manual of veterinary parasitological laboratory techniques, [1357]
Marai, I. F. M., [579]
Marasas, W. F. O., [1402]
Marcus, L. C., [1096]
Market Research Society, 51
Marketing and practice strategies, [1585]
marketing information and market research, 49–50; [297]–[324]; *see also* industry; trade
Marketsearch, 51
Marsboom, R. P., [1007]
Marshall, A. G., [1503]
Marshall's Physiology of reproduction, [1639]
Martin, R. J., [831]
Martin, R. M., [1136]
Martin, S. W., [1291], [1293]
Martin, W. B., [557]
Martindale: the extra pharmacopoeia, [1689]
Marzec, G., [1100]
Mason, I. L., [164], [558], [1653]
Mason, M. M., [894]
Masters abstracts, [155]
mastitis, societies, [2207], [2239]
Mastitis literature survey, 66; [418]
Maton, A., [1255]
Mattison, C., [1097]
Mauritius, national association, [1943]
Maxwell, W. M. C., [1645]
May, C. G., [1059]
May, N. D. S., [559]
Mayhew, I. G., [1409]
Mayr, A., [1343]
Mayr-Bibrack, B., [1343]
Meadowcroft, S., [448]
Meat and Livestock Commission, [2233]
Media resource book: a guide to animal health information, [212]
Medical abbreviations and eponyms, [162]
Medical and health care books and serials in print, [55]
Medical and veterinary entomology, [1544]
Medical history, [1336]
Medical Libraries Association (*and* Veterinary Medical Libraries Section), 31–2
Medical research centres, [187]
medicine: relationship to veterinary medicine, 6–7, 9
MEDLINE, 77–8; [2387]

Medycyna weterynaryjna, [119]
Meek, A. H., [1293]
Mehlhorn, H., [1504], [1505]
Meisch, M. V., [1501]
Meissonnier, E., [4]
Melby, E. C. Jr, [981], [1026]
Menendhall, A. L., [738]
Mengeling, W. L., [639]
Mepham, T. B., [1566]
The Merck index, [221]
The Merck veterinary manual, 86; [362]
Merino-Rodriguez, M., [174]
Merritt, R. W., [1497]
Mersmann, H. J., [650]
Mertz, W., [1431]
Messinger, H., [1068]
Metcalfe, J., [1080]
Methods of Animal Experimentation, [1669]
Mexico
    libraries, [1816]
    national association, [1944]
Meyer, F. P., [1168]
Michel, C., [1171]
Michell, A. R., [832], [1690]
Mickley, L. C., [1755]
microbiology, [1379]–[1395]
    societies, [2059], [2318]
Migaki, G., [1150], [1179]
Miles, A. E. W., [1286]
Miles, J. W., [1500]
Milk Marketing Board, [2234]
Miller, W. H. Jr, [845]
Miller, W. J., [460]
Milligan, L. P., [1450]
Mills, O., [560]
Mills, R., [1175]
Milne, D. W., [739]
Mims, C. A., [1554], [1748]
MIMS: monthly index of medical specialities, [260]
Mineral tolerance of domestic animals, [1434]
Ministry of Agriculture, Fisheries and Food, [1325], [1432], [2479]
Mitchell, D., [481]
Mitchell, J. R., [1619]
Mitchell, W. R., [1291]
Mitruka, B. M., [1303]
Miyasaka, M., [1348]
Miyazaki, T., [1172]
Mloszewski, M. J., [504]
Moberg, G. P., [1775]
Modern veterinary practice, 58; [22]
Mohr, U., [1006], [1012]

Moller, H., [1176]
Moltedo, H.L., [1508], [1509]
Molynaux, D.H., [1602]
Monatshefte für Veterinärmedizin, [120]
Montali, R.J., [1149], [1150]
Montes, L.F., [740]
Montserrat, national association, [1945]
Moore, J.N., [764]
Moore, R.F., [1518]
Morehouse, L.G., [1404]
Moreng, R.E., [1060]
Morgan, J.P., [425], [938], [939], [1629], [1630]
Morgan, J.W.B., [1651]
Morgan, R.V., [833]
Morocco
    libraries, [1817]
    national association, [1946]
Morris, B., [1348]
Morris, D., [883]
Morris, J., [597]
Morris, M.L.Jr, [829]
Morrison, W.I., [1349]
Morrow, D.A., [1643]
Morse, R.A., [1211]
Mortenson, W.P., [454]
Morton, J.K., [511], [1319]
Morton, L.T., [7]
Mosby's Fundamentals of Animal Health Technology, [387]
Mosier, J.E., [917]
Moss, M.O., [1403]
Moulton, J.E., [1463]
Mount, L.E., [640]
Mouwen, J.M.V.M., [1555]
Mowlem, A., [598]
Mozambique, national association, [1947]
MSD AGVET, [1506]
Muir, J.F., [1157]
Muir, W.W., [1221]
Muirhead-Thomson, R.L., [1507]
Mukasa-Mugerwa, E., [678]
Muller, G.H., [834]
Multilingual dictionary of fish and fish products, [181]
multivolume works and series, [364]-[375]
Munoz-Cobenas, M.E., [1509]
Murdoch, D.B., [835]
Murphy, F.A., [1744]
Murphy, H.T., [5]
Murty, A.S., [1177]
mycology and mycotoxicoses,
    [1396]-[1406]
    societies, [2216]

Nabholz, A., [1761]
Namibia, national association, [1948]
National Library of Medicine audiovisuals catalog, [357]
National Office of Animal Health, [2240]
National Research Council, [1416], [1433], [1434]
national veterinary associations, 6, 17-18; [1845]-[2022]
Naude, T.W., [1711]
Navarro Pruneda, G., [180]
Naviaux, J.L., [741]
Neal, J., [599]
Needham, J.R., [1009]
Needham, T., [1173]
Nelson, P.E., [1402]
Nelson, R.W., [808]
Nemeth, F., [409]
Nepal, national association, [1949]
nephrology, societies, [2171]
Nesbitt, G.H., [836]
Nesheim, M.C., [1069], [1535]
Netherlands
    directories, [203], [241]
    journals, [132], [139], [141]
    libraries, [1818], [1819]
    national association, [1950]
Nettles, V.F., [516]
Neumann, A.L., [461]
neurology, [1407]-[1410]
    societies, [2084], [2172]
New England journal of medicine, [147]
New serial titles, [82]
New Zealand
    directories, [204], [242]
    journal, [121]
    libraries, [1820], [1821]
    national associations, [1951]-[1953]
    societies, [2266]
    trade association, [2026]
New Zealand veterinary journal, [121]
Newton, C.D., [837]
Nicaragua, national association, [1954]
Nicholas, D., [1737]
Nicholas, F.W., [1654]
Nicholas, R., [1737]
Nieburg, H.A., [822]
Niemann-Sørensen, A., [375]
Nigeria
    library, [1822]

national associations, [1955], [1956]
Nineham, A.W., [225]
Nissen, N.J., [1722]
Noakes, D.E., [462], [1641]
Noden, D.M., [1240]
Nomina anatomica avium, [1036]
Nomina anatomica veterinaria, [1226]
Nordisk veterinærmedicin, [122]
Norris, D.O., [1570]
North, M.O., [1061]
Norway
    directories, [243]
    libraries, [1823]
    national association, [1957]
*Nottingham University Easter Schools in
    Agricultural Science*, [370]
NTIS, 91; [2389]
Nunamaker, D.M., [714], [837]
Nunez, J.L., [1508], [1509]
nurses, veterinary, *see* ancillary personnel
Nute, G., [1136]
Nute, J., [1136]
Nutrient Requirements of Domestic Animals,
    [1416]
The nutrient requirements of pigs, [641]
The nutrient requirements of ruminant livestock,
    [1435]
Nutrition abstracts and reviews, 60; [1411]
nutrition and digestion, [1411]–[1459]
    societies, [2030], [2060]
*Nutritional energetics of domestic animals and
    glossary of energy terms*, [1433]
Nutting, W.B., [1510]

O'Brien, T.R., [838]
Odend'hal, S., [1749]
Odlaug, T.O., [642]
O'Donoghue, P.N., [1002]
Oehme, F.W., [410]
O'Farrell, V., [940]
Office International des Épizooties, 15;
    [65], [1366], [1377], [2244]
Office of Technology Assessment, [1766]
Official journal of the European Communities,
    93–4
Official methods of analysis of the AOAC,
    [1678]
Ogbourne, C.P., [423], [452], [742]
Okerman, L., [966]
Olds, J.R., [1010]
Olds, R.J., [1010], [1388]
Oliver, J.E.Jr, [1409], [1410]
Olsen, R.G., [884]

Olson, R.G., [1750]
Olsson, L., [752]
Olsson, S-E., [839]
Oltenacu, E.A.B., [1657]
Olusanya, S., [1724]
Oman, national association, [1958]
O'Mary, C.C., [483]
oncology, [1460]–[1466]
    societies, [2270], [2291]
Onderstepoort journal of veterinary research,
    [123]
online services, *see* computerized
    information retrieval systems
ophthalmology, [1467]–[1475]
    societies, [2061], [2076], [2140], [2173],
    [2219]
Organisation for Economic Co-operation
    and Development, [181]
Orlans, F.B., [1773]
Ørskov, R., [1436], [1437]
orthopaedics, societies, [2174], [2299],
    [2301]; *see also* surgery
Osborne, C.A., [840]
Osweiler, G.D., [1646], [1712]
Outteridge, P.M., [1344]
Owen, J., [1438]
Owen, J.B., [463], [561], [562], [579]
Owen, L.N., [1460]
Owen, N.L., [600]
Oxford review of reproductive biology, [1637]

Packer, D.E., [707]
Pagot, J., [1720]
Pakistan, national association, [1959]
Pallaske, G., [1549]
Palmer, S.R., [1610]
Pan American Association of Veterinary
    Sciences, [2247]
Pan American Health Organization,
    [2248]
Panama, national association, [1960]
Papua New Guinea, national associations,
    [1961], [1962]
Paraguay, national association, [1963]
parasitology, [1476]–[1548]
    societies, [2048], [2166], [2203], [2296],
    [2309], [2323]
Parasitology, [1545]
Parasitology research, [1546]
Parasitology today, [1547]
Parker, R.O., [546], [631]
Parker, W.H., [382]
Parry, H.B., [563]

Pascal sigma, [23]
Pascal thema, [23]
Pasquini, C., [464], [743]
patents, 95-6
pathology, [1549]-[1561]
   societies, [2062], [2175], [2262], [2319]
Paton, W., [1767]
Pattengale, P.K., [997]
Patterson, D.S.P., [530]
Patterson, H., [752]
Pattison, I., [1326], [1327]
Patton, N.M., [956]
Pavaux, C., [465], [954]
Pavord, A., [744]
Pawlowski, Z.S., [1535]
Payne, J.M., [466], [1610], [1571], [1572]
Payne, S., [1572]
Payne, W.J.A., [467], [1729]
Pearce, D.T., [527]
Pearson, H., [1641]
Peiffer, R.L.Jr, [841], [1472]
Pelloni, G., [902]
Penny, R.H.C., [639]
Pensaert, M.B., [1740]
People's Dispensary for Sick Animals, [2250]
perinatology, societies, [2220]
Periodika der Veterinärmedizin und ihrer Grenzgebiete, 84
Perrotin, C., [1494]
Perry, T.W., [468], [1439]
Perspectives in Medical Virology, [1742]
Peru, national association, [1964]
The pesticide manual. A world compendium, [222]
Pet Health Council, [2253]
Peters, A.R., [469]
Peters, W., [1603]
Petrak, M.L., [1062]
pets, *see* small animals
   particular species, welfare of, *see* welfare of animals
Pettersson, H., [752]
Petty, C., [1011]
Pfänder, H.J., [1709]
The pharmaceutical journal, [1700]
Pharmaceutical manufacturing encyclopedia, [224]
pharmacology and pharmaceutics, *see* therapeutics, pharmacology and pharmaceutics
PHARMACONTACTS, [216], [2393]

pharmacopoeias, *see* drugs: directories
Pharmeuropa, [216]
Pharr, J.W., [425]
Philippines, national association, [1965]
Phillips, C.E., [1013]
Phillipson, A.T., [383]
Phillis, J.W., [1573]
PHIND, [2395]
Phipps, R.H., [430]
Physiology of the Amphibia, [1098]
Physiology and biochemistry of the domestic fowl, [1039]
physiology and metabolism, [1562]-[1575]
   societies, [2077], [2320]
The physiology of reproduction, [1640]
Physiology of ruminant nutrition, [1451]
Pickering, A.D., [1199]
Piermattei, D.L., [788], [842]
Pig farming, [667]
Pig health and production recording, [643]
Pig international, [668]
Pig news and information, 60; [619]
Pig production and welfare, [644]
Pig unit newsletter, [669]
Pig veterinary journal, [2257]
Pig yearbook, [288]
pigs, [619]-[671]
   societies, [2034], [2212], [2256], [2257]
Pigs, [670]
Pilliner, S., [745]
Pineda, M.H., [1652]
PJB Publications, 50; [316]
Poinar, G.O.Jr, [1212]
Le pointe vétérinaire, [124]
Poland, J., [401]
Poland
   journal, [119]
   libraries, [1824], [1825]
   national associations, [1966], [1967]
Pollak, E.J., [1657]
Pollott, G.E., [539]
Pond, W.G., [645], [646]
Ponting, K., [564]
Popesko, P., [1234], [1241]
Pork '89, [671]
Porterfield, J.S., [1751]
Portsmouth, J.I., [967], [1063]
Portugal
   directory, [244]
   libraries, [1826]
   national associations, [1968], [1969]
Post, G.W., [1178]
Post-Graduate Committee in Veterinary

Science, University of Sydney, 58,
  60, 70, 75, 83; [66], [67], [2258]
Poultry, [1087]
Poultry abstracts, 60; [1035]
poultry and cage birds, [1035]–[1089]
  societies, [2036], [2096], [2135], [2304],
    [2329], [2330]
  trade association, [2101]
Poultry science, [1088]
Poultry science symposium series, [1081]
Povey, R.C., [885]
Powell-Smith, V., [702]
Pozniak, G.I., [179]
Practice, [351]
practice management, [1576]–[1598]
*Practice marketing and management: veterinary
  edition*, [1586]
Practice veterinary video, [358]
Der praktische Tierärzt, [125]
Prasse, K.W., [1308]
*Pratique médicale and chirurgicale de l'animal
  de compagnie*, [868]
Pratt, H.D., [1498]
Pratt, P.W., [395], [396], [886]
*Predicting feed intake of major food producing
  animals*, [1434]
Prescott, J.F., [1691]
Preston, T.R., [470]
preventive medicine, *see* epidemiology and
  preventive medicine
Preventive veterinary medicine, [1301]
Price, C.J., [397], [1064]
Priester, W.A., [1464]
Prieur, W.D., [787]
primates, societies, [2102], [2213], [2259];
  see also laboratory animals
Prince, E.F., [746]
Pritchard, M.H., [1511]
Pritchard, W.R., [383]
private practice, 9, 11
Problems in veterinary medicine, [68]
*Proceedings: first international conference on
  zoological and avian medicine*, [1151]
Proceedings of a deer course for veterinarians,
  [525]
Proceedings of the buffalo seminar . . ., [505]
*Proceedings of the fourth international conference
  on goats*, [611]
*Proceedings of the sixth international congress on
  production disease in farm animals*, [415]
Proceedings of the 3rd world's rabbit congress,
  [972]
Proceedings of the fourth international

reindeer/caribou symposium, [526]
*Proceedings 36th annual Pfizer research
  conference*, [1452]
professional bodies, 13–18
Programme of agricultural and food research,
  [276]
Progress in vaccinology, [1339]
*Progress in Veterinary Microbiology and
  Immunology*, [69]
Prosser, C.G., [1568]
Protozoological abstracts, 62; [1590]
protozoology, [1590]–[1606]
  society, [2296]
Provasoli, L., [1592]
Provenzano, A.J.Jr, [1209]
PROVIDES, 75
public health, [1607]–[1624]
  societies, [2105], [2150], [2177], [2197],
    [2215], [2300], [2316]
publishers and booksellers, 67, 87;
  [2406]–[2530]
Pugh, D.M., [1683]
Pure and applied science books 1876–1982,
  [56]

Qatar, national association, [1970]
*Quarterly index: information access for the small
  animal practitioner*, 60–1; [770]
Quimby, F.W., [1008]
Quinn, A.J., [917]

rabbits, [953]–[974]
  society, [2325]
Rabinovich, M.I., [1692]
Radeleff, R.D., [1713]
radiology, [1625]–[1634]
  societies, [2064], [2136], [2227]
Radostits, O.M., [403], [1294]
Raether, W., [1505]
Rakipov, N.G., [177]
Randall, C.J., [1065]
Randall, D.J., [1156]
Randall, R., [1563]
Rands, M.R.W., [1131]
Raptor management techniques manual, [1137]
Ratcliffe, F.N., [961]
Ratcliffe, N.A., [1312]
Rathore, G.S., [679]
Ratzlaff, M.H., [743]
Rawlings, C.A., [843], [860]
Rawnsley, H.M., [1303]
Recent advances in animal nutrition, [1415]
Recent advances in aquaculture, [1157]

Recent advances in poultry nutrition, [1414]
Recent developments in pig nutrition, [1414]
Recueil de médecine vétérinaire, [126]
Redding, R.W., [844]
Reddy, V.K., [743]
Reedy, L.M., [845]
Referativnyi zhurnal. Veterinariya, 73; [24]
reference books, 85-7; [360]-[363]
Regan, T., [1768]
Registers and directory, 38; [206]
Regulatory affairs bulletin, [1376]
Reichenbach-Klinke, H-H., [1099],
    [1163]
Reid, C.S.W., [540]
Reid, W.M., [1054]
Reinecke, R.K., [1512]
Remington's Pharmaceutical sciences, [1693]
*Répertoire des opérations de recherches dans les
    établissements membres*, [282]
The Report of the Chief Veterinary Officer,
    [207]
Report on the welfare of . . ., [1769]
reproduction and genetics, [1635]-[1663]
    societies, [2054], [2067], [2206], [2208],
    [2220], [2275]-[2277]
reptiles, *see* amphibians and reptiles
research, 41-6
    directories of, 45-6; [274]-[283]
    societies for, [2151]
Research in avian coccidiosis, [1082]
Research in veterinary science, [127]
residues of drugs, societies, [2146]
*Retrospective index to theses of Great Britain and
    Ireland, 1716-1950*, [151]
*Return of proceedings under the Animal Health
    Act*, [295]
review articles, 72-3; [60]-[75]
Review of applied entomology, 62; [1478]
Review of medical and veterinary mycology, 62;
    [1396]
Revista de camelidos sudamericanos, [686]
*Revue d'élevage et de médecine vétérinaire des
    pays tropicaux*, [1733]
Revue de médecine vétérinaire, [128]
*Revue scientifique et technique de l'Office
    Internationale des Épizooties*, [129]
Rew, R.S., [1487]
Reznik, G., [1012]
Reznik-Schuller, H., [1012]
Ribbeck, R., [185]
Ribelin, W.E., [1179]
Rice, M.K., [163]
Richard, D., [680]
Richardson, R.C., [391]
Rickard, J., [872]
Ricketts, S.W., [749]
Rico, A.G., [1694]
Ridgway, S.H., [1138], [1139]
Riemann, H.P., [1297]
Riley, V.A., [1238]
Ristic, M., [1604]
Ritchie, C.I.A., [941]
Robbins, C.T., [1140]
Roberts, R.J., [1157], [1180], [1181],
    [1200]
Roberts, S.J., [1655]
Robertson, Sir A., [1718], [1719]
Robertson, D.E., [580]
Robertson, P., [1128]
Robinson, D.W., [576]
Robinson, M.C., [1066]
Robinson, R., [887]
Robinson, W.F., [1556]
Rochette, F., [1523]
Roe, J.F.C., [1027]
Rolins, A., [942]
Rollinson, D., [1513]
Romania, national associations, [1971],
    [1972]
Rook, J.A.F., [1441]
Rooney, J.R., [747]
Rose, R.J., [697]
Rosenberger, G., [471]
Ross, B., [1182]
Ross, L.G., [1182]
Ross, R.A., [1100]
Rossdale, P.D., [693], [718], [748], [749]
Rossof, I.S., [223]
Rouse, J.E., [472]
Rowan, A.N., [1770]
Rowan Blogg, J.R., [870]
Rowley, A.F., [1312]
Roy, J.H.B., [473]
Royal Agricultural Society of England,
    40-1; [2263]
Royal College of Veterinary Surgeons, 6,
    13-14, 20, 31, 38, 69, 93; [2012]
    library catalogues, [1320], [1321]
    Registers and directory, 38; [206]
Royal Society for the Prevention of
    Cruelty to Animals, [2264]
Royal Veterinary College, 5, 30; [1837],
    [1838]
    library catalogue, [1322]
Rubin, L.F., [943], [1473], [1474]
Rudge, A.J.B., [519]

Rushton, B., [1304]
Russell, A. D., [1687]
Russell, K., [474]
Russell, P. H., [1752]
Russell, W. M. S., [1771]
Russia, *see* Union of Soviet Socialist
    Republics
Rutgers, L. J. E., [409]
Ryan, G. D., [846]
Ryder, M. L., [565]

Sack, W. O., [647], [750], [1232]
*Safety precautions for use in veterinary
    laboratories*, [1781]
Sainsbury, D., [384], [385], [648], [1067],
    [1379], [1779]
St Kitts/Nevis, national association,
    [1973]
St Lucia, national association, [1974]
St Vincent, national association, [1975]
*Salamon's Artificial insemination of sheep and
    goats*, [1645]
San Salvador, national association, [1977]
Sande, M. A., [1390]
Sanderson, J. H., [1013]
Sandford, J., [968]
Sandford, J. C., [969]
Sandys-Winsch, G., [944], [1368]
Sard, D. M., [1782]
Sauer, J. R., [1514]
Saunders, L. Z., [1474]
Savey, M., [407]
Sawyer, D. C., [847]
Sax, N. I., [1703]
Scanlan, C. M., [1268]
Schalm, O. W., [475], [1313]
Schalm's Veterinary hematology, [1313]
Schebitz, H., [751], [848]
Schmidt, G. D., [1515]
Schmidt, P. J., [476]
Schmidt, R. E., [1141], [1014]
Schneidawind, H., [1113]
Schnurrenberger, P. R., [1295], [1618]
Schofield, A. M., [1516]
Scholl, E., [639]
Scholl, P. J., [1530]
Scholtyseck, E., [1605]
schools, veterinary, 5, 18–20, 30–2, 42; *see
    also* education
Schrag, J., [1068]
Schubert, G., [1183]
Schwabe, C. W., [1296], [1297], [1328]
Schwartzman, R. M., [1401]

Schweizer Archiv für Tierheilkunde, [130]
Science citation index, 75; [34]
*Scientific and technical books and serials in
    print*, [57]
Scott, D. W., [411], [834]
Scott, M. L., [1069], [1440]
Seaman, W. J., [1015]
Sedgwick, S. D., [1184], [1185]
Seely, J. C., [990]
Seiferle, E., [902]
Seller, T. J., [1070]
Sellers, K. C., [1405]
Sellers, K. G., [1292]
*Seminars in veterinary medicine and surgery
    (small animal)*, [776]
Senegal, national association, [1978]
Serial sources for the BIOSIS database, [83]
serials, *see* journals
Service, M. W., [1517], [1532]
Sevelius, F., [752]
Seychelles, national association, [1979]
Sharman, G. A. M., [513]
Sharman, R. S., [1295]
Shaw, H. J., [1142]
sheep, [529]–[583]
    societies, [2042], [2241], [2266], [2267]
Sheep and goats in humid West Africa, [612]
Sheep dairy news, [582]
Sheep farmer, [581]
Sheep handling and dipping, [566]
Sheep yearbook, [288]
Shek, J. W., [970]
Shepherd, C. J., [1181], [1186]
The shepherd's guide, [567]
Shifrine, M., [945]
Shirley, R. L., [1442]
Shishkov, V. P., [182]
Shiveley, M. J., [849], [1242]
Short, C. E., [1222]
Short, R. V., [1638]
Shull, L. R., [1706]
Siegel, E. T., [946]
Siegel, P. B., [1271]
Sierra Leone, national association, [1980]
Silvermann, S., [1630]
Simmons, M. L., [1016]
Simpson, A. J. G., [1513]
Simpson, M. E., [904]
Sindermann, C. J., [1187]
Singapore, national association, [1981]
Singh, P., [1518]
Singleton, P., [1379]
Sinn, R., [601]

Sisson, D.D., [855]
Sisson and Grossman's The anatomy of the domestic animals, [1228]
Sittig, M., [224]
Skerritt, G.C., [1243]
Slack, R., [225]
Slater, S., [474]
Slatter, D.H., [850], [1475]
Sliosberg, A., [172]
Sloane, S.B., [162]
Sloss, M.W., [1519]
Sloss, V., [477]
Small, J., [545]
Small, J.D., [994]
Small animal abstracts, 60; [771]
small animals, [770]-[868]
    publisher of handbooks on, [2260]
    societies, [2127], [2232], [2235], [2249], [2253], [2254], [2269], [2326]
    trade associations, [2073], [2251], [2252], [2255], [2306]
    see also cats, dogs etc.
Small ruminant production systems in South and Southeast Asia, [613]
Small ruminant research, [618]
Small ruminants in African agriculture, [614]
Smallwood, J.E., [1627]
Smith, C., [1659]
Smith, E.M., [898]
Smith, F., [1329]
Smith, G.J., [1714]
Smith, J.E., [1403]
Smith, K.G.V., [1484]
Smith, L.S., [1188]
Smith, O.B., [615]
Smith, W.J., [629], [630], [649]
Smithcors, J.F., [1330]-[1332]
Smuts, M.M.S., [681]
Snieszko, S.F., [1155]
Snow, D.H., [753]
SNOVET, 86; [165]
Soave, O., [1369]
Society of Practising Veterinary Surgeons, [2274]
Sodikoff, C., [851]
Sokolowski, J.H., [947]
Solberg, V., [398]
Solomon Islands, national association, [1982]
Soulsby, E.J.L., [1345], [1520]
South Africa
    directories, [245]
    journals, [116], [123]
    libraries, [1827]
    national associations, [1983], [1984]
South West Africa, national association, [1985]
Spain
    directories, [246]
    libraries, [1828]
    national associations, [1986]-[1989]
Sparks, A.K., [1213]
Speckmann, G., [1133]
Spedding, C.R.W., [568]
Speedy, A.W., [569]
Speer, C.A., [1596]
Spiers, I., [522]
Spira, H.R., [897]
Sponenberg, D.P., [707]
Sri Lanka, national association, [1990]
Stahr, H.M., [1704]
Stainer, J.R., [917]
Stamp, J.T., [548]
A standard guide to cat breeds, [888]
The standard periodical directory, [84]
standards, 94; [334]-[337]
Standards in laboratory animal management, [1028]
Standing Committee on Tables of Feed Composition, [1432]
Stansfield, M., [478]
Stanton, H.C., [650]
Stark, B.A., [597], [607]
Starr, J.R., [1257]
Stashak, T.S., [754]
State veterinary journal, [131]
statistical methods, [1782]
statistics, 98-9; [284]-[296], [1777], [1782]; *see also* marketing information and market research
statutory bodies, 13-18
Steiner, C.V.Jr, [1071]
Stephen, L.E., [1606]
Stephens, G., [8]
Stephens, M., [939]
Stevenson, J.P., [1189]
Stickney, R.R., [1190]
Stimson, A.W., [898]
Stock, M.K., [1080]
Stojanovich, C.J., [1498]
Stolen, J.S., [1201]
Strafuss, A.C., [1557]
Straighton, E. (The TV Vet), 88; [479], [480], [572], [651], [758], [890], [949]
Straw, B., [639]

Stromberg, M.W., [1001]
Studdert, M.J., [1744]
Studdert, V.P., [158]
Stunkard, J.A., [1072]
Stünzi, H., [1549]
Sturkie, P.D., [1073]
style, 29–30
Suarez, F.R., [652]
Subject guide to books in print, [58]
Subject headings, 33–4, 53–5
Successful financial management for the veterinary practice, [1580]
Sudan, national association, [1991]
Summerfelt, R.C., [1202]
Summer-Smith, G., [1670]
Sundlof, S.F., [266]
surgery, [1664]–[1674]
    societies, [2065], [2174], [2299], [2301]
Suter, P.F., [852], [922], [1631]
Sutton, C.G., [948]
Sutton, J.B., [915]
Svendsen, E.D., [755]
Swaim, S.F., [853]
Swatland, H.J., [1258]
Swaziland, national association, [1992]
Sweden
    directory, [247]
    libraries, [1829], [1830]
    national association, [1993]
Swenson, J., [1562]
Swindle, M.M., [653], [1671]
Swine in biomedical research, [665]
Swine practitioner, [671]
Switzerland
    journal, [130]
    national association, [1994]
Symons, L.E.A., [1521]
Symposia of the Zoological Society of London, [1152]
Syria, national association, [1995]
Systematized nomenclature of medicine – microglossary for veterinary medicine, 86; [165]
Szabo, K.T., [1656]
Szyfres, B., [1609]

Tacher, G., [1720]
Taiwan, national associations, [1996]–[1998]
Talbot, R.B., [269]
Tams, T., [854]
Tannenbaum, J., [1370]
Tanzania, national associations, [1999],

[2000]
Tatner, M.F., [1198]
Taylor, A.E.R., [1522]
Taylor, D., [889]
Taylor, D.J., [649], [654]
Taylor, M.E., [878]
Taylor, P.M., [818]
Technical Centre for Agricultural and Rural Cooperation, [2283]
technicians, veterinary 13; *see also* ancillary personnel
Technology Management Group, [317]
Telger, T.C., [711]
TELUM, 32
Termouth, J.H., [1426]
The T. G. Hungerford Vade Mecum Series for Domestic Animals, [1676]
Thailand, national association, [2001]
Thear, K., [602], [603], [1074]
Thedford, T.R., [570], [604]
Theilen, G.H., [1465]
therapeutics, pharmacology and pharmaceutics, [1675]–[1700]
    societies, [2031], [2109], [2164], [2320]
    see also drugs
Theriogenology, [1663]
theses, 84–5; [148]–[155]
Thickett, W., [481]
Thienpont, D., [1523]–[1528]
Thoen, C.O., [1267]
Tholen, M.A., [784], [1287]
Thomas, D.G.M., [1259]
Thomas, G.M., [1212]
Thomas, P.C., [1441]
Thomas, R.J., [538]
Thomas, V.M., [482]
Thomas, W.P., [855]
Thompson, D.J., [915]
Thompson, G.B., [483]
Thompson, R.C.A., [1524], [1525]
Thomsett, L.R., [781]
Thomson, R.G., [1558], [1559]
Thorley, C.M., [407]
Thornton, K., [655], [656]
Thrall, D.E., [1632]
Thrusfield, M.V., [1298]
Ticer, J.W., [856], [1633]
Ticks and tick-borne disease control, [1526]
Ticks and tick-borne diseases, [1537]
Tierärztliche Umschau, [133]
Tijdschrift voor diergeneeskunde, [132]
Tilley, L.P., [857]
Timmons, E.H., [963]

Timmons, M.J., [876]
Tizard, I., [1346]
Tobin, T., [756]
Toivanen, A., [1075]
Toivanen, P., [1075]
Tomes, G.J., [580]
Tonga, national association, [2002]
*Topley and Wilson's Principles of bacteriology,
    virology and immunity*, [1389]
tortoises, society, [2284]
Toussaint Raven, E., [407], [484]
Towle, A., [544]
Townson, S., [1102]
toxicology, [1701]-[1716]
    societies, [2028], [2052], [2164]
TOXLINE, 78; [2401]
Toynbee, J.M.C., [1333]
Trabing, M.E., [183]
Trace elements in man and animals, [1453]
trade, 45-50; *see also* industry
trade associations, 46
trade directories, [214]-[273]
trade literature, 67-8, 83
trade marks, 96, 98
TRADEMARKSCAN, 98; [2402]
*Traditional (indigenous) systems of veterinary
    medicine for small farmers*, [1727]
Trainer, D.O., [1120], [1121]
translations, *see* language problems
transport of animals, societies, [2087]
Tribe, D.E., [375]
trichinellosis, societies, [2203]
Trinidad and Tobago, national
    association, [2003]
Tropical agricultural information sources, [191]
Tropical animal health and production, [1734]
Tropical veterinarian, [1735]
Tropical veterinary bulletin, [25]
tropical veterinary medicine,
    [1717]-[1736]
    societies, [2100], [2145], [2285], [2289],
    [2302]
*Tsetse and trypanosomiasis information
    quarterly*, [1479]
tuberculosis, [424]
Tucker, C.S., [1191]
Tuffery, A.A., [1017]
Tunisia, national association, [2004]
Turkey, national associations, [2005],
    [2006]
Turkey production: breeding and husbandry,
    [1077]
Turkey production: health, [1076]

Turner, A.S., [412], [711], [734], [739],
    [757]
Turner, H.N., [571]
Turner, M., [605]
Turusov, V.S., [1018]
The TV Vet, *see* Straighton, E.
Twinch, C., [968]

*The UFAW Handbook on the use and
    management of laboratory animals*, [982]
Uganda, national associations, [2007],
    [2008]
UK, *see* United Kingdom
The UK pet trade year book and buyers guide,
    [261]
UKASTA (The United Kingdom
    Agricultural Supply Trade
    Association), [2286]
Ulrich's international periodicals directory, 84;
    [85]
Underwood, E.J., [1431], [1443]
UNIDO guides to information sources, [9]
Union of Soviet Socialist Republics
    directory, [248]
    journal, [135]
    libraries, [1831], [1832]
    national associations, [2009], [2010]
Unit for Veterinary Continuing
    Education, 99; [352]
United Kingdom
    directories, 38, 40-1; [206], [207],
    [248]-[261]
    journals, [92], [99], [103], [104], [114],
    [127], [131], [134], [138], [140],
    [142], [146]
    libraries, [1783], [1833]-[1838]
    national associations, [2011], [2012]
    statistical sources, [284], [286]-[288],
    [293]-[295]
    theses lists, [148]-[151]
    trade associations, [2089], [2091],
    [2240], [2286]
United Kingdom dairy facts and figures, [294]
United Nations, [1]
United States
    directories, 18, 39, 40; [208]-[213],
    [262]-[272]
    journals, [91], [105], [112], [113],
    [117], [137], [147]
    libraries, [1839]-[1844]
    national association, [2013]
    statistical sources, [286]
    theses lists, [152]-[155]

trade associations, [2080], [2082], [2090]
United States. Government Printing Office, [2508]
United States. National Technical Information Service, 91; [2389]
Universities Federation for Animal Welfare, [2288]
Upson, D.W., [1695]
urology, societies, [2171], [2280]
Urquhart, G.M., [1527]
Uruguay, national associations, [2014], [2015]
US pharmaceutical market: animal and poultry, [309]
USA, *see* United States
USDA-APHIS, [2514]
use of literature, 25-9
The use of nuclear techniques to improve domestic buffalo production in Asia, [506]
USSR, *see* Union of Soviet Socialist Republics

Vaccine, [134]
van Duijn, C., [1192]
Van Gelder, G.A., [1712]
Van Hoosier, G.L.Jr, [1019]
Van Muiswinkel, W.B., [1201]
Van Soest, P.J., [1444]
Van Vleck, L.D., [1657]
Vanden Bossche, H., [1528]
Vanparis, O.F.J., [1523]
Varley, M.A., [635]
Vasseur, P.B., [813]
Vaughan, J.T., [413], [740]
Venezuela
    directory, [273]
    national association, [2016]
Verderame, M., [1529]
Versteeg, J., [1753]
VETAID, [2302]
VETDOC, 62, 78; [26], [2403]
Veterinarian directory, [213]
Veterinariya, [135]
Veterinarski glasnik, [136]
Veterinary and comparative orthopaedics and traumatology, [1673]
Veterinary and human toxicology, [1716]
Veterinary anesthesia, [1225]
Veterinary annual, 73; [70]
Veterinary aspects of fish farming, [1193]
Veterinary biological products: licensees and permittees, [271]

Veterinary bulletin, 53-6, 73; [27]
Veterinary clinical pathology, [1315]
Veterinary clinics of North America, 73, 102; [71]-[73]
VETERINARY COMPUTERISED INFORMATION SYSTEM, 76; [2361]
Veterinary dermatology, [2170]
Veterinary drug formulary, [264]
Veterinary drug registration newsletter, [1377]
Veterinary economics, [1587]
Veterinary encyclopedia: diagnosis and treatment, [363]
Veterinary forum, [1588]
Veterinary history, [1337]
veterinary hospitals, societies, [2033], [2133]
Veterinary immunology. Proceedings of the first international veterinary immunology symposium, [1350]
Veterinary immunology and immunopathology, [1351]
Veterinary investigation diagnosis analysis, [295]
VETERINARY MEDICAL DATA PROGRAM, 99; [2298]
Veterinary medicine, [137]
Veterinary medicine report, [74]
Veterinary microbiology, [1395]
Veterinary multilingual thesaurus, [170]
VETERINARY NETWORK, 60; [2360]
The veterinary nursing journal, [399]
Veterinary parasitology, [1548]
Veterinary pathology, [1561]
Veterinary pharmaceuticals and biologicals 1989/90, [272]
Veterinary practice, 68; [138]
Veterinary practice management, [1589]
Veterinary practitioner's guide to approved new animal drugs, [263]
Veterinary quarterly, [139]
Veterinary radiology, [1634]
Veterinary record, 17-18, 25, 37, 68, 82, 99, 102; [140]
Veterinary research communications, [141]
Veterinary reviews and annotations, [75]
veterinary schools, *see* schools, veterinary
Veterinary serials: a union list of serials held in veterinary collections, 31-2
VETERINARY SERVICES DATA BANK, 79; [2362]
VETERINARY STOCK*FINDER, 79
Veterinary subject headings, [166]

Veterinary surgery, [1674]
Veterinary technician, [400]
Veterinary times, 68; [142]
Veterinary update: clinical abstract service, 56,
    58–60; [22], [28]
*Veterinary viral diseases: their significance in
    South-East Asia and the Western Pacific*,
    [1730]
VETFAX, [259]
Villemin, M., [184]
Vipond, J. E., [520]
*Viral and mycoplasmal infections of laboratory
    rodents*, [1029]
virology, [1737]–[1753]
    societies, [2176]
Virulence mechanisms of bacterial pathogens,
    [1269]
Virus infections of carnivores, [1740]
Vitamin tolerance of animals, [1434]
Vivash Jones Consultants, 50; [318]
Vivian, J., [595]
Vlaams diergeneeskundig tijdschrift, [143]
Vogel, C. J., [753]
voluntary organizations, [2188], [2289],
    [2302]; *see also* charitable
    organizations; welfare of animals

Wagner, J. E., [962], [1020]
Wagner, W. C., [1651]
Walker, D. F., [413]
Walker, R. G., [1665]
Walker, W. F. Jr, [657]
Wallach, J. D., [1143]
Waller, P. J., [1534]
Walshaw, S. O., [798]
Walton, G. S., [444]
Walton, J. R., [658]
Wamberg, K., [363]
Ward, B. C., [983]
Ward, J. M., [997], [998]
Waring, G. H., [759]
Warren, R. G., [387]
Waterman, A. E., [1690]
Watkins, P., [433]
Waynforth, H. B., [1021]
Weatherley, A. H., [1194]
Weaver, A. D., [407], [414], [447], [485],
    [762]
Webbon, P. M., [858]
Webster, A. B., [1271]
Webster, A. J. F., [486]
Webster, C. C., [1728]
Webster, J., [487]

Weems, D. B., [606]
Weindling, P., [1316]
Weisbroth, S. H., [971], [984]
Welch, K. R. G., [1101]
welfare of animals, [1754]–[1775]
    societies, [2035], [2071], [2074], [2093],
        [2106], [2116], [2130], [2144],
        [2154], [2179], [2189], [2190],
        [2235], [2236], [2242], [2250],
        [2264], [2265], [2269], [2288],
        [2327], [2303]
The Wellcome Trust, 44; [283]
Wells, E. B., [687], [692]
Wen, G. Y., [970]
Wenkoff, M. S., [488]
Wensing, C. J. G., [1232]
West, G. P., [157]
West Indies, *see* names of specific islands,
    e.g. Bahamas
Westermayer, E., [1686]
Western Samoa, national association,
    [1976]
What's new in farming, [324]
Whitaker's book list, [59]
White, D. O., [1744], [1748]
White, K., [877], [925]
White, N. A., [760], [764]
Whitlock, R. H., [761]
Whitney, R. A. Jr, [1022]
Whittemore, C. T., [489], [659], [660]
Whittick, W. G., [950]
WHO drug information, [1378]
WHO Monograph Series, [373]
WHO Technical Reports Series, [374]
Who's who in science in Europe, [192]
Wiener tierärztliche Monatsschrift, [144]
Wiesner, E., [185], [711]
Wiggins, G. S., [1620]
wild animals, *see* exotic pets, zoo and wild
    animals
Wildbiologische Informationen für den Jager,
    [1111]
Wildlife disease review, [1105]
Wildlife review, [1106]
Wildt, D. E., [1779]
Wilken, L. O., [268]
Wilkens, H., [751], [848]
Wilkinson, G. T., [859], [891]
Wilkinson, J. M., [490], [607], [1260]
Wilkinson, M., [597]
Willeberg, P., [1293]
Williams, D. J., [1668]
Williams, D. R., [1371]

Williams, R. E., [1530]
Williamson, G., [1729]
Williamson, H. D., [1628]
Willis, M. B., [435], [470], [951]
Wilson, A., [1620], [1621]
Wilson, F. D., [945]
Wilson, N. R. P., [1622]
Wilson, P. N., [491], [1445], [1446], [1728]
Wilson, R. T., [682]
Wingfield, W. E., [860]
Wintzer, H-J., [762]
Wise, G. H., [1295]
Wise, J. K., [298]
Wiseman, J., [661], [1447]
Wisniewski, H. M., [970]
Withrow, S. J., [1466]
Wobeser, G. A., [1145]
Wolf, K., [1195]
Wolff, H. G., [1688]
Wolley, T. A., [1531]
Wolski, T. R., [1278]
Wolvekamp, W. Th. C., [952]
women in the profession, 6
    societies, [2113], [2281], [2331]
Woodbine, M., [1696]
Wood-Gush, D. G. M., [1281]
Woods, G. T., [1299]
Wool technology and sheep breeding, [583]
World animal health, 98; [296]
*World animal health productivity and nutrition
    products market study update*, [318]
World animal science, [375]
World Association for Buiatrics, 15;
    [2311]
A world bibliography of bibliographies, [1317]
*World catalogue of veterinary films/video tapes
    and films/video tapes of veterinary interest*,
    [399]
World Consultation of the Animal Health
    Industry, [2152]
*World directory of schools for animal health
    assistants 1971*, [193]
World directory of veterinary schools 1971, 41;
    [193]
World Health Organization, 91–2; [2324]
World list of scientific periodicals, 84; [86]

WORLD PATENTS INDEX (WPI), 96;
    [2404]
World review of animal production, [1736]
World Small Animal Veterinary
    Association, 14–15; [2326]
World Veterinary Association, 16, 41, 99;
    [2328]
    Bulletin, 41; [326]
World Veterinary Congress, 16, 69, 99
World's poultry science journal, [1089]
Wrathall, A. E., [662]
Wreford, S. M., [693]
Wyatt, H. V., [10]
Wyllie, T. D., [1404]
Wyn-Jones, G., [763]

Yagil, R., [683]
Yeates, N. T. M., [476]
Yerex, D., [521], [522], [608]
Yoder, H. W. Jr, [1054]
You and your vet, NN
Youdeowei, A., [1532]
Young, M. J., [540]
Young, R. J., [1069]
Young, S. S. Y., [571]
Youssef, F. I., [11]
Youssef, M. K., [1574]
Yoxall, A. T., [404], [861], [862]
Yugoslavia
    journals, [87], [136]
    national associations, [2017], [2018]

Zaire, national association, [2019]
Zak, O., [1390]
Zambia, national association, [2020]
Zaslow, I. M., [1672]
Zayan, R., [1078]
Zentralblatt Pferd/Equine abstracts, [688]
Zetner, K., [1284]
Zimbabwe, national associations, [2021],
    [2022]
Zimbabwe veterinary journal, [145]
zoo animals, *see* exotic pets, zoo and wild
    animals
Zoological record, 74; [35]
zoonoses, *see* public health
Zwart, P., [1125], [1126]